When the Focus Is on Care

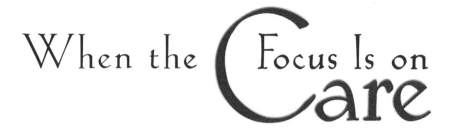

When the Focus Is on Care

Palliative Care and Cancer

Foreword by

John R. Seffrin, PhD
CEO of the American Cancer Society

Edited by Kathleen M. Foley, MD
Anthony Back, MD • Eduardo Bruera, MD
Nessa Coyle, PhD, FAAN • Matthew J. Loscalzo, MSW
John L. Shuster, Jr., MD • Bonnie Teschendorf, PhD
Jamie H. Von Roenn, MD

Published by
American Cancer Society
Health Promotions
1599 Clifton Road NE
Atlanta, Georgia 30329, USA

Interior photographs by Billy Howard Photography, Inc., Atlanta, Georgia;
© 2005 American Cancer Society

Printed in the United States of America
Cover designed by Shock Design, Inc., Atlanta, Georgia

5 4 3 2 1   05 06 07 08 09

Library of Congress Cataloging-in-Publication Data

When the focus is on care : palliative care and cancer / lead editor, Kathleen M. Foley ; editorial panel, Anthony Back ... [et al.].
   p. ; cm.
 Includes bibliographical references and index.
 ISBN 0-944235-53-0 (pbk. : alk. paper)
 1. Cancer—Palliative treatment. 2. Palliative treatment.
 [DNLM: 1. Palliative Care—Popular Works. 2. Adaptation, Psychological—Popular Works. 3. Neoplasms—psychology—Popular Works. 4. Neoplasms—therapy—Popular Works. 5. Terminal Care—Popular Works. WB 310 W567 2004]
 I. Foley, Kathleen M., 1944- II. Back, Anthony, MD. III. American Cancer Society.

 RC271.P33W48 2004
 616.99'4029—dc22
                        2004014736

A Note to the Reader

The information contained in this book is not intended as medical advice and should not be relied on as a substitute for talking with your doctor. This information may not address all possible actions, treatments, medications, precautions, side effects, or interactions. All matters regarding your health require the supervision of a medical doctor or appropriate health care professional who is familiar with your medical needs. For more information, contact your American Cancer Society at 800-ACS-2345 or http://www.cancer.org.

Brief Contents

Contents

Chapter 8

Managing Your Symptoms

Foreword

New Directions for the American Cancer Society

EACH YEAR MORE THAN HALF A MILLION AMERICANS die from cancer. That's over 1,500 persons per day. Cancer is the second leading cause of death in the United States, with about 1 in every 4 deaths caused by cancer. But as important as the number of people who die from cancer is the number of people who live with it.

With modern advances in cancer treatment, millions of people are conquering the disease and living longer, better lives. The American Cancer Society has played an important role in this change. More than 9 million people in this country are currently living with a diagnosis of cancer. That's 3 percent of our population. Now, with a welcome downward trend in mortality rates for the past few years, the Society is increasing its emphasis on survivorship research, quality of life, and the delivery of palliative care.

While continuing to serve our constituency by delivering services and funding research to conquer cancer and save lives, the goal of measurably improving the quality of life for people with cancer, their loved ones, and their caregivers is increasingly important to the American Cancer Society. Our 2015 goals and nationwide priorities acknowledge that we must sensitively address the comfort and well-being of patients and families throughout the course of the disease. Assuring quality care—not just in prevention, early diagnosis, and treatment, but also for those facing the end of life—is a real challenge, and the American Cancer Society is working to meet that challenge.

We believe it is time for organizations like the American Cancer Society to take the lead in guiding others in the private, public, and nonprofit sectors to commit to making palliative care a priority. This includes carrying out research, delivering excellent palliative care to all segments of the population, training professionals to provide palliative care, providing accurate and complete information to the public, and advocating for changes in the policies that govern payment for palliative care in public and private sector insurance.

The Role of Palliative Care in Improving Quality of Life and Diminishing Suffering

The concept of palliative care is somewhat new for Americans, and the term *palliative care* may be unfamiliar, but the philosophy of palliative care is one shared by many: *that people with cancer need not suffer.* The goal of palliative care is to help people with cancer and their families experience the best quality of life possible throughout the course of the disease, even when there are symptoms to manage, grave concerns for survival, and practical issues to attend to. Palliative care focuses on the patient and the family, assuring that they are well informed and that they receive state-of-the-art care. This approach includes competent and compassionate management of symptoms such as pain, sleep loss, fatigue, and functional change. It can help families cope and adjust to changes in their lifestyle over time.

Palliative care specialists are emerging as important team members in many health care settings. All patients deserve and should reasonably expect to have their care delivered by knowledgeable and sensitive health care providers. They need only work together with their health care team to understand the options for symptom management and use the resources that are available. Managing the challenge of cancer can sometimes seem like a daunting task, but palliative care can help ease the burden.

Fulfilling Our American Cancer Society Mission

This new book, *When the Focus Is on Care*, is just one example of the many ways the American Cancer Society is striving to fulfill its formal mission: to save lives and diminish suffering from cancer through research, education, advocacy, and service.

This book offers information and resources designed specifically for the person with cancer, as well as chapters that focus on topics of concern to a family caregiver. People with cancer and their families are better equipped to maintain their quality of life, to plan for the future, to reduce their worries and concerns, and to cope effectively with the disease and its treatments when they are well informed and well supported. *When the Focus Is on Care* offers guidance to be used throughout the course of a person's illness, from diagnosis through the end of life, and addresses the myriad issues confronting people with cancer and their families as they seek and receive cancer care.

When the Focus Is on Care empowers patients and families with the information they need to make educated decisions that will result in quality cancer care and support throughout all stages of cancer illness.

About the American Cancer Society

Represented in more than 3,400 communities throughout the country and Puerto Rico, the American Cancer Society is a nonprofit health organization dedicated to eliminating cancer as a major health problem and improving quality of life for people with cancer and their loved ones and caregivers. The Society is the largest private source of cancer research dollars in the US. Approximately 2 million Americans volunteer their time to the Society to work to conquer cancer.

I invite you to contact the American Cancer Society by calling 800-ACS-2345 or visiting our Web site at http://www.cancer.org to learn more about what we can do for you.

JOHN R. SEFFRIN, PhD
CEO, American Cancer Society

Preface

OUR CULTURE AND OUR SOCIETY FIND IT DIFFICULT TO TALK ABOUT illness, dying, and death. In part, our silence has fostered an information void that prevents people with cancer from knowing about and accessing the resources they need as they face the last years, months, and days of their lives. This guide seeks to address the concerns, fear, and anxiety of those people with advanced illness by providing information and support. *When the Focus Is on Care* also educates and supports family members, loved ones, and caregivers by introducing the concept of palliative care.

Palliative care is an approach to caring for people with cancer that focuses on improving their quality of life. It is a response to patients' and families' needs for symptom management and psychological, spiritual, and social support. As emphasized throughout this book, palliative care is not just about end-of-life care; rather, palliative care is about quality cancer care throughout all stages of illness.

In 2001, the National Cancer Policy Board (NCPB) issued a report entitled *Improving Palliative Care for Cancer* (available online at http://www.nap.edu/books/0309074029/html/). In order to reduce the needless suffering of people with cancer and their caregivers, the NCPB report stressed that both the public and the professional community need to be better educated about how to improve patient and physician communication, how to manage symptoms, and how to access and provide psychological support. *When the Focus Is on Care* is one part of a broad American Cancer Society strategy to address these needs. Conceived as a helpful resource and a practical guide to palliative care for cancer patients and their loved ones and caregivers, this book responds to NCPB's challenge to educate patients and caregivers about the care that people with cancer deserve from diagnosis to death, and provides them with tools to access that care.

When the Focus Is on Care will help readers understand choices and options for care, and make use of the resources and expertise available. It was designed from the start to help people with cancer and their loved ones, to encourage them to communicate about these issues, and to provide them with the support and information they need to begin the conversation.

KATHLEEN M. FOLEY, MD
April, 2004

Introduction

Who This Book Is For

IF YOU ARE READING THIS BOOK, CHANCES ARE you or someone you care about has been diagnosed with cancer. This book is designed primarily for people who are living with cancer. Although loved ones and caregivers will benefit from reading the entire book, the "you" in chapters 1–10 is the person with cancer. A special collection of chapters (11–13) is written expressly for caregivers and loved ones, and addresses issues unique to the important roles they play in the life of someone with cancer.

Additionally, *When the Focus Is on Care* is tailored to people with cancer who have metastatic or advanced cancer (cancer that has spread many places or has greatly harmed tissues and important organs). If this is your diagnosis, you face special challenges that are different from the issues faced by those whose cancer is more easily treated.

Even if cure is no longer a possibility, some people can live many years with metastatic or advanced cancer. Others may experience a more rapid decline. The focus of this book is on making the most of the time you have left, however long or brief that time may be.

What This Book Is About

This book is about palliative care. Palliative care is a comprehensive, family-centered care approach that addresses the physical, psychological, social, and spiritual needs of the seriously ill person, as well as the needs of their loved ones and caregivers. Its goal is to achieve the best quality of life for the person with a serious disease like cancer by relieving suffering, controlling pain and other symptoms, and enabling that person to function as fully as possible. Respect—for the person's culture, beliefs, and values—is an essential component.

While palliative care can and should be delivered at any time during a person's experience with cancer, in this book we tend to focus on the role of palliative care toward the end of life, when a person's need for symptom control and comfort care are typically greatest.

Why We Wrote This Book

We wrote *When the Focus Is on Care* because as doctors and nurses and social workers, and as children and parents and spouses/partners and siblings and caregivers, we felt there was a need for it. Our own professional and personal experience has shown us that there are things people with advanced cancer and their loved ones can do to improve their quality of life, to plan ahead, to reduce their worries, to access information, to get the best medical care possible, and to cope with a serious illness like cancer and its far-reaching effects. Yet this information isn't always readily available, or easy to understand, or collected in one place.

We wrote this book to acknowledge the importance of palliative care throughout the course of a person's experience with cancer, from diagnosis through the final moments. There is much that we know about how to improve the care of people with cancer that is not being applied, and this book takes on the difficult task of trying to ensure that all people with cancer and their loved ones understand that a wide range of approaches for care are available, that symptoms can be managed, and that psychological supports are available for people with cancer and their loved ones and caregivers.

Discussing the possibility and the eventual inevitability of death is not easy. Yet national surveys of people living with serious illness, studies of the patterns of their care, and a series of government reports have all emphasized the need to improve the care of individuals with serious life-limiting illness whose diseases are not responsive to current therapies. We hope this book helps meet that need.

What You'll Get From This Book

People with cancer increasingly have the opportunity to participate in treatment and care decisions. This opportunity brings with it responsibility—to be educated about your disease, to communicate openly with your medical team and your loved ones, and to consider both the quality of your life and the possibility of your death.

When the Focus Is on Care is designed to help you through the issues most important at different phases of your cancer treatment and care, from diagnosis to the end of life. Because we want to demystify the topic of end of life and explain what you're likely to experience throughout the course of a progressive disease like cancer, we've taken a fairly matter-of-fact approach. However, we humbly acknowledge that many of these topics are difficult to read about (we know they weren't always easy for us to write about), but are necessary nonetheless. Therefore, we'll take a practical but sensitive look at how cancer treatment and palliative care may affect your body, your emotions and your spirit, your family, your legal and financial situation, and your life in general. You'll learn valuable information, connect with helpful resources, and get tools to help you determine what choices are available and what decisions are best for you.

This book is designed to give you the tools to live your life—even through its final years, months, weeks, days, and minutes—on your own terms.

How This Book Is Organized

Throughout this book, we focus on the importance of quality care and treatment, symptom management, and psychological support throughout the course of cancer, and provide practical discussions about preparing for the end of life.

In the first two chapters, we provide an introduction to palliative care, and explain what it is and how it can help you throughout the course of your illness. Next, we provide insights that will help you navigate the sometimes-confusing health care system and ensure you receive the best care possible. We also share ideas and strategies for coping with the stresses and emotions that a disease like cancer can cause.

This book is also focused on the practical aspects of dealing with advanced cancer, including decision-making about care and medical intervention at the end of life, and dealing with the variety of work, insurance, legal, and financial matters that are sure to come up. We also address what to expect and how to manage symptoms as the cancer progresses and the end of life nears. Finally, we consider the personal, emotional, and spiritual aspects of death and mortality.

For caregivers and loved ones, we offer 3 chapters at the end of the book. These chapters address learning to be a caregiver, coping with the stresses, joys, and responsibilities of caregiving, and dealing with grief.

Acknowledgments

The American Cancer Society is enormously grateful to the book editors and authors for providing the substantive information that forms the core material of this text. We would like to acknowledge the vision and leadership of Kathleen M. Foley, MD whose stewardship made possible the transformation of this book from idea to reality. We also thank the editorial board members Anthony Back, MD, Eduardo Bruera, MD, Nessa Coyle, PhD, FAAN, Matthew J. Loscalzo, MSW, John L. Shuster, Jr., MD, Bonnie Teschendorf, PhD, and Jamie H. Von Roenn, MD, who embodied a spirit of collaboration and interdisciplinary teamwork in their passionate commitment to educating people with cancer about palliative care. Teresa Caldwell, MSW, Youngmee Kim, PhD, and David S. Landay, JD, also helped in the preparation of specific chapters.

The American Cancer Society would also like to thank the many people who contributed their time and expertise to provide reviews and feedback on the drafts of this book as it was being developed: Terri Ades, RN, MS, AOCN; Stephen R. Connor, PhD; Leticia Flores DeWilde, JD; Ronit Elk, PhD; Ted Gansler, MD, MBA; Herman Kattlove, MD, MPH; Jonathan N. Kromm; and Jerome W. Yates, MD, MPH.

The editors would like to express their gratitude to the American Cancer Society for its vision and commitment to improving the quality of life for people with cancer and their loved ones, and for advocating on behalf of the importance of high quality, accessible palliative care throughout all stages of the disease.

The editors would also like to thank their patients and their patients' families and caregivers for providing them with the inspiration and experience to advocate for public awareness and quality care.

In addition, we would like to acknowledge the more than 65 members of the American Cancer Society Cancer Survivors Network whose stories and experiences appear throughout the book. We have relied on the voices of these American Cancer Society constituents to honestly illustrate the real-life challenges and triumphs people with cancer and their loved ones and caregivers experience on a daily basis. We are very grateful to them for generously sharing their stories in order to help and support others facing similar situations. Several of the people who were interviewed for the Cancer Survivors Network project have since died as a result of their cancer, and we offer this book as a tribute to their lives.

Photographer Billy Howard also deserves special mention for generously sharing his time and talent, as do the amazing people whom he photographed for this book. We are also grateful to the Hospice Atlanta Center, the Winship Cancer Institute of The Robert W. Woodruff Health Sciences Center at Emory University, and the American Cancer Society's Hope Lodge, all in Atlanta, Georgia, where the photography took place.

In addition, leading national organizations who focus on palliative care such as the American Academy of Hospice and Palliative Care (AAHPM), the Association of Oncology Social Work (AOSW), Hospice and Palliative Nurses Association (HPNA), Last Acts and the Partnership for Caring, and the National Hospice and Palliative Care Organization (NHPCO), also deserve kudos for their ongoing efforts to advocate on behalf of quality palliative care and make information about palliative care and cancer available to the public.

We also acknowledge the many, many sources from which we have drawn to prepare this text: the multitudes of books, Web sites, and patient education materials, as well as the personal experiences of so many individuals whose lives have been touched by cancer and palliative care. This book is a cumulation of the ever-evolving literature from across the discipline of palliative care, and we are very grateful to all who have advanced the field by contributing to the conversation. It is our hope that in providing this book, we will continue to further the science and the cause of palliative care, and encourage better patient-doctor communication so that all people with cancer receive the care they require and deserve.

About the Editors

LEAD EDITOR

Kathleen M. Foley, MD, is an attending neurologist at Memorial Sloan-Kettering Cancer Center and professor of neurology, neuroscience, and clinical pharmacology at Weill Medical College of Cornell University. She is a previous chief of Memorial Sloan-Kettering Cancer Center's Pain and Palliative Care Service and one of the editors of the Institute of Medicine Report *Improving Palliative Care for Cancer.*

EDITORIAL PANEL

Anthony Back, MD, is an associate professor at the University of Washington and affiliate member at the Fred Hutchinson Cancer Research Center. He is founder and director of the Palliative Care Service at the Veterans Affairs Puget Sound Health Care System in Seattle, Washington. His research focuses on doctor-patient communication and communication skills education for clinicians.

Eduardo Bruera, MD, is professor of medicine and the F.T. McGraw Chair in the Treatment of Cancer at the University of Texas M. D. Anderson Cancer Center. He is the current president of The International Association for Hospice and Palliative Care.

Nessa Coyle, PhD, FAAN, is director of the Supportive Care Program of the Pain and Palliative Care Service, Department of Neurology, at Memorial Sloan-Kettering Cancer Center. She works with highly symptomatic advanced cancer patients who are being cared for at home, their families, and community nurses responsible for their care.

Matthew J. Loscalzo, MSW, is director of patient and family support services at the Rebecca and John Moores University of California San Diego Cancer Center with his appointment at the UCSD Medical School. He is internationally known for his contributions to psychosocial oncology relating to palliative care and problem solving.

John L. Shuster, Jr., MD, is a research physician at the Tuscaloosa Veterans Administration Medical Center and teaches at the University of Alabama. He practices both palliative medicine and psychosomatic medicine. Formerly, he was the founding director of the University of Alabama Center for Palliative Care and led the Alabamians for Better Care at Life's End initiative.

Bonnie Teschendorf, PhD, is director of quality of life science at the American Cancer Society in Atlanta, Georgia. Her interests include quality of life, needs assessment among cancer survivors, and interventions to assist cancer caregivers. In her earlier work as director of outcomes analysis at Memorial Sloan-Kettering Cancer Center, she interacted with the disease management teams and served as cochair of the Quality of Life Committee and member of the Surgical Quality Assurance Committee. She was a caregiver for her husband during his extended struggle with cancer.

Jamie H. Von Roenn, MD, is professor of medicine, medical oncologist, at Northwestern University, Robert H. Lurie Cancer Center in Chicago, Illinois. She is director of the Hospice and Palliative Medicine Program at Northwestern Memorial Hospital. She is a practicing oncologist, clinical researcher, and educator. She is editor-in-chief of the *Journal of Supportive Oncology* and serves as an editor for the *Education in Palliative and End-of-life Care Project* for oncologists.

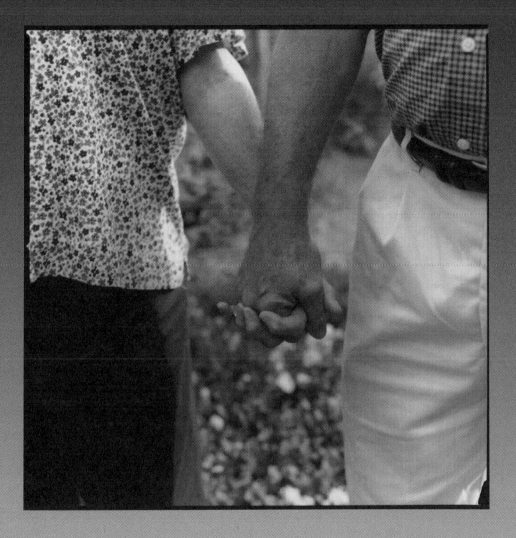

Chapter 1

What Is Palliative Care and How Can It Help?

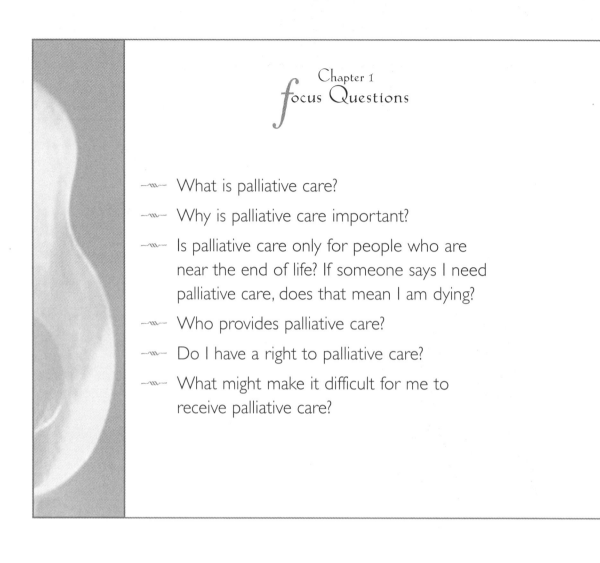

Chapter 1
*f*ocus Questions

—⧓— What is palliative care?

—⧓— Why is palliative care important?

—⧓— Is palliative care only for people who are near the end of life? If someone says I need palliative care, does that mean I am dying?

—⧓— Who provides palliative care?

—⧓— Do I have a right to palliative care?

—⧓— What might make it difficult for me to receive palliative care?

"Chuck was 34 years old when he was diagnosed with cancer, and in addition to being young, he was very healthy and physically fit. He was an active-duty army officer, so he ate right, he went to the gym 5 days a week, he was very healthy, very active, and then very young on top of that. Which, of course, caused some problems with diagnosis and dealing with things initially. And so he was diagnosed in March and fought the colon cancer. When he was initially diagnosed, within a week of his initial diagnosis, they found out through a CAT scan that it had already metastasized to his liver and both lungs, so he was stage IV pretty much right away at diagnosis. He battled the disease for just over a year, and passed away the first of April. So he was just 35 years old when he died. From the very beginning, it was palliative treatment as opposed to curative treatment. From the very beginning we were dealing with life or death."

— Ann I.

FACING CANCER CAN BE DIFFICULT FOR EVERYONE INVOLVED—the person with cancer, his or her family and other loved ones, and health care providers, too. But there are ways to make life better for people who are sick or dying and for their loved ones. It is called *palliative care*.

In this chapter, we'll explore the concept of palliative care in greater detail, describe state-of-the-art palliative care in action and explain how it can help, and let you know what you can do to receive the palliative care you deserve.

What Is Palliative Care?

A person with an illness like cancer needs a variety of types of care. While standard care for a chronic illness focuses on treatment of the disease, palliative care is a comprehensive approach to treating serious illness (in this case, cancer) that focuses on the physical, psychosocial, and spiritual needs of the patient and the needs of his or her loved ones. Its goal is to achieve the best quality of life available to the person with cancer by relieving suffering, controlling pain and symptoms, and enabling the patient to live as normal a life as possible. Respect for the person's culture, beliefs, and values are essential components.

In other words, the goal of palliative care is to prevent, reduce, or relieve the symptoms of a disease like cancer. The focus is on care, independent from efforts to cure the disease. But the two are not exclusive, and palliative care integrates both symptom control and anticancer treatment.

But good palliative care is more than just an emphasis on symptom management and quality of life; it is also an attitude toward patient care. Palliative care means treating and caring for the whole person, including the body, mind, and spirit. It means looking at the person with cancer in context—not only as a patient with a disease and specific symptoms, but as a husband, wife, or partner; father or mother; son or daughter; neighbor, friend, or coworker—and caring for the needs of loved ones too.

> "I am living while I am here. I'm not dying. I try to spend my life, how much or how little might be left, living it. And I want other people to look at me that way as well, and I want them to live with me."
>
> – Catherine

The goal of palliative care is for people with life-threatening diseases like cancer to have the best quality of life possible throughout the entire course of their illness, so that they can enjoy every day to the fullest possible extent.

Palliative care can help a patient at any stage of illness. Early on, when curing the disease is the goal, palliative care focuses on reducing symptoms, managing patient distress, and providing support. Pain management, control of nausea and vomiting, and counseling for anxiety and depression are examples of palliative care approaches that can help people with cancer live as well as possible.

The palliative care team can also educate the person with cancer about decision making, such as the role of living wills and advance directives (see chapter 5).

Figure 1-1. **A Brief Palliative Care Glossary**

Many of the following terms we define can have multiple meanings. For the purposes of clear communication, the authors of this book have settled on these definitions to anchor you as we proceed with our discussion of palliative care and cancer. You will find a complete glossary of terms at the end of this book.

palliative care: a team-oriented approach to care that seeks to improve the quality of life of people with serious illnesses like cancer and their families through the prevention and relief of suffering.

palliative medicine: the study and treatment of patients living with life-limiting or severe advanced illness where care is focused on relieving suffering and promoting quality of life. Major components of this specialty are pain and symptom management, information sharing, advance care planning, and coordination of care, including psychosocial and spiritual support for patients and their loved ones.

anticancer treatment: all medical interventions (regardless of curative or palliative intent) directed against the growth and spread of cancer. Also called anti-tumor treatment.

end of life: the period of time before death.

dying: 1. those who are likely to die within a few days to several months; 2. those who have a life-limiting illness or advanced progressive disease whose "timetables" for death are less predictable.

death: legally, the irreversible cessation of circulatory and respiratory function, or of all functions of the entire brain.

hospice: palliative care, delivered by a multispecialty team in the last stage of life, that most often takes place at home, but can also be delivered in a hospital, in a nursing home, or in residential care homes.

quality of life: health as perceived and valued by people for themselves rather than by clinicians; a broad term that can involve physical, mental, and social dimensions, ability to fulfill daily roles and responsibilities (sometimes called *role functioning*), freedom from bodily pain, satisfaction with health care, and an overall sense of general health and well-being.

As the disease advances, the number and intensity of symptoms a person with cancer experiences tend to increase. At this stage, members of the palliative care team try to relieve pain and other distressing symptoms, and to provide care that supports a person's comfort in a way that is consistent with his or her values and expressed desires. As the end of life nears, the team guides and supports people with cancer and families through transitions in care and helps patients address issues of life completion. Even after a person dies, the palliative care team responds to the needs of those left behind by providing support and bereavement counseling.

Palliative care is sometimes called *comfort care*, *hospice care*, or *supportive care*. These terms are sometimes used interchangeably, and while they have much in common, they can mean slightly different things, especially to medical professionals.

Illness and dying are natural and personal processes. As a discipline, palliative care recognizes this. Palliative care does not hasten or postpone death, but pledges that people with cancer will have the opportunity to make choices and actively participate in their care, and say and do what matters most to them, even in their final moments. Overall, palliative care is a relationship between people with life-limiting illnesses and their caregivers that aims to positively influence the course of the person's illness at every step of the way, enhance his or her quality of life, and—when the time comes—ensure a comfortable death.

> "I remember when I first figured out that I needed a whole group of people helping me plan how I was going to live well for the rest of my life. And I didn't know at the time that was called palliative care, but I really needed palliative care."
>
> — Ric

Is Palliative Care the Same as Hospice Care?

Is palliative care the same as hospice care? Yes and no. *Palliative care* is the overarching term that includes palliative services, palliative medicine, and hospice care. Both palliative care and hospice care share the same philosophy and principles of care. Palliative care is more generally thought of as the care itself that is delivered, or an *approach* to care, one that is responsive to personal needs, wishes, and values and aims to prevent, reduce, or relieve the symptoms of a disease like cancer and improve quality of life for a patient and loved ones and caregivers.

Hospice care is a model of care within which palliative care is delivered. It can take place at home, in a hospital, or in a nursing home or residential care facility.

The term hospice is often used to describe the *Medicare hospice benefit,* a program for people over the age of 65 or for those who are currently receiving Medicare disability benefits, and who are expected to live fewer than 6 months. The Medicare hospice benefit includes a very modest amount of money (approximately $120 a day) to provide care to the patient at home, including medications needed for symptom control, medical appliances and supplies, physician services, 24-hour on-call availability for nursing care, and social services and counseling, such as bereavement services for the family after the death of the patient, for example. Cancer patients receiving anticancer therapies with curative intent are usually *not* eligible for hospice care. New models for simultaneous hospice care and cancer therapies that aim to improve patient symptoms and quality of life are currently being developed.

It is important to note that hospice care is not limited to those receiving the Medicare hospice benefit. Many health care insurance programs provide palliative care outside of the Medicare hospice benefit.

Palliative care teams in hospitals and home care programs address the needs of people with life-threatening illness, significant symptoms, and/or psychological or social distress who are usually not candidates to receive the Medicare hospice benefit. They may be ineligible under the Medicare eligibility criteria or because they choose to continue aggressive medical care. Care by such teams is currently covered financially through existing health care insurance programs.

Most often, hospice care takes place in a person's home, and while intermittent nursing care is available, most responsibility still falls to family or other caregivers. When choosing amongst care options at end of life, and considering the importance of remaining at home in your final days, it is important to recognize the major role that the family or other caregivers have in caring for the person with cancer under the hospice model.

Please see chapter 6 for a more detailed discussion of hospice care and the Medicare hospice benefit, as well as other insurance-related issues.

Palliative Care and Its Special Role at the End of Life

Many think that palliative care is only for people who are dying. However, we want to make clear that palliative care is an approach to treatment and care that can take place at any time throughout an illness, from diagnosis to end of life.

Palliative and supportive measures naturally tend to play a greater role in the care of a person with cancer as the disease progresses and symptoms or side effects from treatment intensify. Therefore, palliative care plays an especially important role for cancer patients with advanced illness as the end of life approaches.

In a recent survey of seriously ill persons, bereaved families, and health-care practitioners, Americans listed the following goals for their end of life: pain and symptom management, preparation for death, achieving a sense of completion, being in charge of decisions about treatment preferences, being treated as a "whole person," and most of all, avoiding a prolonged and painful death. As evidenced by these findings, many people fear the process of dying more than they fear death itself; they fear dying alone, dying in pain, and dying without dignity. Palliative care acknowledges those concerns and addresses them head-on, by attempting to ensure that the care a person receives at the end of life is administered according to his or her wishes, and that death takes place in accordance with his or her personal, emotional, and practical preferences as well as religious or spiritual beliefs.

> "I think that when people hear the word 'cancer', or if they're told they have cancer, they immediately think of death. And that is, I believe, what the big scare of cancer is, 'Oh, my God, I'm going to die!' And I tried to try to make myself more comfortable with that concept of death. Of course, I wasn't really public about that, that I was trying to become okay with the concept of death, but I think that that helps to resolve some of the fear."
>
> – Greg

A Team Approach

The success of palliative care depends upon the participation and cooperation of many individuals. Your palliative care team might include physicians, nurses, nurses' aides, psychologists, pharmacists, pastoral caregivers, social workers, volunteers, and family members. For this reason, the palliative care team is sometimes described as *multidisciplinary*. This team coordinates your care to ensure your changing needs are met, and to ensure there is continuity in your care and treatment through each clinician who treats you, each setting in which you receive care (hospitals, home care, hospice, long-term care, adult day services), and each stage of your illness.

In some countries, such as the United Kingdom and Australia, palliative care is a medical specialty. In the United States, this specialty designation for doctors is currently being developed. For now, there are more than 1,800 physicians who have been certified by the American Board of Hospice and Palliative Medicine.

Over 10,000 nurses have completed a certifying examination by the Hospice and Palliative Care Nursing Association. Certifying exams for palliative care are in development for social work, pastoral care, and hospital medical directors.

The Whole Person

Earlier in this chapter, we mentioned that palliative care embraces the whole person in his or her own context. You may wonder what this means, exactly. Simply stated, it means that if you are sick, the palliative care team will look beyond your clinical case —the physical pathologies and symptoms you present—and will consider all aspects of your being. For example:

- **Your physical comfort:** Are you in pain? Are you receiving the most effective treatment for your illness, and are the treatments being administered in ways that minimize potential side effects?
- **Your emotional health:** Has a cancer diagnosis or an extended struggle with the illness caused you to become anxious or depressed? Are you and your loved ones having difficulty coping?
- **Your personal relationships:** Have you made peace with those who matter most to you, tried to heal old wounds, and expressed your love to those dear to your heart?
- **Your religious beliefs:** Do you want a religious advisor or leader involved in your care? What about members of your house of worship? Are there religious services, prayers, or rituals that would be helpful to you?
- **Your spiritual dimension:** Have you reflected on the meaning of your life and come to terms with your death? Have you considered spiritual questions about why you became ill or what may happen after you die? Have you made arrangements with your family to carry out your wishes regarding appropriate memorials after you are gone?
- **Your cultural context:** Are you receiving culturally competent care? That is, is the care you are receiving consistent with your culture's values? Are your doctors and nurses sensitive to your ethnic or cultural background?
- **Your financial well-being:** Has your illness prevented you and/or your caregiver from working? Have medical bills put a strain on your finances? Are you on top of all the paperwork that insurance companies require?
- **Your legal situation:** Have you put your estate in order?

- **Your thoughts on medical care and intervention:** Have you written a living will? Have you made your wishes about artificial nutrition, hydration, and resuscitation known?
- **Your personal preferences:** Is your goal of care to achieve relief from symptoms? To extend your life? To maintain your quality of life? To remain alert? To "fight" your illness until the end? Not to be a burden on your loved ones? To receive care at home? (Your feelings about which of these preferences are most important may change and evolve over time.)

Palliative care embraces all of these realms. We'll talk more about how palliative care relates to each of these topics in greater detail in later chapters of this book.

A Family Affair

When someone is seriously ill, it affects everyone around him or her—family members, friends, coworkers, neighbors, and members of his or her house of worship, for example. So it makes sense that when professionals treat someone who is sick they take into consideration the entire constellation of people affected by that person's illness.

The palliative care team can provide physical, psychological, social, and spiritual support to help the person with cancer and his or her loved ones adapt to the decline often associated with progressive disease.

FAMILY CAREGIVERS

It can be difficult for a caregiver to balance caregiving responsibilities while still meeting his or her own personal needs. Research shows that family caregivers (also called *informal caregivers*) can be at higher risk for fatigue, physical illness, and emotional distress. Families may also bear an additional financial burden when caring for a loved one who is ill.

The members of the palliative care team are aware of the substantial physical, emotional, and economic

> "Because of the loss of our daughter, I've been on both sides of the ledger, being the person laying there getting the surgery, getting the treatment, and I never had any idea what my family was going through, until our daughter was diagnosed… how difficult it is for the spouse and the caregiver, the kids, and everybody in the family. It's a very difficult journey for them…they're going through as much trauma as you are as a patient."
>
> – Keith

Figure 1-2.   **Possible Barriers to Palliative Care**

It may help you to be aware of some potential barriers to receiving palliative care you might encounter, but don't let these barriers get in your way. You have a right to palliative care. Your physician and your health care institution should provide you with resources for adequate symptom management and psychological support.

1. Forced Choice: The current Medicare hospice benefit forces people with advanced disease to choose between curative therapies (care that might prolong a person's life) and hospice care. Currently, for a person to enter hospice, a doctor must certify that he or she is expected to live 6 months or less. Once in hospice, the person receives palliative care, but can no longer receive therapies that are focused on curing cancer. This "either/ or" choice has led many people with cancer to only choose hospice care in the last 2 to 3 weeks of their illness, thus reducing the full benefits that they might receive from earlier help from a hospice program.

2. Knowing When to Say "Enough Is Enough": People with cancer and their physicians can be reluctant to address the reality that at some point, cure is no longer a possibility and additional treatments with curative intent will be ineffective, and perhaps even detrimental. People with cancer often cannot acknowledge the failure of curative therapies because they lack the education or the will to do so; if they can, sometimes their loved ones cannot. Well-intentioned but misguided family members may insist that the person with advanced disease participate in futile therapeutic interventions. Physicians may not want to be seen as powerless or ineffectual, and may continue to prescribe treatments so as not be seen as "giving up" on their patients.

3. Death—A Difficult Subject: There are strong cultural and societal attitudes against talking about death. Some people with cancer and their families view discussions about end-of-life care as giving up hope. These attitudes can prevent people from receiving the care that they require and deserve.

4. Limited Professional Training and Education for Health Care Providers in Palliative Care: Fewer than 1 in 3 medical schools and residency programs currently integrate palliative care into their professional training, and the same is true of schools of nursing and social work. However, the number of professionals with expertise in palliative care is growing and more and more hospitals and cancer care centers provide these services.

5. Unequal Access and Disparities in Care for Underserved Populations: A thorough discussion of this problem and the variety of potential solutions for it is beyond the scope of this book, but the fact remains that this barrier is profound, significant, and needs to be addressed by the health care system both locally and overall. Current efforts to ensure that every person in need has access to quality palliative care regardless of race or ethnicity, geographic location, or socioeconomic status—such as those spearheaded by the National Resource Center on Diversity in End-of-Life Care (866-670-6723 or http://www.nrcd.com)—are a good start.

6. Other Barriers: A lack of standards of accountability in caring for dying persons, inadequate information on palliative care services for the public, and lack of government support and funding for research and training on end-of-life issues can complicate matters as well.

demands placed on families caring for someone at home. To alleviate some of these stresses, the palliative care team can provide supportive services to caregivers such as respite, round-the-clock availability of expert advice and support by telephone, grief counseling, personal care assistance, and referral to community resources. See chapters 11–13 for more information; these chapters were written especially to address the needs of caregivers and loved ones of someone with advanced cancer.

Personal Choice and Self-Determination

Palliative care is person centered and family centered. That means the palliative care team encourages participation from the person with cancer and his or her loved ones in important decision-making processes about care, treatment, care settings, living situations, and services. It also ideally means that once a person has expressed desires about care and treatment, the clinicians will honor that person's unique choices and preferences through careful attention to his or her values, goals, and priorities.

The palliative care team can help people with cancer in establishing goals of care by facilitating their understanding of their diagnoses and prognoses, clarifying priorities, promoting informed choices, and providing opportunities for negotiating care plans with providers.

Conclusion

Palliative care is an approach to treatment and care that can take place at any time along the continuum of an illness, from diagnosis to end of life. This approach is responsive to personal needs, wishes, and values, and it aims to prevent, reduce, or relieve the symptoms of a disease like cancer and improve quality of life for a person with cancer and his or her loved ones and caregivers. Hospice care is a model for providing palliative care. The Medicare hospice benefit helps cover the costs of hospice care for people who meet certain eligibility criteria.

Palliative care can help you embrace your life and improve its quality throughout your cancer experience—whether you have days, weeks, months, or years to live.

"I think one of the things that being diagnosed with cancer has done for me is to make me realize that for whatever reason, there may not be a tomorrow. Whether it's a car accident or it's the cancer or something. There are things I want to do with my family, there are places that I wanted to travel with my husband, and we're doing all those. …There are just things that today I ought to go ahead and do and not look for the excuses not to do them."

— Patti

"Life is a process of moments. It's not years. It's the magic, and it's what we choose to do in terms of the living part of life as opposed to the dying part of life."

— Michael

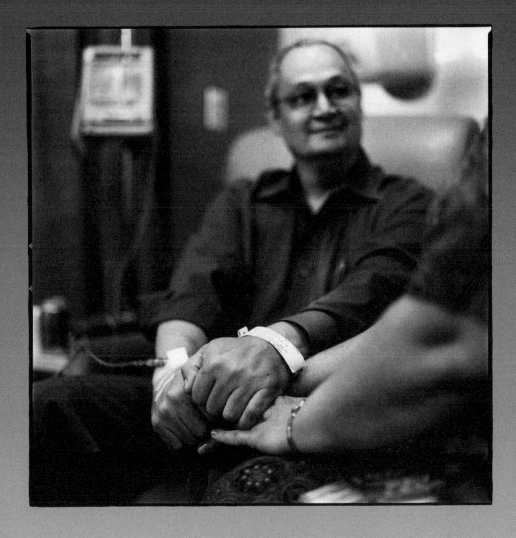

Chapter 2

Care Throughout the Course
of Your Illness

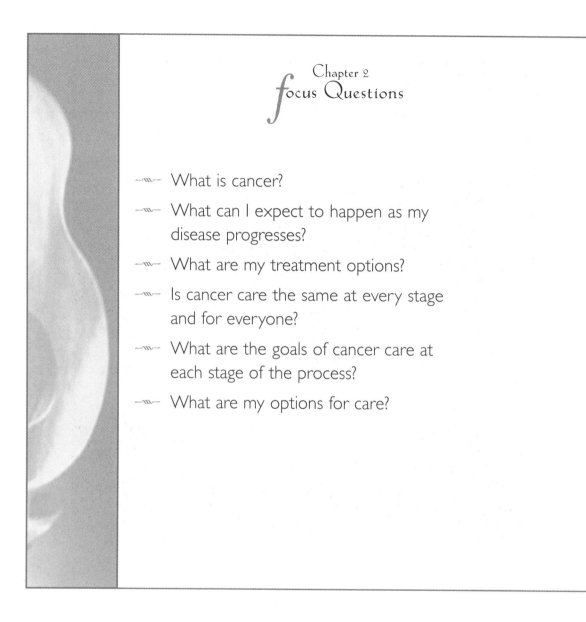

Chapter 2
focus Questions

--∿-- What is cancer?

--∿-- What can I expect to happen as my disease progresses?

--∿-- What are my treatment options?

--∿-- Is cancer care the same at every stage and for everyone?

--∿-- What are the goals of cancer care at each stage of the process?

--∿-- What are my options for care?

"I went to a 50th high school reunion and I overheard a couple of classmates talking about cancer and saying it was the best thing that ever happened to them, and that almost knocked me over. I thought, what in the world are these people saying, but then I discovered a little bit more about them—these are people I knew 50 years ago in high school, and ours was a small high school, but the stories of several of these indicated to me that they were demonstrating the ultimate courage by turning this adversity into a major victory. You know, the idea of crisis into opportunity.

"It's not an understatement to say that cancer is a crisis of unparalleled proportions, for both the individual and his family. Over the next several months I came to terms with my own situation and began to see that in the crisis of this prostate cancer were the seeds of an incredible opportunity for me, not how long I might extend my life, although I was hoping for something about that, but how I might expand it…For me that was the beginning of trying to do something constructive for myself."

— Robert A.

MORE THAN 1 MILLION AMERICANS WILL BE DIAGNOSED with cancer this year. Nearly 1 out of every 2 American men and a little over 1 out of every 3 American women will have some type of cancer at some point during their lifetimes.

Years ago, a diagnosis of cancer was almost equal to a death sentence. As a result, the main focus of cancer medicine and research was on a cure—for everyone and at every stage of the disease. Today, millions of people are living with cancer. Early detection strategies have allowed many more cancers to be found and treated early, when a good outcome is most likely. With more and more people living with cancer, the importance of symptom control, quality of life, and other aspects of palliative care from diagnosis through end of life have become even more important.

Palliative care allows for a balance of both anticancer treatment and symptom management, in varying degrees, throughout the course of the disease (from diagnosis through long-term survival or death).

What Is Cancer?

Cancer is not just one disease but a group of diseases. Although there are many kinds of cancer, they all start because of the out-of-control growth of abnormal cells. Normal body cells grow, divide, and die in an orderly fashion. But cancer cells do not—instead of dying, they outlive normal cells and continue to form new abnormal cells.

Most types of cancer cells form a lump or mass called a *tumor*, which can invade and destroy healthy tissue. Some cancers, such as blood cancers, do not form tumors. Left untreated, cancerous cells can travel to other parts of the body and can grow in new places. This spreading process is called *metastasis*. (When cancer spreads, it is still named after the part of the body where it started. For example, if breast cancer spreads to the lungs, it is still breast cancer, not lung cancer.)

Doctors often use a number of different words that mean the same thing when they are talking about cancer. For example, a growth, lesion, nodule, or tumor that is *malignant* can be cancer. A *benign* tumor is not cancerous. If it is not clear to you what the members of your health care team are talking about when you discuss your illness with them, ask.

Cancer can arise from virtually any site in the body. Cancers that begin from the surface of organs, such as the lining of the lung or colon, are generally called *carcinomas*. A second group of cancers, called *sarcomas*, begin in the bone and cartilage, joints, fatty tissue, and muscles. Carcinomas are more common than sarcomas. *Lymphomas* arise in the lymphatic system, which filters bacteria, fights infections, and carries fluid from the limbs and internal organs back into the blood. *Leukemia* is cancer that begins in the bone marrow.

Phases of Illness

Recent advances in technology and medicine—many of them in the past few decades—have made it possible for many more people who have been diagnosed with cancer to be cured, or at least experience a period of one or more remissions.

Diagnosis, Staging, and Prognosis

Doctors diagnose most cancers with a *biopsy*, in which a sample of abnormal tissue is removed and examined under a microscope to see if cancer cells are present. Once a diagnosis of cancer has been made, the next steps are to determine where the cancer came from and whether the cancer has spread. This will probably involve a physical examination and a series of diagnostic tests, such as blood tests, a chest x-ray, and possibly other tests such as computed tomography (CT) or magnetic resonance imaging (MRI).

The process of determining how far the cancer has spread is called *staging*. Staging is important because it helps your health care team communicate clearly with one another about the extent of your cancer and also dictates what treatments are most appropriate for you. A cancer's stage is based on:

- the tumor's size
- whether the tumor has grown into other nearby areas
- whether the cancer has spread to nearby lymph nodes
- whether the cancer has metastasized (spread) to distant areas of the body

The lower the number assigned to the stage of your cancer, the better your predicted outcome, or *prognosis*, is. Your prognosis is the physician's estimation of how your cancer is likely to behave, how likely it is to get better with treatment, and how it will affect your overall survival.

Stage I disease is generally a small cancer that is found only in one spot and is often curable. Stage II and/or III disease generally is a larger tumor and/or involves lymph nodes near where the tumor began. For most cancers, stage IV means metastatic cancer or cancer that has spread to parts of the body not close to the original cancer.

In addition to stage, other clinical information helps your physician predict your prognosis. *Performance status* is a measure of how active you are and how well you feel. For example, are you able to do all of your usual activities or are your symptoms so bad that you spend most of the day in bed? While this may not sound very scientific, many studies have confirmed the relationship between performance status and survival. The better your performance status, the better your outcome is likely to be.

Some symptoms are associated with a poorer prognosis, including confusion, breathing problems, or losing weight without trying. These symptoms are most often seen with advanced cancer. Finding the cancer in many different places (for example, lung, liver, and bones) or finding that the cancer has spread to the nervous system (the brain and/or spinal cord) also indicate a poor prognosis.

Determinations of prognosis are based on experience with many people who have had similar cancers and/or symptoms similar to yours. Remember, though, statistics—which you may or may not want to hear—are based on groups of people, not individuals. You may fall on either side of a statistic, and the doctor is not able to predict exactly what will happen for you. Furthermore, your prognosis changes with time. If the therapy keeps the cancer away or makes it disappear, the prognosis is *very* different from when the cancer fails to get better with treatment. (See chapter 3 for more information on prognosis.)

> "Regardless of what human endeavor you seem to be involved with, when you have this kind of a diagnosis, it's always right in your face. So, regardless of what you do, if you're out driving a car, if you go to an event, you go shopping, whatever it is, your mind always comes back to the fact that you have cancer and that it's stage IV."
>
> — Dan

Recurrence

Recurrence of a cancer—that is, a return of the cancer after it has been away for some period of time—can be devastating. It raises all the fears of dying of cancer that were probably dealt with to some degree (and put in the back of your mind) with the original diagnosis. For many, recurrence is more difficult to cope with than the original cancer diagnosis. Unfortunately, recurrence does suggest a higher risk of death from cancer, but recurrence is not a death sentence and should not be mistaken for one.

When cancer recurs, cure is still the obvious goal. More often, however, treatment for recurrent cancer can shrink the cancer and/or make it go away for some period of time, but not forever. Complete disappearance of the recurrent cancer is associated with better survival than when the cancer can be only partially controlled. As with your initial diagnosis and treatment, this is a period of time when people need at lot of support, and it is important to let your health care team know if you are feeling distressed. Distress is common, and it is appropriate to address the emotional distress of recurrence. The better you feel physically and emotionally, the better you are able to get through another round of treatment. As with your original cancer treatment, it is important to control any symptoms during the treatment of recurrent cancer.

> "When cancer recurs, you at least know what's in store for you somewhat. You've been through the initial treatments of chemo, radiation, surgery, whatever it's been, and as a whole you're probably much better prepared to handle this. You know what to expect. It's no longer this big mystery."
>
> – Linda S.

Advanced and Metastatic Disease

The phrase *metastatic cancer* is sometimes used interchangeably with the term *advanced cancer*, but they are not necessarily the same. Cancer is called metastatic even if only a small amount of the cancer has spread. In many cases, metastatic cancer can be treated successfully if it has not already done a lot of damage. But metastatic cancer may be advanced if it has spread many places and cannot be removed or has greatly harmed tissues and important organs.

With the exception of certain types of cancer that are especially responsive to specific treatments, advanced cancer is not curable. But even if cure is no longer a possibility, treatment can sometimes shrink the cancer, help relieve symptoms, and help you live longer. (We'll talk more about this later in this chapter and throughout the book.) The goal of treatment in this setting is to prevent or slow down further spread of the cancer, improve symptoms related to the cancer, and, ideally, shrink the cancer and increase the expected length of time you will live. Some people can live many years with advanced cancer.

The first treatment for metastatic or advanced cancer may improve symptoms, shrink the cancer, and improve survival. However, the more drugs a cancer is exposed to, the more likely it is to become resistant. Similar to the way bacteria can become resistant to antibiotics, cancer cells can bypass the effects of anticancer drugs. When this happens, the cancer is likely to continue to grow and, as a result, cause more symptoms.

Talking to your health care team about treatment choices and the goals of treatment is important at all stages of cancer. However, when the cancer is advanced or metastatic, it is especially important to ask how likely a particular treatment is to make you feel better and whether or not it will make you live longer. Some drugs make cancers shrink and make you feel better overall, even if the treatment does not offer cure.

Treatment

Based on the type of cancer you have, the stage of your disease, your overall health, and your symptoms, your health care team will make recommendations regarding treatment. Different types of cancer can grow at different rates and respond to different treatments. A different stage of disease generally leads to a different recommendation for treatment as well. Additionally, not every person goes through every cancer stage. Finally, a single type of treatment can be administered with different purposes. For example, radiation may be given to try to destroy the cancer or to control symptoms such as pain.

Treatment Options

The most common treatment options prescribed for people with cancer are surgery, radiation, and chemotherapy. These can be prescribed to treat both the cancer itself and the symptoms it causes. We'll discuss these at greater length here.

Depending on the type of cancer you have and its stage, your health care team may also recommend *hormonal therapy* (drugs that change the hormone environment in your body or react with hormone-sensitive substances in the cancer cell) or *immunotherapy* (treatments that use the body's own immune system to fight disease by stimulating it to work harder, or using an outside source, such as manmade immune system proteins) as well. Other treatments, such as *gene therapy* (which involves inserting a specific gene into cells to restore a missing function or to give the cells a new function), have shown promise in research studies and clinical trials but are not yet widely available.

SURGERY

Surgery is an operation performed with the general purpose of restoring health (see below for specific types and purposes of surgery). Surgery is the oldest form of treatment for cancer. Advances in surgical techniques have allowed surgeons to successfully operate on a growing number of patients using less invasive techniques. Surgery offers the greatest chance for cure for cancers that have not yet spread to other parts of the body. Most people with cancer will have some type of surgery.

Preventive surgery is done to remove body tissue that is not malignant (cancerous) but is likely to become malignant. For example, this type of surgery may be used if you have a precancerous condition such as polyps in the colon. *Diagnostic surgery* is used to get a tissue sample (also called a biopsy) to identify your specific cancer and make a diagnosis. *Staging surgery* helps determine the extent and the amount of disease. *Curative surgery* is the removal of a tumor when it appears to be confined to one area. This type of surgery is done when there is hope of taking out all of the cancerous tissue. *Debulking surgery* is done in some cases when removing a tumor entirely would cause too much damage to an organ or surrounding areas. In these cases, the doctor may remove as much of the tumor as possible and then try to treat what's left with radiation therapy or chemotherapy. *Palliative surgery* is used to treat complications of advanced disease. This is not intended to cure the cancer, but can be used to correct a problem that is causing discomfort or disability. For example, some cancers in the abdomen may grow large enough to obstruct (block off) the intestine. This may require surgery for effective relief.

RADIATION THERAPY

Radiation is energy carried by waves or a stream of particles that damages cells. Radiation therapy targets cancer cells, but it can also affect cells of normal tissues; this damage to normal cells is what causes side effects. Each time radiation therapy is given it involves a balance between destroying the cancer cells and sparing the normal cells.

Radiation may be used in early stage cancers to cure or control the disease. It can be used before surgery to shrink the tumor or after surgery to prevent the cancer from coming back. Radiation may be used to treat symptoms such as pain caused by the cancer that has spread from the original site. In certain types of cancer it may be used along with surgery and/or chemotherapy. Radiation may also be used to prevent growth of cancer in some situations. If a type of cancer is known to spread commonly to a particular area, doctors often assume that a few cancer cells have already spread there, so that area may be treated to keep these cells from growing into tumors. For example, people with some types of lung cancer may receive radiation to the head because this type of cancer frequently spreads to the brain.

CHEMOTHERAPY

Chemotherapy uses medicine to treat cancer. As you have learned, cancer is a broad name for many different diseases that affect your body in different ways. But these diseases have one thing in common: they involve cells growing out of control. Chemotherapy is targeted to your unique medical situation and the specific type of out-of-control cells that are growing in your body.

Depending on the type of cancer and its stage, chemotherapy can be used to cure cancer, to keep the cancer from spreading, to slow the cancer's growth, to kill cancer cells that may have spread to other parts of the body, or to relieve symptoms caused by cancer.

Chemotherapy drugs attack actively dividing cells, but they cannot tell the difference between the actively dividing cells of normal tissues and cancer cells. The resulting damage to normal cells can cause side effects. Each time chemotherapy is given, it involves a balance between destroying the cancer cells (in order to cure or control the disease) and sparing the normal cells (to lessen undesirable side effects).

Chemotherapy drugs can be administered in a variety of ways: you might swallow a pill, receive a shot, or have chemotherapy medicines administered intravenously.

Unlike radiation therapy or surgery, chemotherapy drugs can treat cancers that have spread throughout the body, because they travel throughout the body in the bloodstream. Often, combinations of chemotherapy drugs are used.

For some people, chemotherapy is the only treatment used in an attempt to cure, control, or palliate their cancer. In other cases, chemotherapy may be given in combination with other cancer treatments.

TREATMENT AND STAGING

Although it is difficult to generalize about the approach to all cancers, there are some basic principles that you might find helpful. If you have stage I cancer, the primary approach to treatment is likely to be a local therapy (a treatment that treats only the site where the cancer started). This is usually accomplished by surgery and/or radiation therapy. When surgery is used to treat an early cancer, the lump of cancer is removed along with some normal tissue. For example, if the cancer is in the skin, such as a melanoma, the cancer itself is removed along with some surrounding normal skin. Similarly, if a cancer occurs in the breast, the lump of cancer is removed along with some surrounding normal breast tissue. It is important that no cancer cells are left behind. This lowers the chance that they will regrow in the place they started. In some cases, removing an entire organ (such as an ovary, testicle, kidney, or lung) offers the best chance for a cure. Radiation therapy is sometimes added to surgery, because radiation can kill tiny amounts of cancer cells in the spot where the cancer started and help prevent recurrence (regrowth of the cancer).

Stage II cancers suggest that there is more cancer (the cancer may be bigger or may have spread to the lymph nodes), and therefore, more treatment may be needed. Depending on where the cancer started, your doctor may recommend multiple therapies, including surgery, radiation therapy, and/or chemotherapy. Stage III disease also is usually best controlled by multiple types of treatment.

Surgery is not usually part of the treatment for metastatic, or stage IV, cancers. Because by definition these cancers have spread through the bloodstream and gone to many places, they require *systemic therapies* that also go to multiple places. Drug therapies—such as chemotherapy, hormonal therapy, or immuno-therapy—are generally necessary. These drugs may be given as pills, put into your bloodstream *intravenously* (through your veins, or "by IV"), or sometimes given as shots under the skin. All these drugs, however, are absorbed into your bloodstream and therefore can go wherever the cancer may be.

PALLIATIVE CARE FOR IMPROVED QUALITY OF LIFE

As we discussed in chapter 1, palliative care is an approach to care that seeks to improve the quality of life of people with cancer and their families facing the problems associated with life-limiting illnesses. It aims to prevent, reduce, or relieve the symptoms of a disease like cancer. You can receive palliative care at the same time as treatments designed to cure cancer.

As your cancer progresses and cure is a less likely possibility, you may experience an increasing number of symptoms, and palliative care will likely play an increasingly important role in your treatment plan. To support your physical comfort, the palliative care team will help provide relief from pain, fatigue, lack of appetite, nausea and vomiting, shortness of breath, or other distressing symptoms. You may also experience emotional symptoms (feeling sad, nervous) and feel distressed over financial concerns due to mounting medical bills or prolonged time away from work. You may even begin to reflect on your spiritual or religious well-being. Your palliative care team can help address all these issues. If you have made your preferences about care known (see chapter 5 on advance decision making, including advance directives such as a living will), the palliative care team will help ensure your wishes are followed as well.

Palliative care is also an attitude toward care. Members of the palliative care team will treat and care for your body, your mind, and your spirit. They will try to see beyond your disease and look at your unique needs in the context of your life, your loved ones, and your values, culture, and personal preferences. The goal of palliative care is to ensure you have the best quality of life possible throughout the entire course of your cancer, including when a cure is no longer possible.

RESEARCH STUDIES AND CLINICAL TRIALS

There are many reasons people with cancer consider participating in research studies and clinical trials. Perhaps their cancer is progressing despite their having tried all conventional treatment options, or perhaps there are no known effective treatment options. In other cases, people with cancer may decide to forego standard options because of severe side effects or other reasons. In addition, many participants express an interest in helping future patients.

Research studies and clinical trials help the medical community to find out if a new treatment is safe and effective. There are 3 phases of study every new cancer treatment needs to go through before it can become a standard treatment.

- **Phase I Studies:** Only a small proportion of drugs tested in laboratory studies on tissue cultures or in animals will be judged promising enough to warrant phase I clinical research in humans. The purpose of phase I studies is to find out how safe these treatments are and the dose patients need, not to find out if the drug is effective for the treatment of cancer.
- **Phase II Studies:** The purpose of phase II studies is to find out if this treatment is capable of shrinking or eliminating a given type of cancer. Phase II studies are offered to patients who have not benefited from standard treatment.
- **Phase III Studies:** The main purpose of these studies is to find out if this new treatment is better than what is currently available. At this point, investigators already know about the different side effects and they already know that this treatment is capable of shrinking some cancers. In most cases, phase III studies are designed so that some

randomly selected patients will receive standard treatment and others will receive the new experimental treatment. This random assignment helps scientists minimize the factors that might confuse the results, helping them learn rapidly if the new treatment is good enough to outperform and replace the existing standard treatment.

Rewards of Clinical Trials

Some of our most powerful advances in cancer treatment have been made as a result of participation in clinical trials. Generally, participation in clinical trials offers benefits such as access to treatments that are not otherwise available, careful monitoring of your condition and the possible side effects of treatment, and the possibility of payment for part or all of the medical care received during the study by some study sponsors (this is not true for all clinical trials, so be sure you are aware of the costs of your participation).

Most compelling, however, especially for individuals with advanced cancer who no longer have reason to believe their cancer can be cured, is the opportunity to possibly help others who have the same condition in the future by contributing to cancer research.

Risks or Burdens Associated With Clinical Trials

The ultimate goal of all cancer research is to give cancer patients more effective and less toxic treatments. Even though the federal government, granting agencies, universities and hospitals, and investigators take great care in ensuring that the cancer research protocols are as safe as possible, there are always uncertainties regarding the effectiveness and the side effects of these treatments. So success is not a certainty.

But risks are a part of any medical test, drug, or procedure. The risk may be greater in a clinical trial because some aspects of any new treatment are unknown. This is especially true of earlier phase clinical trials. When a clinical trial is in phase I, scientists don't know the effect the treatment may have on humans or the treatment's side effects. But by the time a drug or treatment reaches a phase III clinical trial, it is generally less risky.

There may be a financial burden if care during the study is not paid for. There is also the possibility that the patient may have to travel long distances to receive treatment. However, clinical trials are not limited to major cancer centers in large cities; many are available in community oncology practices and community hospitals.

When making a decision about clinical trials, a key question is whether the risks or burdens are outweighed by the possible benefits. People with advanced cancer are often willing to accept a certain amount of risk or burden for a chance to be helped, but it is always important to have a realistic idea about the actual chance of being helped. Some people decide that any chance of being helped is worth the risk or burden, whereas others choose to be more cautious. Weighing all of these factors will help you make a more informed decision —one that is right for you.

Finding Out More

There are a large number of research studies covering almost all types of cancer. Some research studies involve entirely new drugs, and others involve a combination of already known drugs or a different way of administering them. Other clinical trials involve radiation therapy or surgery. Most patients with advanced cancer will have access to phase I or phase II clinical trials of new treatments.

To find out more about ongoing cancer clinical trials, ask your doctor. The American Cancer Society (ACS) offers a free clinical trial matching and referral service. For more information, visit the ACS clinical trials Web site at http://www.clinicaltrials.cancer.org or call 800-ACS-2345. You can also learn more by calling 800-4-CANCER or visiting the National Cancer Institute (NCI) Web site at http://www.cancer.gov/clinicaltrials.

COMPLEMENTARY AND ALTERNATIVE THERAPIES

Complementary and alternative therapies involve the use of treatments other than those we have already described in an attempt to fight disease, reduce symptoms, or otherwise improve quality of life.

Complementary therapy refers to supportive methods that are used to complement, or add to, mainstream treatments. Complementary methods are not given to cure disease; rather they may help control symptoms and improve well-being. Examples of complementary methods include meditation, yoga, massage, and acupuncture. *Integrative therapy* is a term that refers to the combined offering of evidence-based standard treatments and complementary therapies. *Alternative therapies* are treatments that are promoted as cancer cures. They are unproven (they have not been scientifically tested) or were tested and found to be ineffective. If alternative therapies are used *instead of* evidence-based treatment, the person with cancer may suffer, either from lack of helpful treatment or because the alternative treatment is actually harmful. Some are toxic and dangerous, and some can also interfere with the treatment prescribed by your doctor. Talk to your health care team about any complementary or alternative therapy you are considering.

Resources such as the American Cancer Society, the NCI Office of Cancer Complementary and Alternative Medicine (http://www3.cancer.gov/occam/information.html), the National Center for Complementary and Alternative Medicine (http://nccam.nih.gov/), the Memorial Sloan Kettering Cancer Center "About Herbs" Web site (http://www.mskcc.org/aboutherbs), and the M. D. Anderson Web site (http://www.mdanderson.org/departments/CIMER/) all provide reliable information on complementary and alternative treatments that is regularly updated.

Response to Treatment

When your doctor talks about what to expect from treatment, the discussion will include information about response rates (how likely the cancer is to get better with a particular treatment), the risk of recurrence (how likely the cancer is to come back), and survival (will the cancer shorten your life). What do these terms mean? *Response rate* can be divided into *complete response* and *partial response*. A complete response means technically that the cancer completely goes away by physical examination and all diagnostic tests (x-rays, bone scans, etc.) and stays away for at least 4 weeks. A partial response means that all of the cancer shrinks by at least 50 percent and, again, stays away for at least 4 weeks. Response is *not* the same as cure. However, if you get a complete response with treatment, you have a better prognosis by far than if you don't. That is, a cancer that goes away completely is very likely to stay away for many months or years. Although you may want to hear your doctor say the word cure, doctors are more likely to use the word remission. A *cure* means that all cancer cells are gone and that the cancer will not come back. Such a pronouncement is difficult to make with certainty. Complete response or *remission* is a more conservative statement that simply means tests and examinations have not detected any remaining cancer cells.

Stable disease means that the tumor has not grown bigger or smaller by more than 25 percent and no new tumors have developed. By definition, *progressive disease* means that the cancer is worse—specifically, the tumor has increased in size by 25 percent. *Recurrence* occurs when the cancer has been gone for some period of time and then reappears. Sometimes, recurrent cancer can be treated with local therapies (such as surgery and radiation therapy), resulting in complete resolution of the problem. However, once a cancer recurs, the risk of it returning either in the same place or in another organ is greater.

Goals of Treatment

Some people are able to manage cancer as a chronic or recurrent condition and still maintain their quality of life for years. However, about half of people with cancer will eventually die of the disease. Everyone with cancer hopes that their cancer will be cured, but when a cure is not possible, people begin to think about their life in terms of years, months, or days that they have left. When it is apparent that a person's cancer is advanced and not responsive to available treatments, the goal of quality cancer care is to control symptoms caused by the cancer or the cancer treatment, so that the person can continue to be as active as he or she chooses and die free of pain and needless suffering. When a person's cancer is advanced, increasing symptoms are often a sign of advancing illness. For these persons, the focus of care is on their quality of living and activities of daily life, emphasizing the need to control symptoms and to make the persons as comfortable as possible.

The fact that an illness is no longer curable does not mean it is not *treatable*. Cancer can be treated for long periods of time, but the goal is to manage the symptoms of progressive disease without expecting to get rid of it entirely. With increasing symptoms, the focus of care will change from treatment with curative intent to care that relieves suffering, controls symptoms and side effects from cancer or its treatment, and makes the person with cancer as comfortable as possible.

The goals of cancer care are different at each stage of the disease. When cancer is first diagnosed, particularly if it is caught at an early stage, people with cancer and their loved ones seek treatment focused on a cure and expect to return to normal life soon. The first goal for everyone is cure. It is important to ask your doctor if this is a reasonable expectation. If cure is a possibility, it is likely that you will be willing to tolerate more side effects from your treatment than if cure is not an option. If the cancer returns, treatment is directed at conquering the cancer once more, or at least holding it at bay and prolonging survival.

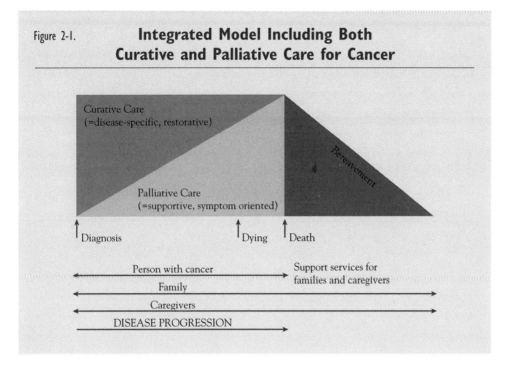

Figure 2-1. **Integrated Model Including Both Curative and Palliative Care for Cancer**

Curative Care
(=disease-specific, restorative)

Bereavement

Palliative Care
(=supportive, symptom oriented)

Diagnosis   Dying   Death

Person with cancer

Family

Caregivers

DISEASE PROGRESSION

Support services for families and caregivers

But what happens when the disease is not curable, when it appears that your time is limited and you will die from cancer? Once the cancer is advanced, you may wonder: *what is the point of care if I'm going to die anyway?* But you have care options, even at the end of your life. A cure for your cancer is not the only reason to seek treatment. Your health care team and those who love and care for you can help you focus at this point on the *quality* of your life rather than its *duration*.

For example, despite your advanced cancer, you may want to continue working, or at least continue to be active with family and friends. You may find that weakness prevents you from going out very often. But you may still want the continued enjoyment of the people you love and the ability to join them at the dinner table, read together, or watch movies. When your symptoms are worse still and you are bedbound, the definition of quality of life may change again, and as long as you are able to enjoy those around you, there is meaning—and therefore quality—in your life.

Realistic expectations of what will happen to you depend on the stage of your disease, the type of cancer, and available treatments. It is important for you to speak with your health care team about their goals and yours. However, no matter what the goal of the treatment is, you should expect the doctor and your health care team to work hard to prevent and treat expected side effects of your treatment, such as nausea and vomiting. The more you tell your doctor about how these problems affect your day-to-day life, the more help you can get.

It is important that throughout treatment your *quality of life*—that is, your ability to enjoy your life and do your usual activities—is maintained as much as possible. The treatments now available to control symptoms and prevent side effects of treatment have improved dramatically, just as the treatments for cancer itself have gotten better over many decades.

UNDERSTANDING THE PURPOSE OF TREATMENT

As your disease progresses, you will certainly have to make decisions about continuing or discontinuing certain treatments and beginning others. As you make these decisions, it is important to know the purpose of each treatment intervention. Sometimes this can be confusing because some treatments used to cure cancer are also used to relieve symptoms. For example, radiation therapy can be used to try to cure cancer, but it can also be used to control symptoms such as bone pain. Ask your doctor to clarify if the recommended treatment is anticancer treatment to fight the cancer or to diminish symptoms.

Knowing When to Say "When"

Some people with advanced cancer feel that if they stop their cancer treatment they are "giving up." However, as with all treatment decisions, you should consider the benefits and the drawbacks of each possibility. Ask yourself, for example, if it is worth it to continue with chemotherapy with curative or life-prolonging intent even if your cancer is not responding to the treatment and the side effects are immobilizing. You may have to make a difficult decision about whether you want to continue efforts to cure cancer, or if you would rather focus on making the time you have left the best it can be. Your answer will depend on many factors and is a personal decision.

This doesn't necessarily have to be an either/or decision. You can receive treatment with curative intent and still receive palliative care, for example. But you should know that there may come a time when the option to continue curative treatment no longer exists. We'll talk more about making these decisions in chapter 3.

—Λλ—

"When am I going to know enough is enough? I don't know. I have no answer for that. But what I think is, as long as today is a good day and my doctor has come up with some new 6-month chemotherapy that he wants to try, I'll probably do it. If they ask me on a bad day, I probably won't. I don't know. My doctor says that I'm going to know when I'm tired and I don't want to do any more. I hope he's right, but I don't know. I don't worry about it. I mean, my goal is living well every day, and whether it happens 6 months from now, well, I'll deal with it then."

— Ric

Care Options for People With Advanced Cancer

As your disease progresses, not only will you be faced with new decisions about your treatment options; you will also need to consider care options. Especially as your symptoms increase and your mobility and functional status decrease, you will need to rely more on others for care. In what environment do you want this care to take place? Would you prefer to receive care in your own home, for example, or would it be easier for all involved if you were moved to a skilled nursing facility?

A wide range of facilities can provide care to people who are ill, and it is beyond the scope of this book to address them all. In the following sections, we'll look at some options that are specific to people receiving cancer care. Refer to chapter 6 for a fuller discussion of insurance and Medicare benefits and their coverage of these and other care options.

Outpatient Care

Outpatient care is the type of care you are most likely to receive when your cancer is in its earliest stages, or if your cancer is in remission and is being monitored. You will visit a doctor's office, clinic, or hospital outpatient department for office visits and/or to receive treatment, with the expectation that when the consultation or therapy is complete, you will return home.

Home Care

When your disease progresses, occasional treatment on an outpatient basis may no longer be an option. You may need to be in an environment where you can be closely monitored on a regular basis. People with advanced cancer often feel most comfortable when they can receive this type of care at home. The familiarity and comforts of home can add a peace and security during a time that may be particularly difficult or stressful. Most people want to be able to sleep in their own bed, eat home-cooked food as their appetite allows, and be surrounded by loved ones and friends without the restrictions of visiting hours. If you share these preferences, home care can help you achieve this.

> "Hospice is an extraordinary gift we have in our society for people with terminal illness, but hospice comes late in the process. From the time you're diagnosed with a terminal illness until you're ready for hospice, there's a long period of time, hopefully, and our resources are few and far between."
>
> — Ric

Your loved ones may assume the primary caregiving role, but involving personal care assistants from private home care agencies is also an option. These agencies offer personal care assistants for home-based services such as in-home laundry and meal preparation. Usually these agencies are able to provide staff for part of the day or around-the-clock. If you turn to a private agency, be certain to find out if the staff is bonded and how they are trained. Referrals from professional staff at the hospital or your physician will help to ensure that you are provided with personnel that are well trained and reliable.

Services provided by home care agencies may include access to medical equipment (such as a hospital bed, wheelchair, or a variety of assistive devices designed to enhance independence); visits from registered nurses, physical therapists, and social workers; help with running errands, meal preparation, and personal hygiene; and delivery of medication. Not all home care agencies offer palliative care, but some agencies offer both home health and hospice care services.

Home care services can be expensive, and your insurance may or may not cover this type of care. Medicare may offer limited reimbursement for some home care services, so call 800-MEDICARE or visit http://www.medicare.gov to check if you receive Medicare. You may also be eligible for other help in paying for home care. States must provide home care services to people who receive federal income assistance such as Social Security Income and Aid to Families with Dependent Children, and disabled veterans can receive home care services through veterans hospitals (contact the Department of Veterans Affairs at 877-222-VETS or http://www.va.gov/health_benefits/). The Older Americans Act provides federal funds for state and local social services programs that help people older than age 60 maintain independence. (Contact your local Area Agency on Aging or call the Eldercare Locator at 800-677-1116.)

One other issue to keep in mind when considering the option of home care is the demand it will place on your family, your loved ones, and your caregivers. While a nurse, physician, or other allied health professional may help with home care, it is usually the family member who is responsible for around-the-clock supervision and care of the person with cancer. The stress and responsibility of in-home care on other members of your household can be considerable, and can tax family relationships. Caregivers can also suffer burnout or experience feelings of guilt, anxiety, and helplessness (see chapters 11–13 for more information about and resources for caregiving). On the other hand, many loved ones and family members want to play a role in your care. Many will look upon caregiving not as a burden, but as an honor and a gift they can give to you as your life draws to a close. Talk with those who would participate in your at-home care to determine their feelings before making any decision. The important roles your loved ones will play in caregiving at home should not be overlooked.

Skilled Nursing Facilities

People with advanced cancer have many medical and emotional needs. Sometimes these needs are too many or too complicated to be adequately addressed in a certain setting. If being cared for at home is no longer possible, skilled nursing facilities offer another option for care.

A skilled nursing facility may be necessary if someone needs around-the-clock nursing care; needs help with meals, bathing, personal care, medications, and moving around; needs more help than the current caregiver can possibly give; or cannot live alone. Skilled nursing facilities supply 24-hour services and supervision, including medical care, to people living there.

Hospitalization

This care setting, also called *inpatient care* or *acute care*, is typically engaged during health care crises, when a patient's medical needs cannot be met in another environment.

> "When we realized that Bob was not going to win the battle, we contacted hospice. What they can offer is so tremendously important. Taking so much of the paperwork, if nothing else, off your shoulders. Offering immediate access to health care professionals, all of that advocacy, aside from the social work type benefits they can also offer....It's an incredibly, incredibly wonderful service. I recommend it highly."
>
> — Janet

Hospice Care

Both palliative care and hospice care seek to create a comfortable environment for the person with cancer by preventing, reducing, or relieving the symptoms of disease. Recall from chapter 1, however, that palliative care is more generally thought of as an *approach* to care, while hospice is a *palliative care delivery system* that takes place at home, in a hospital, in a residential care facility, in a nursing home, or in a freestanding hospice care facility.

Hospice services are generally targeted to people who have advanced disease and limited life expectancy. About three-quarters of a million Americans a year use hospice services; over half of Americans who died of cancer last year used hospice programs.

Services typically include physician services, nursing services, and services from allied health professionals such as physical therapists. Psychological or spiritual counseling and social services are also a part of hospice. Grief counseling and bereavement follow-up are available on an as-needed basis as well. Medical equipment and supplies (hospital beds, bandages, etc.) and drugs for symptom control and pain relief are usually covered. Additional services may also be available, such as help around the house (preparing meals, running errands), personal care (bathing, eating, dressing), and *respite care* (relief for the at-home caregivers).

FOUR LEVELS OF HOSPICE CARE

People who choose hospice services may require different types of care during the course of their cancer. These are the 4 levels of care generally associated with hospice and outlined by Medicare:

1. **Routine Home Care:** Routine home care is the care provided in the home of the person with cancer. Most patients, with the assistance of the hospice team, are able to remain in their place of residence, whether it is a private home, assisted living facility, or nursing facility, for the duration of the illness.

2. **General Inpatient Care:** If the person with cancer requires aggressive treatment for symptoms that cannot be controlled in a home environment, inpatient care (referred to earlier as hospitalization; also called acute care) is provided. This care usually takes place in a hospital setting but may also be provided in a nursing facility.

3. **Continuous Home Care:** If the person's symptoms are out of control, but he or she does not want to leave his or her residence, continuous care may be initiated. Continuous care is provided by certified nursing assistants and nurses from several hours a day up to 24 hours a day until the crisis is resolved (usually a maximum of 3 days). The hospice nurse assists in determining when continuous care is needed.

4. **Respite Care:** Caregivers occasionally need to take short breaks to maintain their own health. Inpatient units, as well as nursing facilities, are available to provide family caregivers a much-needed rest. Respite care may be given for up to 5 days at a time with no out-of-pocket expenses according to Medicare guidelines.

See chapter 6 for more specific information about the Medicare hospice benefit.

HOME: THE PREFERRED CARE SETTING

Hospice care can be delivered in a variety of locations, but most people with cancer choose to receive hospice care at home. In fact, more than 90 percent of the hospice services provided in this country are delivered in home settings.

Home-based hospice programs allow many people to be able to accomplish some of their end-of-life objectives. For example, 3 out of 4 Americans in the last stage of their lives express a wish to die at home, yet only about 1 in 4 of them actually does so. In contrast, among those who used hospice services in 2001, more than half died at home.

While a nurse, physician, and other professionals staff the home care hospice program, the primary caregiver is still the central figure responsible for full-time supervision of the person with cancer. To handle crises, Medicare-certified hospice programs have a staff of nurses and other health care professionals who are on call 24 hours a day to make home visits. The roughly 10 percent of US hospice patients who do not have a primary caregiver remain at home (sometimes with a hired caregiver) or stay at home until they have to go to a hospital or skilled nursing facility for end-of-life care.

Conclusion

No matter what the stage of your cancer—early cancer, recurrence, or advanced cancer—you are in charge of your care and treatment. Ask questions, make it clear what is important to you, and expect that your symptoms will be controlled throughout the course of your cancer care. (If your symptoms are not being well controlled, ask for referral to a palliative care expert.) With early disease, it is likely that care will focus on curing the cancer more than on symptom control. If your cancer is advanced, you should expect that your sense of well-being and the control of symptoms will take priority. Symptoms and side effects should be aggressively treated, whether they are a result of the cancer or the treatment. You have the right to palliative care at all points during your cancer experience.

In the next chapter, we'll talk about how to choose among the many treatment and care options that are available to ensure you find the ones that are best for you.

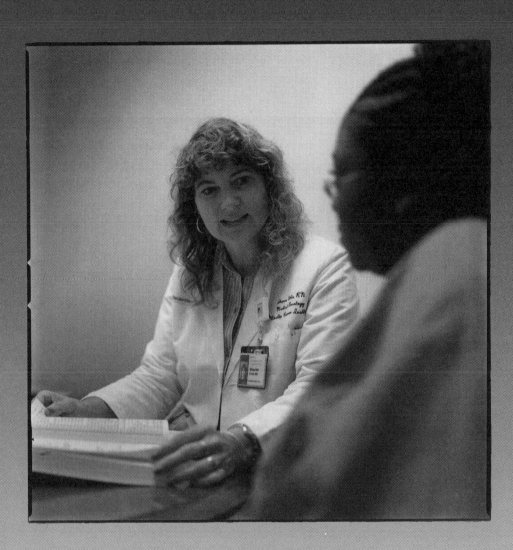

Chapter 3

Making Informed
Treatment Decisions and Getting
Good Medical Care

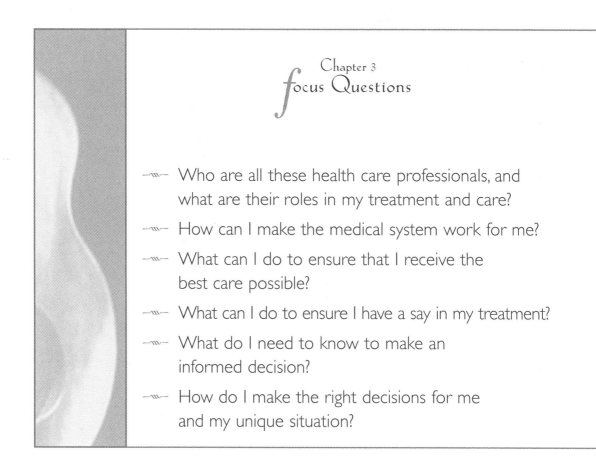

Chapter 3
*f*ocus Questions

—∞— Who are all these health care professionals, and
what are their roles in my treatment and care?

—∞— How can I make the medical system work for me?

—∞— What can I do to ensure that I receive the
best care possible?

—∞— What can I do to ensure I have a say in my treatment?

—∞— What do I need to know to make an
informed decision?

—∞— How do I make the right decisions for me
and my unique situation?

"The most important thing I would say to somebody is to really understand what your diagnosis means, and at every step of the way keep asking your doctors how this disease will impact your ability to live well until the end of your life. To have a dialog about that, because we need to understand that our cancer and our treatment are going to make us tired. It's going to make us sick. But that doesn't mean that life is over, just because your diagnosis is terminal. You need to be able to play. You need to be able to enjoy time with the people that you love most, and the only way that you're going to be able to do that is to really understand what's ahead for you."

— Ric

THE INFORMATION IN THIS CHAPTER WILL FAMILIARIZE YOU with strategies and tips for working within the health care system to get the medical care you need and to obtain reliable information and support for making treatment decisions throughout the course of your cancer, from early stages of disease to end of life.

Making the Medical System Work for You

You may have already discovered that finding your way through the medical system can be a pretty big job. Your diagnosis probably seems overwhelming enough without having to worry about how to navigate the maze of health care providers, treatment and care options, and paperwork. However, we believe that you can improve your quality of life as well as the quality of the medical care and treatment you receive if you understand more about how the system works and know what questions to ask.

Your Diagnosis

When a doctor tells you that you have cancer or advanced cancer, she should be able to explain exactly how she made the diagnosis. Usually she has run some tests, which might include blood tests, x-rays or scans (like a CT scan or MRI scan), and a biopsy (which involves getting a little piece of tissue that will be examined under a microscope by a specialized doctor called a pathologist). Feel free to ask lots of questions (see the list of questions to ask your health care team about your cancer diagnosis in Figure 3-1) and expect clear answers from your doctor about how your cancer was diagnosed.

Choosing Your Doctor

Because of your insurance coverage or your financial situation, you may be limited in your choice of doctors. If you do have the opportunity to choose your doctor or the other members of your health care team, there are a variety of issues you may want to consider.

Finding the doctor who is right for you is very important. You want someone who is experienced treating your type of cancer, but you also want someone you are comfortable with. Communication is an important issue for your relationship with your doctor.

It may seem intimidating, but do not be embarrassed to ask questions about the doctor's background, training, and experience. You can ask about the number of procedures the doctor has performed, the number of people he or she has treated for this type of cancer, and the doctor's patient load, for example. (See Figure 3-2 on page 45.)

> —m—
> "A proactive relationship with your physicians is the best thing you can do for yourself."
>
> — Richard

Figure 3-1.

Questions to Ask Your Health Care Team
About Your Cancer Diagnosis

- What is the exact type of cancer I have? How frequently is that type of cancer seen?

- What should I expect with this type of cancer in terms of the disease, the treatment, and the symptoms and side effects?

- Would you explain my pathology report?

- What is the stage of my cancer? What does that mean in my case?

- Has my cancer spread to lymph nodes, internal organs, or my bones?

- What is your opinion of my prognosis?

- How does the stage of my cancer affect my treatment options?

- Did a pathologist experienced in diagnosing this type of cancer review my slides?

- Should someone else—a second pathologist, for example—look at my slides?

- Were any other tests done on my biopsy sample?

- What other tests will I need to undergo?

- What are my treatment and care options?

- What treatment or care option would you recommend for me and why?

- What are the side effects of the treatment?

- What symptoms or complications can I expect from the treatment and from the cancer itself?

- What will we do to manage these symptoms or complications?

- Are there any complementary treatments I should consider to help manage my symptoms or help me cope?

- How will I stay up-to-date as my condition changes or progresses?

> "My doctors have always been extremely willing to work with me…I have a very strong feeling that if you are trying to work with a doctor who doesn't want you involved with anyone else or isn't willing to listen to what you've discovered, then you need to hike yourself to a new doctor. That's my feeling."
>
> — Catherine

A solo practice means that a person sees the same doctor on each visit, which provides continuity in your care. In a group practice, which is made up of several doctors, you will likely see the same doctor on each visit, but you may occasionally see other doctors instead. A group practice may offer more resources, expertise, and availability of care. Board certification means that a doctor has been trained and has taken certification exams in a specialty. Fellows are specialists who have completed training in a general area of medical practice (such as internal medicine, surgery, or gynecology) and are undertaking additional specialized training in cancer care.

Because doctors can send patients only to those facilities where they have admitting privileges, people seeking treatment should know where doctors are affiliated—meaning which hospitals and/or institutions patients will go to for surgery or other care. A teaching affiliation, especially with a respected medical school, may indicate that the doctor is a respected leader in the field. Physicians with teaching affiliations who maintain practices often are in close touch with experts around the country and are usually well versed in the latest therapies.

Once you have identified the specialist you would like to see, don't be surprised if it takes several weeks to get an appointment. If you have been diagnosed with cancer and are seeking a second opinion, ask your doctor if you can afford to wait. Finding someone with an excellent reputation who will provide you with the care you desire and deserve is worth the research and a short delay if your situation permits.

Who Your Health Care Team Is and What It Does

Building a qualified and supportive health care team can increase your chances of having a positive treatment experience. Cancer care is an interdisciplinary endeavor, and while your oncologist may be the doctor you see most often, you will also see a variety of different professionals.

Questions You May Want to Ask a Doctor

- Experience: What is your experience and training? Are you board certified? How long have you been in practice? What is your specialty? What training have you had in treating this type or stage of cancer? How many patients with this type or stage of cancer have you treated in the past year?

- Office Visits: What can I expect from our office visits? Can you be contacted outside regular office hours? Who sees your patients when you are on vacation? May I tape-record our conversations so that I can review the details later or bring someone to my appointments to take notes?

- Members of the Team: What other types of doctors will be on my care team? What hospitals are you affiliated with? Will you handle referrals to specialists? Can you suggest an expert in this type or stage of cancer who can offer me a second opinion? Who on my health care team should I consider my main contact, and how do I get in touch with that person if I have questions or concerns?

An *oncologist* is a doctor who specializes in diagnosing and treating cancer. You may have been referred to the oncologist by your *primary care physician*, the doctor you would normally see first when a problem arises. (Your primary care doctor could be a general practitioner, a family practice doctor, a gynecologist, or an internal medicine doctor/internist). The oncologist will help determine the diagnosis, establish the treatment plan for your cancer, prescribe and supervise chemotherapy, and do some of your medical follow-up.

A *pathologist* is a doctor who uses laboratory tests to diagnose and classify diseases like cancer. The pathologist determines whether a tumor is benign or cancerous, and, if cancerous, the exact cell type and grade. A *radiation oncologist* is a doctor who specializes in radiation therapy that is given to treat cancers. A *surgical oncologist* is a doctor who specializes in cancer surgery. Usually these doctors focus on one part of the body, like the abdomen or the head and neck. A *neurologist* treats diseases of the nervous system. A *neuro-oncologist* is a neurologist with expertise treating brain tumors and the neurological complications of cancer.

An *oncology clinical nurse specialist* is a registered nurse who is an expert at caring for people with cancer. Oncology nurse specialists may administer treatments like chemotherapy, monitor patients, prescribe and provide supportive care, and teach and counsel patients and their families. An *oncology social worker* coordinates and provides non-medical care to people with cancer and their families, especially counseling and assistance in dealing with financial problems, housing (when treatments must be taken at a facility away from home), child care, and emotional distress. An oncology social worker is an expert in matching services and resources to a person's unique needs.

A *psychologist* assesses a person's mental and emotional status and provides counseling. *Psychiatrists* (medical doctors who specialize in mental health and behavioral disorders) provide counseling and can also prescribe medications. A *psycho-oncologist* is a psychiatrist with expertise dealing with people who have cancer.

You might also work with *pain specialists*, who may be doctors or nurses that make recommendations about the best treatments for controlling different kinds of pain. A *physical therapist* is a health professional trained to educate and assist you with exercises and other methods to restore or maintain your body's strength, mobility, and function. A *home health nurse* can give medications in the home, teach patients how to care for themselves, and assess their conditions to see if further medical attention is needed A *home health care aide* can assist with day-to-day household tasks such as bathing and preparing or feeding meals, but such services may not be covered by insurance plans or Medicaid/Medicare. A *nutritionist* or *dietician* assesses your nutritional state and recommends ways to eat that will help you deal with having cancer and cancer treatments. A *pastoral care expert* will provide spiritual care that is not limited to a single religion, and can address your spiritual concerns even if you are not religious. Sometimes throughout this book, we will refer to spiritual or religious leaders, or leaders of your faith or house of worship. The emphasis in this book is not on a particular religious denomination or school of thought, but on the ability of these individuals (be they ministers, priests, pastors, chaplains, rabbis, imams, etc.) to listen without judgment and provide spiritual counsel in times of need. See chapter 10 for

> —ɯ—
> "I think the most important question is, 'Am I going to be part of this team?' Where I work, our philosophy is that all of the members of the medical profession are part of the team and the patient is the captain."
> — Susan S.

more information on religion and spirituality, and the role of the pastoral care expert.

As mentioned earlier in chapter 1, *palliative care specialists* (usually members of a team consisting of a physician, nurse, social worker, and chaplain, all of whom have special training in palliative and supportive care) focus on providing comfort, controlling physical symptoms such as pain, and giving emotional or spiritual support to you and your family members, especially as the end of life nears.

Don't forget that you and your loved ones and caregivers are also important parts of the interdisciplinary care team. The information you can provide to clinicians about your life experience, your illness, and your culture and belief system is an essential contribution.

Talking to the Members of Your Health Care Team

Communication is a vital part of your medical care. You should feel comfortable talking with your clinicians and asking questions about your treatment and care. Here are some tips for talking to members of your health care team.

- **Tell your doctor how much you want to know.** Some people want detailed information about their medical status, including all their lab tests, and want to learn the medical language used to describe their condition. Other people want to know what is happening to them, yet don't want to learn about all the medical details. Some would even feel burdened or worried unnecessarily by knowing all the details. Many oncologists will allow you to be the guide to how much information you want (and when you want it) according to the questions you ask.

- **Be clear about your expectations.** For example, if you are having a test like a CT scan, be sure to make another office appointment or set a date or time when it would be best for you to call to discuss your test results.

- **Be honest.** Being honest with your doctor is critical too. In addition to allowing your doctor to gauge how much detail you want to know, most doctors find it helpful when their patients are upfront and straightforward about their preferences, questions, and concerns. For example, if you don't think you'll remember to take your antibiotic 4 times a day, you should tell this to your doctor. She might be able to substitute an antibiotic you only have to take twice a day.

—m— **Ask for a "plain language" explanation.** Don't hesitate to say: "You know, I think you just lost me. Could you explain that again?" or "I don't think I understood all the terminology there. Could you explain it again with words that will make sense to me?"

—m— **Consider what environment you need to have a productive conversation.** You should expect to talk about your medical issues in a place that is quiet and confidential. You may need to be sure the right people in your circle of family or friends are present.

—m— **Prepare a list of questions to ask.** Write your questions down before you visit the doctor. You may have questions about symptoms you are experiencing or about cancer information you have read or heard. If you bring your list of questions in when you see the doctor, your questions will more likely be answered. If you have a large number of questions, it is good to prioritize them in case your doctor does not have time to answer them all. You may be able to show your list of questions to a nurse, who can help you figure out which questions you should ask the doctor and which questions can be answered by another member of your health care team.

—m— **Figure out a strategy for retaining and sorting through information.** You'll want to keep track of the details of your treatments and care, both for your own information and to help assist others who participate in your caregiving. Hearing unpleasant, unexpected, and unwanted news is often overwhelming and may leave you feeling confused, numb, and angry. Most people only hear a fraction of what is being said at a time like this and therefore need to take steps to make sure they absorb and understand what was said. Taking carefully written notes of the conversations or having a dependable loved one with you can be helpful when hearing scary and complex information. Repeating back to the physician what you have just heard also helps you to better understand what is being said. If a family member or friend cannot be with you, ask that a

—m—

"You have to be your own advocate. I think you need somebody else in the room with you and you need to be taking notes, and don't let a doctor, he or she, put a hand on the doorknob to leave until you're through. You're the customer, and you ask all the questions and make sure you get them answered in a layperson's language so you can comprehend what they're saying."

– Keith

Figure 3-3. **Questions to Ask Yourself to Ensure
Good Communication with Your Health Care Team**

—~— How much information do I want to be told about my diagnosis or
health status?

—~— How do I want my health care team to communicate with me about these
issues (for example, don't beat around the bush, or break it to me gently)?

—~— What are the conditions I need when speaking with my health care team
(such as a quiet place, an adequate amount of time, no interruptions, a
tape recorder or personal advocate present to capture information)?

—~— How does my doctor like to make decisions, and how does he or she
present information to me?

—~— How will my doctor keep me posted about new developments in my care?

—~— What is most important to me when I consider treatment and care options
(for example, I want to live longer, minimize side effects, avoid pain, and/or
stay alert) and how can I communicate this to my health care team? As
my priorities change, how can I keep my health care team informed?

—~— Is there anything I can do to make communication with my health care
team easier?

—~— How can I reach my health care team in an emergency?

nurse be present when you receive medical information, and ask him or
her to help you sort through the information after the doctor leaves. You
may want to ask your physician if he or she minds if you tape-record your
visits. If you start this system of information gathering early, you will be
able to maximize your time with the health care team.

—~— **Communicate your goals.** Communication is a two-way street. By
telling your doctor what *your* most important goals and values are, your
doctor will come to know how she can best help you.

49

We've talked about discussing treatment and care options with your health care team. Reporting your symptoms is an essential part of that discussion as well. We'll talk more about this in chapter 8 as part of our discussion of identifying and coping with common symptoms experienced as a result of advanced cancer and its treatments.

Your Prognosis

A *prognosis* is a prediction of the probable course and outcome of a disease and an indication of the likelihood of recovery from that disease. When doctors discuss a person's prognosis, they are projecting what is likely to occur for that individual based on their own and others' experience with patients who have similar diagnoses. A particular prognosis does not necessarily indicate what is going to happen in your case. A person's cancer prognosis is determined by many factors, including the type of cancer, its stage, and its grade. Other factors that may also affect a prognosis include a person's age, general health, and the effectiveness of treatment.

> "I don't know what my outlook for the future is, but one of the things I do know about my outlook for the future is that I'm never going to know. And, that I have to learn to live with that. So, the uncertainty is just going to be part of my life."
>
> — Mary

DISCUSSING YOUR PROGNOSIS

Maybe you're wondering whether to ask your doctor about your prognosis. First, you should decide whether you want or need this information. Some people want to know as much detail as possible, so they can make plans and be very active in leading their health care team. On the other hand, some people would simply rather not know.

Some people feel that having lots of detail about their illness and prognosis could add to their burden or make them worry. Some might think, "If I can't change anything, why worry about all the details?" If you'd rather not know, you can expect that your health care team will respect your wishes, but you may need to take the lead to tell them that you're not a "give-it-to-me-straight" kind of person. Be honest with your team and with yourself when it comes to your preferences for this information. This way information can be shared with you in a manner that is tailored and made manageable specifically for you. Being truthful about how you cope best with the health care team and with yourself is always the best policy.

When deciding whether to ask about your prognosis, keep in mind that our experience tells us that people who are able to openly talk about their prognosis are much better able to make plans for the future and to create an atmosphere where communication is possible. In situations where there is an unspoken rule that prognosis is not to be talked about or even mentioned, energy is misdirected into maintaining the secret rather than talking about how to best care for the person with cancer during this difficult time. It takes a lot of energy to maintain a secret, especially one that is obvious to all concerned.

Requesting prognostic information is a personal decision. It is up to you to decide how much information you want, how you will cope with it, and what decision you will make next. You may have to take the lead, initiate the conversation, and ask your oncologist about your prognosis directly. Some doctors are reluctant to give a prognosis for fear of worrying you or taking away your hope.

If you feel you can cope with the information, it can be quite helpful to know your prognosis. First, knowing (in general terms) about the potential for recovery, remission, or how much longer you are likely to live can help you set priorities about your care, your goals (in treatment and in your life), and your time. You and your loved ones may be comforted by knowing whether or not certain symptoms (such as pain or shortness of breath) are likely to occur or intensify as your illness progresses, and that if these symptoms do occur, they can be managed. Even more importantly, you will likely be comforted to know some detail about the plan to control those symptoms if they do arise. Unless you tend to be a worrier, you may find that having more information makes you feel more in control and therefore more calm and soothed.

THE POSSIBILITY OF AN UNFAVORABLE PROGNOSIS

There may come a time when your oncologist tells you that efforts to cure your cancer have failed. When you hear this news, it may be difficult to muster the courage to ask your doctor to predict how long you have left to live. You should know that estimating this type of prognosis is difficult for your doctor as well as for you. These predictions are very hard to make with accuracy, and many doctors fear that putting a specific time estimate on the time a person has left to live can only be harmful, by taking away hope or encouraging a focus on dying instead of living. However, for most people, knowing at least an estimate of their prognosis can help them make decisions about their care,

> "At first when they said I had colon cancer stage IV, I didn't know what stage IV was....I said, 'Well, what is stage IV,' and they said, 'Metastatic cancer.' And I said, 'Well, what are you talking about here?...What are we talking here time wise?' And they said, 'Well, in your case, less than a year.'"
>
> — Sally

make plans for the time they have left, and begin the process of adapting to their new situation.

Being able to accurately predict exactly when a person is going to die is somewhere between tough and impossible. Many variables are important here, such as the extent of the disease, how rapidly it is advancing, and the impact of the disease on other illness processes not directly related to cancer. Of course, other important factors also include age and overall relative health. Generally, it is much easier to predict when one will die when the person is very near death (within hours or a very few days of death). If a person is on artificial life-support systems, such as a ventilator for breathing, the prediction is sometimes easier.

Don't expect a very specific estimate of prognosis, such as an exact date. You'll more likely be given a general range of times ("hours to days," or "days to weeks," or "several months at most," or "probably no more than a year or two"). While such time ranges are not specific, these estimates are more reasonable, given how difficult such predictions are to make.

Research suggests that both physicians and patients have a tendency to overestimate the amount of time people with advanced cancer have left. Sometimes this means that people with cancer don't access hospice care as soon as would be optimal.

And remember that your prognosis can change over time, depending on how the disease progresses, for example.

THE ROLE OF STATISTICS IN YOUR PROGNOSIS

Statistics is the collection, study, and interpretation of facts and figures to learn more about a certain event, experience, or group of people. Doctors use statistics to help estimate prognosis. Survival statistics indicate how many people with a certain type and stage of cancer survive the disease. It is easier for some people to cope if they know the survival rates for their cancer type, stage, and grade; others become confused and afraid when informed of statistics for their cancer. Your doctor is familiar with your individual situation and is most capable of accurately providing you with a prognosis.

Although statistics reflect how long very large numbers of individuals will live with any given condition, these are averages. Within those averages, there is a great deal of variation. Some people may live much, much longer than average, and others may not.

Getting a Second Opinion

Many people who receive a serious diagnosis like cancer, cancer recurrence, or metastasis find it helpful to have a second opinion. A second opinion involves going to see a different doctor who can take your history, do a physical exam, look at your test results, and give you her assessment of what is going on and what your treatment options are.

Getting a second opinion can reassure you that your cancer diagnosis is correct and that your treatment options are clear. Some people are scared to take the time to get a second opinion, worrying that their cancer will progress at a dangerously rapid rate. Your oncologist should be able to tell you if a few days or weeks will make a difference in your care. Although there is always a sense of emotional urgency relating to cancer, ask your oncologist: "Will it make a significant difference to the possibility of cure or meaningful extension of life if we wait a week or 2 so we can get a second opinion?" Except in those situations where there is an immediate medical crisis, it is quite rare that a few days or even a week or 2 will make a meaningful difference to long-term survival in persons with cancer.

"I went for a second opinion, and both doctors pretty much gave me choices. …I think there is a good feeling about knowing that you have looked into it, and you've decided. Then you accept that that's the one, whatever the outcome is, rather than someone else saying, 'Do this,' and not having a voice in it yourself. It gives you a little bit of power in the situation, I guess."
— Jeanne

The benefit of getting multiple opinions in terms of peace of mind can be immeasurable. Sometimes doctors disagree, and it helps to be able to gain a professional consensus.

You should not feel hesitant about seeking a second opinion, or even a third. Most doctors expect and welcome this step.

Taking an Active Role in Your Cancer Care

People have different feelings about how much space in their lives they want to give over to their cancer treatments. Some people want to rearrange their whole lives around their cancer treatments; other people want to keep part of their life totally free from any thinking about cancer and the treatments. Sometimes hard choices have to be made.

> "Health care these days, I think, is seen, generally speaking, as a partnership between doctor and patient; but sometimes it's the patient who has to be the aggressor, if you will."
>
> — Patty

Active participation can mean many things when it comes to cancer. However you decide to do this, taking charge of a part of your treatment can help you feel more like you have some control over what is happening.

Most people want to take the medication their doctors prescribe, and sometimes this can be a challenge if you are taking a number of different pills or shots. You can take charge of this by keeping track of when you take your pills and knowing when you will need refills or new prescriptions.

Some people keep track of their symptoms as a way of taking charge. You might want to keep a log of your pain experience, for example, that you can show to your doctor or nurse—they might even have log sheets that you can use to track symptoms. You can download logs for tracking pain and symptoms from the American Cancer Society Web site (http://www.cancer.org/docroot/MON/MON_1.asp).

Some people keep track of their lab and test results. This can get to be pretty complicated, but for some people is an important way of keeping on top of their cancer treatments. It's a good idea for everyone with cancer to keep track of any and all test results and keep medical information readily available. (If this task feels too daunting for you to undertake, you may want to ask a trustworthy friend or family member to help you organize this information.) You never know when you will be in a situation when your medical facts will need to be explained to another heath care provider.

"I wanted to be part of the process. So I found a surgeon who would make my husband and I part of the process, would explain everything to us, would give us options….I think you [take control] through reflective listening. You just say, 'I hear that you're saying that I need to have such and such done. In order to feel comfortable with that and to be the best patient that I can be for you, I need to have such and such.' Education, resources, I need to investigate insurance, and just spell it out in that way. 'I understand that you have my best interest at heart, that you want to do this procedure for me. I will be certainly willing to go along with all that, but first of all I need to have basic information and perhaps counseling.'"

— Ann F.

Finally, preparing for your visits with your doctors and nurses can enable you to get the most out of those visits. Asking questions, getting the information you need, and understanding what your doctors and nurses are recommending is a way of participating in your treatment. Having your questions answered and understanding the plan for your treatments will help you to cope better. And it will help you to be ready for the questions your friends and family might ask you.

Getting the Best Care Possible

How can you be sure you're getting the best care possible? For most people, what constitutes the "best" care depends on a number of things: how easy it is to get access to the care, how the doctors and nurses treat you as a person, how knowledgeable the doctors and nurses and other clinicians are in dealing with your medical issues, and whether the office, hospital, or medical center has the resources you need. While there are now many lists of "best" doctors, clinics, and cancer centers, the most important thing is how confident you feel in the treatment you are getting.

Depending on your health insurance, your financial situation, and your location, you may not have a great deal of choice in who treats your cancer or where that treatment is administered. But even if you cannot hand-pick your health care team, there are some steps you can take to ensure that you end up with a treatment setting and doctors and nurses that you feel confident about.

"I think the most important thing is to bring somebody in with you that can listen. Because one of the things that I found out was…that I didn't actually even realize 'til much later on after my treatment, was that things that I heard my doctor say were not the same things that my husband heard the doctor say.

"I think it's very, very important before you go to see a doctor to write down on a piece of paper a list of questions that you want to have answered. And as those answers are given to you, to write down what the answer is, and if more questions come up that you hadn't written down, ask those, write those down, and write down those answers as well."

— Susan S.

For example, you may have the experts at a cancer center in the nearest major urban center set your treatment plan, and then have the treatment administered locally. Good communication is the key.

You or your loved ones and caregivers may need to be prepared to advocate for you to ensure you receive the best care and treatment. While some organizations talk about "patient rights," it may be more productive for you to think about your relationship with your doctor and health care team as a collaboration rather than a battle of rights. If you don't feel like you have a good partnership, bring it up with your doctor. This will allow you to say what you would like in your medical care. Focus on what you need, because that will help you negotiate what could be changed in the future.

If that doesn't work, you may want to tell your oncologist that you would like to change to a different doctor. This happens to all doctors occasionally, and you do not need to worry about hurting his or her feelings. If you are able to mention this to your doctor, she might be able to refer you to another doctor who matches you better. Your primary care doctor can also be a very good source of information, because primary care doctors often deal with cancer specialists in working with their other patients. Of course, you can also get ideas for other doctors from your friends or other people you meet in the clinic or a support group.

A very helpful way to know you are getting the best care is to get a second opinion about the cancer care you should be getting (see the section on second opinions on page 53). In most cases, especially with rare cancers, it may be

"Many times we do not understand the medical terminology that has been initially used in giving us a diagnosis or a plan for treatment. And I think to cope with cancer, to make knowledgeable judgments on treatment, we need to get as much factual information that we understand as quickly as possible, in order to move forward with treatment. I tell the patients that I work with every day that they are consumers; that they have a right to ask questions of the physicians that they are seeing and to demand answers.

"My feeling is that it's the unknown that makes us anxious. Therefore, we need to expect information. So I not only asked the surgeon, I contacted the American Cancer Society. I used any resource I could to get specific information related not only to my diagnosis, but to the surgery that I was told I needed to have."

— Mary Jane

worth considering a trip to a cancer center where that particular kind of cancer has been treated numerous times.

Making Informed Treatment and Care Decisions

Once you have lined up your team of professionals, it's time to move forward with your treatment and cancer care. But with so many options available, lots of hard-to-understand medical terminology involved, and so much at stake, how can you be sure the treatment and care decisions you make are the right ones?

First of all, *there are no right or wrong answers*. There are only right answers and wrong answers *for you*. The decisions you make about treatment should be dictated by your type and stage of cancer. While the medical situation is generally the most important factor in decision making, you may also want to consider other issues. For example, how does the recommended treatment or care decision fit with your lifestyle, your self-image, your priorities, and your life goals? Does it mesh with your moral and spiritual beliefs and make sense to your loved ones and caregivers as well? Work with your health care team to try to make a treatment decision that is medically sound and that works for you.

—⁂—

"I think that it's important for all of us to make our own decisions when we are discussing treatment. It's very important because we are the ones that have to live with that treatment and the result of that treatment. And so, although I love my doctor, I choose not to just jump on anything that he or anyone else would say. So for me it's very calming and reassuring and helpful to research the information and discuss it with my oncologist, but ultimately to make the decision for myself....You're the one that has got the problem, and so it doesn't help to be able to say, 'Well, I didn't make the decision, it was my doctor.' So it's very important, I think, to be able to assess the information and feel comfortable. I think you have to feel that this is the best option that I can choose for myself."

— Greg

Making medical decisions can be a daunting task. But there are some essentials in the decision-making process that will maximize your abilities to make the best choices possible. First and foremost, you need to decide if decision making will be a solo endeavor or a collaborative effort. You must have clear and accurate information that you can understand, and that comes from reliable sources. You should always have someone with you (a loved one, a friend, a nurse) that you can count on to help you ask questions and push for clarification of information as needed. And you should be clear about the benefits and burdens of each treatment or care option. If the information you desire simply does not exist, then you need to know that as well.

Your Role in Decision Making

Earlier in this chapter, we talked about how not everyone with cancer wants to know the same amount of detail about their disease. Similarly, although most people want to know how their cancer can be treated, not everyone wants to play the same role in decision making. Different people have different decision-making styles. These styles vary widely and can be influenced by personality, culture and ethnicity, age, gender, level of education, and even mood on a current day. Some people want the oncologist to simply explain what the best treatment should be. Other people want the oncologist to describe all the possible treatment options, think about the options, and then make a shared decision with the oncologist. Finally, some people want to read the medical research themselves and want to have the primary decision-making role. Whatever your preference, make sure you express to your oncologist which decision-making style you prefer, so your health care team can respond to you in the most appropriate way. (See Figure 3-4 on page 60.)

THE ROLE OF OTHER PEOPLE IN YOUR DECISION MAKING

Obviously, your doctor's recommendations will carry a lot of weight in your treatment decisions. But there can be other people's opinions that you might want to take into account as well.

> "I'm the kind of person who wants all the information that I can get. I want to be able to make a decision as an equal partner with my providers. If I don't have the information, then I feel very uncertain and not reassured."
>
> — Ric

Consider the role you want your family or loved ones to play in the decisions about your treatment and care. First, you will want to make sure that they understand what you are facing. You may want to have one or two people be especially involved with your decision making. These "key supporters" might be a spouse, a friend, or an adult child. They might go to your medical appointments, so they hear all your conversations with your doctor and can help remind you of things that you talked about with the doctor, or even clarify things that you didn't quite understand. They might take notes to help you remember what the doctor talked about, or might take a recorder so that you could listen to the conversation with the doctor again later. They might help inform your other family members and/or friends about what is going on so that you do not have to tell the same information over and over again, which can use up a lot of your energy. They might help you make priorities and goals based on what they know about you. And they can tell you how the whole situation is affecting them, so that you can take that into consideration too.

There may be the opinions of others to consider as well. Do you routinely rely on fellow members of your house of worship or a member of the clergy to help you make big decisions? Is there anyone else who might be affected by your decision making that you want to discuss your options with, such as your employer? Figure 3-5 on page 60 lists some questions you may find helpful as you consult others and gather information to help you make decisions about your treatment and care.

Figure 3-4. **What Is Your Preferred Role in Decision Making?**

What role you want	What you say to the oncologist
Oncologist is primary decision maker	"I would like you to make a clear recommendation."
Shared decision making between you and the oncologist	"I would like you to tell me about the treatment options, so I can think about the pros and the cons, and then I would like us to make a decision together."
You are the primary decision maker	"I would like to hear about the treatment options, so that I can make a decision about what would be best for me."

Figure 3-5.   **Questions to Ask Others When Deciding on Treatment**

Questions for your family and/or close friends	• What is your opinion about the treatments? • How do you think this will affect our relationship? • Can I talk to you as a sounding board when I'm feeling unsure about things? • What are the ways you want to be involved with the treatments I'm thinking about?
Questions for your social worker	• What kinds of resources are available to help me and my loved ones? • Are there support groups that we could attend? • How can I cope with having cancer and having to deal with the treatment?
Questions for your chaplain, priest, minister, rabbi, imam, or other spiritual leader	• How can I stay connected to my faith during this time? • Are there practices or prayers that could help me? • Would you ask the faith community to pray for me (intercessory prayer)?

Gathering Information to Make Informed Decisions

If you want to share decision making with your doctor, or if you want to be the primary decision maker, you will need to gather information on your options. There are many ways to learn about the treatment and care options for the cancer you are dealing with, and several steps you should follow when gathering information leading up to a decision.

WHERE DO YOU GO FOR INFORMATION?

First, talk to your health care team. Your oncologist and the other professionals involved in your care have extensive knowledge about your treatment options and also have lots of hands-on experience with persons who have undergone those treatments. Have your team members explain the possible treatment options for your type and stage of cancer, and be sure each explanation includes the pros and cons of each option. As noted, it may be helpful to record the conversation, or have a friend or family member take notes while the oncologist is talking. Getting a second opinion is another way for you to gather information about treatment options.

Don't overlook sources in print or online. Your public library can be a valuable resource. Many people find the Internet useful for learning about treatment options, although the amount of information available on the Internet can be overwhelming and not all of it is scientifically accurate or current. The American Cancer Society (800-ACS-2345 or http://www.cancer.org) and the National Cancer Institute (800-4CANCER or http://www.cancer.gov) are reliable sources of up-to-date information. Both are great places to start.

> "I always imagined my feeling about hearing the words 'You have cancer' would be that I would just shrivel up and die on the spot, and I didn't. I immediately said, 'What is this, and tell me about it, and where can I get information?'"
>
> — Catherine

Naturally, talking to other people with cancer is very useful, especially to learn what it is like to undergo a particular type of treatment. Sometimes others are dealing with a situation that is different than yours, and you will want to check out this information with your nurse or doctor.

WHAT DO YOU NEED TO KNOW TO MAKE
AN INFORMED DECISION?

First, you should know what type of cancer you are dealing with and what stage it is. This information is in your pathology report and should be clear to you from your conversations with your health care team. If it isn't, seek clarification before proceeding any further. Next, you should know the treatment options, including their potential side effects, how often each treatment will be given, and what it is like to get each treatment. You will also want to know what impact the treatment will have on your quality of life and how often the treatment is successful in shrinking a tumor and in curing cancer. Note that some cancer treatments will shrink the cancer but are not expected to cure the cancer. Finally, you will also want to know how the treatment will impact the length of time you may live. Some cancer treatments can help people live for years longer; other treatments are expected to help people live for months longer. You may want to know this before you make a decision about starting treatment.

> "For me, fear—I guess for most people—comes from lack of information. I think that if you can get information on your particular cancer and the treatments and the success of those treatments, that it can alleviate some of that lack of information and fear. For me, it's done that."
>
> — Greg

Knowing what your oncologist expects from the treatment is important in helping you make plans and develop goals. Admittedly, asking for this information can be scary. Yet, if you can have a conversation about this with your doctor, this knowledge can be extremely valuable for you and your family. In the next few sections, we'll look at some questions you may want to keep in mind as you consider your treatment options. Honest and open communication with your loved ones and caregivers and your health care team can ensure you make the right treatment decisions for your unique situation at this particular time.

Can This Treatment Prolong Your Life?

For people with advanced cancer, treatments directed at curing cancer are not likely to completely eliminate their disease. However, some types of cancer treatment can sometimes help persons with advanced disease live longer than those who do not receive treatment. When considering any treatment options at this stage, ask your oncologist how likely this treatment is to prolong your life, and for how long.

Ask your doctor to consider your unique situation and estimate the approximate expected survival improvement with the treatment *for you*. If you are having trouble understanding the statistics or percentages involved with this kind of prognostication, ask your doctor questions like "How likely am I to be alive 6 months or 1 year from now if I decide to receive this treatment or if I decide to decline this treatment?" "How about 2 or 3 years from now?"

Can This Treatment Make You Feel Better?

One of the most important questions to ask when considering cancer treatment at this stage is "Can this treatment make me feel better?" Chemotherapy, radiation therapy, and other cancer treatments may still be useful for some persons even if there is no significant chance their lives will be lengthened by the treatment. In these cases, the main purpose of the therapy is to temporarily slow or retard the growth of the cancer, while minimizing the potential side effects from the treatment. Ask your doctor how likely each treatment is to help you live longer and what side effects you can expect to experience—this information will help you make an informed decision.

In some cases the oncologist may prescribe a treatment as a way of preventing a problem from happening rather than treating a problem that is already there. For example, sometimes doctors administer radiation therapy to the spine to decrease pressure on nerve tissue, which can cause paralysis of your legs as well as bladder and bowel problems. In these cases it is useful to ask the doctor how likely this treatment is to prevent the problem from happening and also to consider how bad the problem would be if it is not prevented. For example, weakness in your legs might be much more of a problem if you are now functioning well than if you are already spending most of your time in bed.

What Are the Potential Side Effects?

All cancer treatments have some side effects. It is important to consider the benefits and the risks of each treatment, as well as your overall quality of life when making a treatment decision. The frequency and severity of side effects can be very different for some treatments as compared to others. Study the situation and have your doctor make recommendations based on your specific case. If you are concerned about treatment-related symptoms and side effects as they relate to your quality of life, express these worries to your health care team so that you can work together to decide upon the best course of treatment.

What's Involved in This Cancer Treatment?

If you are considering a cancer treatment, you should be aware of the logistical arrangements for receiving this therapy. For example, one particular cancer treatment may require you to travel a long way to a cancer care center, while another may require you to give up your usual activities. Sometimes treatments can be very expensive, and if they are considered complementary or experimental, they may not be covered by insurance.

It is completely appropriate for you and your loved ones and caregivers to consider the logistic arrangements when deciding if you will receive a certain cancer treatment. Discuss these arrangements with your oncologist, since it may be possible to change the treatment to better suit the logistical needs of a given person with cancer and his or her family. For example, some treatments can be administered at a local hospital so that the person with cancer doesn't need to travel to a cancer care center. Or, it may be possible to replace multiple lower-dose radiation therapy treatments with 1 or 2 stronger doses, so that the person receiving care does not need to travel to the hospital many times.

Your oncologist may not be familiar with the specific logistical difficulties you may be facing, so be sure to discuss how any cancer treatment you are considering will affect your living arrangements, transportation, family support, caregiver responsibilities, or finances. Then you can work together to decide on a treatment that meets all of your needs.

Weighing the Benefits and Burdens of Each Treatment Option

Studies show that many people with cancer simply pick a treatment option based on their oncologist's recommendation. This approach works well for many, but other people may want to independently consider the benefits and burdens of each option. By *benefits*, we mean the reasons that the treatment will be helpful. A benefit might be that the treatment helps 50 percent of the people who get it to live longer compared to those who do not receive the treatment. Or a benefit might be that the treatment helps relieve pain. (A *survival benefit* is a very specific term used by doctors and statisticians to describe relative prognoses. Here, we're just talking about general benefits or advantages to choosing a certain treatment.) By *burdens*, we mean the side

Figure 3-6.

Weighing the Benefits and Burdens
of Treatment Options
(Sample Comparison Chart)

Treatment Option	Burdens	Benefits
Chemotherapy	• Can cause nausea • Requires weekly visit to clinic, with weekly blood tests • Requires IV line • Will probably cause some fatigue	• Can help me live longer, in the neighborhood of weeks to months longer • Can help control pain • Weekly visits enable me to get support at the clinic • I feel like I'm fighting the cancer
No chemotherapy	• I might not feel as hopeful because I'm not taking medicine to fight the cancer	• Will give me more time to spend with family and friends • No nausea or other chemo-related side effects • No need for weekly clinic visits, blood tests, or IV

effects of the treatment. For instance, some types of chemotherapy cause hair loss. Another kind of burden is how much the treatment requires in terms of clinic visits, lab tests, and scans. Some people will count the impact of the treatment on their family as another burden; for example the time off work a spouse might need to travel to the cancer treatments.

It can be very helpful to make a chart of the treatment options and the related burdens and benefits so you can see them all in one place and study the big picture (see Figure 3-6). Another type of chart can help you put the cancer in perspective with all the other issues you have in your life. This second chart was developed by medical ethicists who work with people facing difficult decisions (see Figure 3-7 on page 66).

Figure 3-7. Examining Other Issues Prior to Decision Making
(Sample Chart)

Medical issues	• Chemotherapy won't cure this cancer but it can slow the cancer down for some people.
	• The chemo has helped people with my types of stage of cancer live from weeks to months longer.
	• The chemo has side effects including nausea and fatigue. These side effects can be treated.
	• The chemo requires a weekly clinic visit.
Patient preferences and priorities (goals)	• To live as long as possible with a reasonable quality of life.
	• To make sure my family is taken care of during this difficult time.
Quality of life	• The chemo will definitely affect my quality of life, but I think I can still have a reasonable quality of life even during the chemo.
	• The nausea and fatigue won't interfere with my ability to enjoy my favorite pastimes, such as reading mystery novels and watching TV. However, it might affect my ability to enjoy my favorite foods and the amount of energy I have to play with my grandson.
Contextual issues	• My insurance will cover the chemo and the clinic visits so that the financial impact on my family and me will be manageable.

Tools for Decision Making: Advanced Cancer and Palliative Care Treatment Guidelines for Patients From NCCN/ACS

Originally developed for cancer specialists by experts at 19 of the nation's leading cancer centers in the National Comprehensive Cancer Network (NCCN), the *Advanced Cancer and Palliative Care Treatment Guidelines* have been translated for the general public by the American Cancer Society (ACS). This collaboration between the NCCN and ACS provides an authoritative and understandable source of cancer treatment information for the general public.

Presented in the form of background information on key topics followed by charted illustrations of "decision trees," these guidelines can help you better understand how to make decisions about your cancer care that are important to you. Call the American Cancer Society at 800-ACS-2345 to request a copy or visit the Web site at http://www.cancer.org to view or print the document. Ask or search for the latest version of the *Advanced Cancer and Palliative Care Treatment Guidelines for Patients*.

What Happens When What You Want Is Different From What Your Oncologist or Health Care Team Recommends?

Sometimes, what the person with cancer and his or her loved ones wants is different from what the health care team thinks is advisable. These situations may occur at any stage of illness and care. If this does happen, you and your loved ones and the members of your health care team should talk openly with one another to describe why each one feels a particular course of action is the best one. The better informed you are about one another's reasons, the more likely it is that you will be able to reach an acceptable solution or compromise.

When your oncologist or health care team makes a recommendation and you want to do something different, it can be stressful. Many people feel some pressure to do what the doctors and nurses recommend, because these people are considered the experts. However, it is equally important that you do what is right for you and your life. Your doctor or nurse may not completely understand what issues or circumstances you are facing.

If you want to choose a different course of treatment or a different care option than your team recommends, you may want to consider the following steps.

1. **Try explaining to your nurse or doctor why you want something different than what they are recommending.** Admittedly, some nurses and doctors will be more open to having this kind of conversation than others, and it is okay to choose the person that you find easiest to talk to. The goal of this talk should be to see if they can understand your point of view and also to make sure you understand the reasons for their recommendations.

2. **Consider getting a second opinion to see how another doctor or health care team would view your decision.** This can help you because you may learn something new that might influence your decision.

3. **Decide whether you can continue to work with that oncologist or health care team.** Most of the time, people with cancer can work with their health care team even if they do not share exactly the same opinion

about decisions. However, once in a while, a person with cancer will find that she does not feel comfortable with her oncologist or health care team. In this case it would be worth looking for an oncologist and health care team that you feel comfortable working with. This may mean switching institutions or clinics as well as oncologists. All oncologists have had patients who ultimately decided that they would like to work with someone else, and you do not need to worry about what your oncologist will think about you.

The Treatment You Have Decided on Works—What's Next?

When your treatment is effective in combating your cancer, then it is time to celebrate! Dealing with cancer has probably made you see your life, your relationships with loved ones, your work, and your spiritual dimension in new ways. Now you have the opportunity to appreciate and act on these new insights.

As you look back on your recent experience with cancer, it is also important to keep looking ahead. If you did not talk about prognosis with your doctor before, you may want to do this now. It may be important for you to understand how long the treatment will keep the cancer away. For some cancers, the treatments are expected to cure the cancer. For other cancers, the treatments will cause the cancer to regress temporarily. It may be important for you to know what to expect, because the time you have to celebrate may be a time you should use wisely. Many people with cancer have been dismayed when their disease returned, only to find out that their doctor only expected the treatment to last for specific period of time. Those people tell us they would have spent their time differently if they had known they had not been cured indefinitely, but had only won a temporary reprieve from illness.

What Happens If the Treatment You Have Decided on Doesn't Work?

Just because you spend time and energy gathering information, weighing the benefits and burdens, and deciding on the best course of treatment for your unique situation *doesn't mean the treatment will work*. You may undergo surgery, radiation, and/or chemotherapy only to find that your cancer has progressed despite medical intervention. What happens next?

Your doctor may have another anticancer therapy to offer, or perhaps he will know of a clinical trial involving an experimental treatment. But sometimes there are no clinical trials for your type of cancer, and no other treatments that are proven to work.

A SHIFT IN THE FOCUS OF CARE

As your disease progresses and the anticancer treatments are no longer effective, your oncologist may redirect your treatment toward a greater emphasis on comfort care and symptom management. If you haven't already been working with a palliative care team, your oncologist may put you in touch with one. A palliative care team is an interdisciplinary team of professionals who have special training in symptom control and addressing your psychological, social and spiritual needs. You can, of course, opt to continue to receive anticancer treatment alongside palliative care, and you may already be receiving both. You do not have to choose one or the other.

> —ᴍ—
>
> "The toughest time in the last 7 years has been when I've reached a new stage. Either treatment didn't work and we had to look at other options, or finally the doctor said, 'Okay, there's no cure possible. It's not even possible to live with this disease indefinitely. All we're doing is buying time. That's all we can do.'"
>
> — Ric

If your need for symptom management and supportive care warrants it, your oncologist may refer you to a palliative care physician. You and your oncologist may jointly decide that it makes the most sense for the palliative care physician to become the primary doctor coordinating your care at this point. However, change can be difficult, especially when the change means making adjustments to the health care team you know and trust. Meeting new people and having to manage the difficult and unwelcome news about disease progression is seldom easy. The palliative care team will have expertise and resources for dealing with these special issues that your oncology care team may not possess.

MAKING END-OF-LIFE TREATMENT AND CARE DECISIONS

Facing your mortality and contemplating your death can be very frightening. If you decide to continue with anticancer treatment such as chemotherapy or to try experimental therapies in the face of advanced cancer, it is important to think about—and to share with your family and health care team—what matters most to you. How many weeks or months of added survival is treatment with chemotherapy worth? Will the treatment make you feel better?

Will the treatment allow you to do or complete activities that are important to you? Will the treatment require too many trips to the oncology office, or can it be given by mouth? You need to weigh the pros and cons of treatment in the framework of your personal goals.

You do not need to do things to please anyone but yourself and those most important to you. For some people, experimental therapy—"doing everything"—is an important way of contributing by adding to our knowledge and understanding of new treatments and helping future persons with cancer. For others, being home with family and friends, saving energy for the people they love, makes much more sense. For each individual, these decisions are personal, and what's right is what feels right to you. When the time comes to make these decisions, it is important to focus your attention and your energy on what matters most to you. Regardless of your decisions regarding experimental therapy, everything possible should be done to improve your sense of well being by aggressively treating symptoms and preventing them when possible and getting emotional support for you and your loved ones.

> —ⁿⁿ—
>
> "My family absolutely thought I was giving up when I decided that I did not want to do chemo again….I went and told everyone that I wasn't going to do it anymore, and I would just let whatever happened happen. My friends and family thought that I had given up—that I just was going to go home and lie down and die. And I said, 'No, that's not it at all!' I said, 'I know who I am.'"
>
> — Karen

QUALITY OF LIFE AND END OF LIFE

Treatment decisions are usually a balancing act between what is most desired and what is realistic. It is generally accepted that with each treatment that fails to show benefit, the next treatments are less and less likely to offer a significant chance to extend either the length of your life or improve the quality of daily living. Our experience consistently shows that those people who get accurate information and have realistic expectations can make decisions that are best for themselves and their unique circumstances.

When there is no real chance of cure and precious time that can never be recovered is spent pursuing futile anticancer treatments, the costs can be high for all concerned. Meaningful time that could have been spent with family and close friends may be lost forever. Squandered time can never be regained. The statement that "we have nothing to lose" by continuing such therapies, no matter what, is not accurate. There is much to lose. Almost all anticancer

> "We live in a culture, in Western culture, that does not want to talk about death and doesn't have much to support those of us who are dying at younger ages, or even for the elderly who are dying….Everything is about youth and looking great until you're 900 years old! So, for someone who's 49 or 56, we're facing death, and yet it's all about fighting cancer…. So what happens when you decide not to fight it anymore, and you just decide to accept the fact that you're dying?"
>
> — Karen

treatments have unpleasant side effects and may be expensive. Once the balance of benefit and burden is clearly understood and openly discussed, an informed decision can be made. When the costs and risks of additional disease-directed therapies outweigh the benefits, all energies are best directed at humanizing the time remaining among loved ones. Remember that even if you discontinue treatments that are designed to try to cure cancer or stop its spread, you do not have to give up all treatments—supportive care and symptom management are still treatments. Palliative care can be especially helpful at this time. Ask your health care team about treatments that can make you more comfortable, such as taking medications that can control symptoms such as pain, bleeding, or shortness of breath.

ARE YOU GIVING UP?

When cure is no longer a reasonable expectation, it is easy to feel like a failure, rather than to acknowledge that medicine is limited and that science has not yet mastered all cancers. This is a hard fact of life. Openly sharing these realities of life can be a way of bringing you and your loved ones closer together and enabling you to feel both truly human and deeply connected to each other. Avoidance and keeping secrets wastes vast stores of energy and time that can be better used by you to provide caring and comfort. When there is no longer a cancer treatment that realistically holds promise for meaningful extension of life, the time you have left to share becomes even more valuable. Fears are helpful in alerting you to potential danger, but sustained fear interferes with peaceful, meaningful living.

When anticancer treatment shifts to palliative care (comfort-directed treatments aimed at maximizing quality of life), there can be a sense of fear and concern over abandonment. Whether it is a palliative care team in the hospital or a hospice team that comes to your home, you will need to learn how to relate to the new team of professionals. Palliative care and hospice teams are always comprised of a team of at least a physician, nurse, social worker, and pastoral care expert. They will focus on the cancer symptoms and also attend to the emotional, psychological, and spiritual needs of the person with cancer as well as his or her family members, caregivers, and loved ones.

RECEIVING THE NEWS

Coping with bad news, especially when it comes to a prognosis that your time is limited, can cause you to feel sad, frightened, and emotionally overwhelmed, at least at first. If you need some time to regain your composure before you get further information, ask for it. You can help your doctor know the pace you need to absorb the information you need and handle the emotions you may feel.

> "When I was first told that I was terminal, it was like bullets hitting me. I mean, at that point I couldn't have heard a thing that anybody was saying."
>
> – Karen

If your doctor says, "There's nothing more to be done to treat your cancer," you may feel like giving up. Once you digest this news (which can be a very difficult mental and emotional task and may take some time), you may want to approach your health care team with questions like, "Can you tell me about what our new plan will be?" or "Can you help ensure that I receive good supportive care in this next phase of my illness?" For many people, coping with their own mortality is the hardest task they will ever encounter. For some people who are facing their death, there is a strong desire to protect loved ones, to understand death within the larger context of a life lived, to control their fear about the unknown, and to ensure that they will not be abandoned. For others, their own needs and concerns are all they can possibly concentrate on. We'll address these issues and more in the next chapter on talking about and coping with cancer.

MAKING NEW PLANS AND SETTING NEW GOALS

As you absorb the information about the progression of your disease and deal with its emotional effects, you will gradually go through a process of making new plans and setting new goals based on your new situation. This can be a very important time for you and your family to reflect on what has transpired and what is yet to come. You can leave a legacy, renew connections with your loved ones, perhaps even go to some of your favorite places. See chapter 9 for information on making the most of the last stage of your life.

>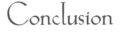
> "You are facing every single day with the fact that you need to put as much life as you can in every moment that you possibly can."
> – Michael

Accepting any sort of change takes good coping skills (see chapter 4) and a certain amount of work. But the payoffs can be rich.

Conclusion

One of the challenges for persons with advanced cancer and their loved ones is determining whether continued anticancer treatment is appropriate for them at the present time, and if so, what is the expected outcome. For example, will you choose to continue chemotherapy with curative intent despite severe side effects, even when it appears that the treatment is no longer effective? Will you choose to undergo treatments that will not cure your cancer, but might be able to prolong your life?

Making decisions about treatment for progressive disease can be stressful for people with cancer and their loved ones. Keep in mind that no decisions are final: being willing to receive therapy now does not mean that you need to continue receiving therapy indefinitely. On the other hand, the decision to not receive anticancer treatment today does not mean that you cannot revisit and review this decision days or weeks later.

Medicine is an art as much as a science. Caring for others is a calling as much as a job. Finding the right team of professionals who can help you balance hard science with humanity as you gather information for making treatment and care decisions can help make your experience within the medical system a positive one.

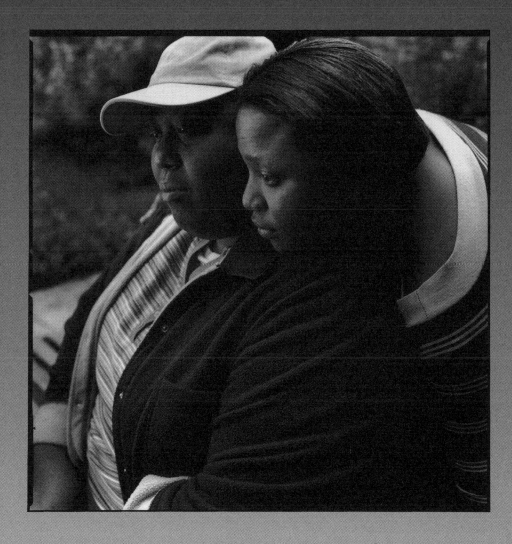

Chapter 4

Coping With
a Life-Limiting Illness

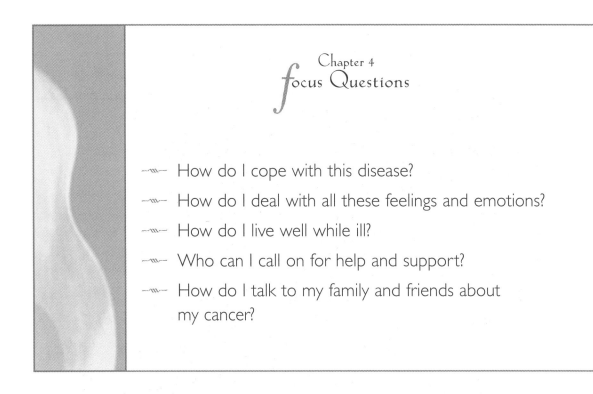

Chapter 4
focus Questions

—∽— How do I cope with this disease?

—∽— How do I deal with all these feelings and emotions?

—∽— How do I live well while ill?

—∽— Who can I call on for help and support?

—∽— How do I talk to my family and friends about
my cancer?

"I'd like to offer a definition of 'positive attitude.' It wouldn't be a happy, upbeat, definitely-everything's-going-to-be-okay attitude all the time. A positive attitude is one that helps you get good medical care, helps you relate to the people in your life, and helps you live as fully as possible no matter what is happening. If you can look for the silver linings, if you can try to put a positive spin on difficult times, if you work really hard to find and nourish hope, that feeds a positive attitude. But it also means allowing the unpleasant, negative, painful emotions to surface in safe places so that you can deal with them and move on."

— Wendy

A DIAGNOSIS OF ANY SERIOUS ILLNESS IS DIFFICULT to understand and manage. Most people will feel overwhelmed at first with the very idea of cancer and what lies ahead. The path can become rockier when you are going through the struggles of a recurrent or second cancer, metastasis, or when you discover that cure or long-term remission is no longer likely.

There is no single formula for coping when you are seriously ill or approaching death. However, we do know a lot about caring for cancer patients with advanced disease. In this chapter we will share this wisdom with you. The information that follows has helped us and others to manage the challenges of a serious illness and of dying well. We cover a broad range of topics in this chapter, and it may be that not all of them apply to you and your unique situation, so feel free to focus on the sections that most closely pertain to your needs. Also, your needs may change throughout the course of your illness, so you may want to return to this chapter as new challenges arise.

What Is Coping?

Coping means managing problems and difficulties and attempting to overcome them. Coping is relatively easy when challenges are small and problems can be solved. But when the problem is cancer, and cure does not seem to be a likely possibility, coping is about managing the cancer and its progression in a way that focuses on your quality of life each day. In other words, it means living today to the fullest.

> —⁓—
> "Something that works wonderfully for one person can be damaging to another, and there is no right way or one way to go through cancer."
>
> — Wendy

Why Is Coping Important?

Developing good coping skills will help you accept and deal with difficult situations. Managing the challenges you face with grace is also helpful to those around you. When you are at peace, it makes those around you feel calmer. In this way, you are also teaching your loved ones how they can cope with the serious problems *they* may encounter. Whether the challenge is learning how to best manage the news of a new cancer diagnosis or learning how to die well, you will benefit from trying the methods of coping other people with cancer and their loved ones have found helpful.

Strategies for Coping

Although the implications for managing difficult news can be quite different depending on the specific circumstances, the ways in which you can best cope with life's challenges are essentially the same. Think of how you have gained control of other difficult situations and serious problems in your life. How did you surmount those challenges? What strategies worked for you? What resources were you able to call upon to help you through the most difficult times?

The steps to best manage the challenges before you will be same whether you are coping with the news of your initial diagnosis, a recurrent or second cancer, metastasis, or the news that your cancer is not responding to treatment and your time is limited.

—⟨⟨⟨—

"Cancer caused a tidal wave of changes! And they were very difficult. There were practical issues to address. I had a lot of emotional issues. I wasn't functioning as a doctor. I couldn't take care of my children. I was afraid of dying. I was sick....

"I was 36 years old, there were many things that, I think partly because of my age, I wasn't comfortable with or I didn't have the tools for dealing with it. Because I was willing to discuss these difficult things and share my genuine emotions of fear or anxiety or sadness, I developed tools. I learned tools that made me stronger than ever."

— Wendy

In the next few sections of this chapter, we'll outline some specific coping strategies you can use to help manage your situation wherever you are in the course of your cancer care. These strategies include, but are not limited to: identifying and managing emotions, taking action, making plans, building your support network, and talking to others.

Identifying Your Feelings

A first step in coping is to try to identify your feelings. Next, determine if these emotions and sensations are new or familiar, and if they represent an increasing level of distress. Be honest with yourself. Are you someone who tends to have a short temper? Are you someone who tends to worry or be fearful? Are you someone who easily gets overwhelmed in stressful situations? Look at the pattern of your whole life. Ask someone you trust who knows you well for an outside perspective. If what you're feeling is a familiar emotion or trait with "the volume turned up louder" because of the stress of the situation, this is helpful information. You may be soothed to know that this is likely to settle down once you adapt to the stressful situation you're in.

On the other hand, if your feelings are new or unfamiliar, if they represent a change from your usual inner world, then consider your situation. Have you just heard some bad news or found out about some new challenge you'll have to face? Though these feelings are distressing and can be very intense, they may simply be normal reactions to sudden stresses. You may want to talk things over with someone you trust. Reflect on the activities that can help reduce your distress such as listening to music, meditation, and prayers. Make a conscious effort to do things that you enjoy and that bring you pleasure—watching movies, arranging photographs in an album, playing cards or doing crossword puzzles, spending time with loved ones, or engaging in a favorite hobby. And most of all, be gentle with yourself. Give yourself permission to experience the spectrum of emotions that are likely to present themselves. Allow yourself time and the space to adapt to this latest challenge.

One way to do this is to engage in an internal dialogue, sometimes also called self-talk. Everyone engages in self-talk, either spoken out loud or silently noted. The things we say to ourselves are often task oriented, such as "don't forget to pick up that new prescription at the drugstore on the way home." But self-talk can also be positive (such as, "I know I can get through this") or negative (for example, "I might as well just give up"). Communication and medical professionals have researched the psychological components of self-talk, and they have concluded that what people say to themselves affects their ability to cope. Individuals can tap into the power of their own self-talk by recognizing it for what it is, and replacing negative internal messages with positive ones.

> "I think that it helps to have a positive attitude because it makes your days worthwhile. I'm not convinced that it will change how long I live, but it will certainly change the quality of my life."
>
> — Jeanne

If any troubling or unfamiliar feelings don't go away, or if they keep getting more intense, you may need more specific attention or professional intervention. We'll talk more about handling emotions like fear, anger, guilt, grief, anxiety and depression, and hopelessness in the next few sections.

FEAR

What if you are scared to die? This is a specific example of a fear that, for most people, becomes less of a problem when it is talked about. Find someone you trust and talk with them about your fears. Try to articulate what exactly you are frightened of. What do you fear in particular about dying: the process of dying, or what will happen to you after your death?

Your health care team can help you know what to expect as disease advances. Often, knowing that those who are caring for you know what complications and problems are likely to arise, if any, is reassuring. Even more reassuring is hearing that there are already plans in place for how to manage these problems if they do emerge. Ask questions, get answers, and know the plan ahead of time.

Mental health professionals can also offer a great deal of support to you and your loved ones as you try to come to terms with your fears about advancing illness, death, and life after it. Don't hesitate to ask your doctor to recommend a social worker, psychiatrist, or psychotherapist to help you address these concerns.

A trusted clergy person, chaplain, or pastoral care counselor can also help you work through existential and spiritual issues related to confronting your illness and seeking peace and meaning at end of life (see chapter 10).

If your worries have to do with what will happen to those you love after your death, help them prepare. Are there documents such as a will that need to be prepared? (See chapters 5 and 7.) Are there conversations you need to have to pass on instructions? Are there conversations you need to have to pass on blessings? Are there conversations you need to have to ask for and offer forgiveness for past hurts? (See chapter 9.) Now is the time to resolve unfinished business—for your peace of mind, your quality of life, and for the quality of your relationships with those you love most.

> "It's kind of like the stock market, you know, your feelings really fluctuate."
>
> — Dan

ANGER

Anger, though frequently justified, can be a signal that something is wrong and needs attention.

People often displace their anger onto those who are close to them. If you are feeling angry, consider the source of your anger and who you are taking it out on. Because you cannot express your anger to the disease itself or to a different source of your frustration and sadness, you may find yourself feeling angry and irritable with family and friends, or whoever happens to be nearby. Try not to lash out in anger because you are overwhelmed, frustrated, afraid, and upset about your situation.

Anger itself is not a bad thing; how you handle it is the key. Anger can be a productive emotion if it is harnessed and channeled toward productive ends. Try redirecting your anger into positive action, such as making positive changes in aspects of your life and your cancer care that you can control. If you are having difficulty coping with your anger, and you find yourself "taking it out" on those around you, seek the help of a mental health professional.

"I remember her being so angry and taking this tissue box and with her good arm, her right side, and flinging it at me. It was just a tissue box, so it wasn't anything, but she just started picking up things and throwing them at me, and I went in the bathroom and I closed the door and I just wouldn't come out until, like, she kind of calmed down…I was not so much angry with Wendy. I mean, I was angry that she was dying. I was angry at the whole situation."

– Joanne

GUILT

Both people with cancer and those who provide them with emotional support and care may experience feelings of guilt. You might feel guilty about being ill, even if you know it isn't your fault. You may feel guilty that you are leaning so heavily on others, or that your illness is using up family resources. You may feel guilty that you cannot meet the responsibilities you used to be able to meet, or fulfill promises you made when you were in better health.

Caregivers—especially loved ones and family members who assume this primary role—are likely to experience some guilt as well (see chapters 11–13 for more information and resources for caregivers). They might feel guilty about opportunities they are missing because of their caregiving responsibilities, about being healthy when someone they love is sick, about not doing enough for their loved one, or even for having feelings of frustration or resentment stirred by the challenging task of caregiving.

The best things you can do to alleviate guilt on all sides are to clear the air and be open about your feelings. Acknowledge that everyone is doing what they can to make the best of a difficult situation and that some sacrifices are involved. Express your gratitude to one another. When possible, primary caregivers should share the work of providing care with others—family members, friends, even professional nurses or paid companions—who can help.

GRIEF

Grief isn't only experienced after someone dies. Grief is a deep and poignant distress caused by the loss of something dear. It encompasses feelings of sorrow (sadness) or regret, especially for the loss of someone or something you love. You may be grieving the loss of the life you used to have before cancer. You may

"When my daughter first heard, she was just getting married and they had only given me like 4 months to live. Her immediate reaction was, 'You won't see my babies.' And I said, 'Michaela, I can't go there.' I said, 'I really can't go there.' I mean, she was so upset—you know, the thought of me not being able to see her children, and then also the fact that I wasn't going to be a part of her life ongoing. And I said, 'We just have to stay here in the present moment. We have to be able to live our life right now, day by day by day, and not worry about things in the future, because the future may not be there.'"

— Karen

be grieving over "what could have been," the loss of opportunities to experience things in the future. You may even be grieving on behalf of your loved ones for their loss of you. This grieving should not be discouraged; it must be acknowledged and worked through to gain peace of mind and acceptance of your situation. While different people deal with grief and sorrow differently, there are some common steps in the grieving process and some things you can do to help ease your suffering.

Caregivers and loved ones may experience grief while a person is ill as well as after they pass away. See chapter 13 for more information on how loved ones and caregivers may experience and manage grief.

ANXIETY AND DEPRESSION

Under the stress of advanced illness, some people develop emotional distress. Anxiety and depression are types of that distress and are common complications of advanced cancer like pain or fatigue. Like other complications, there are effective medical and non-medical treatments for depression and anxiety, and you should not have to carry the extra burden of these complications when you are battling advanced cancer.

Depression might make you feel very sad or negative about yourself or others, diminish your ability to enjoy the good things in life, interfere with your sleep or appetite, or even make you feel like giving up altogether or ending your life. Anxiety may manifest itself as excessive worry, inability to relax, physical or mental tension, or full-blown panic attacks. Your distress makes the suffering caused by physical symptoms (pain, breathing problems, insomnia) worse, and may even make the experience of these physical problems more intense. Your health care team can help to assess your situation, provide medication to relieve these symptoms, and/or make a referral to someone who counsels people experiencing these symptoms. If depression or anxiety complicates this time in your life, don't just try to "tough it out." You don't have to struggle with these extra burdens. Seek treatment for these problems and get the most out of this precious time with the ones you love. See the Coping With Depression and Managing Anxiety sections of chapter 8 on pages 175 and 176 for more information on managing these conditions.

HOPELESSNESS

What if you feel like giving up? If you have trouble shaking a feeling of hopelessness, tell a trusted family member, friend, spiritual advisor, or member of your health care team right away. *If you feel you have no options other than to end your life now, seek help immediately.* You do not have to bear these feelings alone. These kinds of thoughts and feelings are very commonly a manifestation of distress and difficulty coping. People with feelings of hopelessness may have other problems (pain, nausea, shortness of breath) that worry and distress them to the point that they feel their only escape is to escape this life. Non-physical problems (a serious family fight or conflict, a spiritual crisis, or financial worries) may also leave a person feeling hopeless. Your family and treatment team can help you in addressing these underlying problems directly, but only if you make them aware of the situation.

Also, efforts aimed at finding and strengthening hope in specific areas where you have control and can look forward to good things happening can help reduce general feelings of hopelessness (refer to the Finding and Maintaining Hope section in chapter 10, page 226).

Taking Action/Doing Something About It

Sometimes, there's no better way to cope with a problem than to *do something about it*. You may not be able to stop cancer in its tracks, but there are lots of things you can do to take control of your situation and cope with your disease.

EDUCATE YOURSELF

Oftentimes, we are scared of what we don't understand. Learning as much as you can about your disease may help you and your family address fears about what could happen as your cancer progresses. Check out books from the library and search reputable Web sites for information (see Figure 4-1 on page 86). Talk with other people who are going through similar experiences.

Don't hesitate to ask your doctors, nurses, and other health care providers if there is something you want to know. Don't be embarrassed to ask the doctor to repeat or explain something or spell unfamiliar words. Don't worry that your doctor will be upset if you question his or her treatment recommendations.

Your health care providers may seem hesitant to offer information. They may not be able to explain exactly what to expect. Or they may be waiting until you seem ready for the information. You can signal your readiness by asking specific questions about your life, your illness, and what will happen to you. Most health care professionals know that coping with treatment is easier when people with cancer understand what is happening and why, and that the learning process itself is an effective coping mechanism.

TAKE AN ACTIVE ROLE IN YOUR TREATMENT AND CARE

Taking an active part in your care can help you regain a sense of control. There are many ways to get involved. For example, do what you can to keep your doctor informed. Make notes about your symptoms and report honestly how you feel. If problems arise, describe them as specifically as possible. Take notes on conversations you have with your health care team, and ensure you get copies of your medical records. Ask your health care team to share all options with you, even complementary methods or the possibility of participating in

Figure 4-1. **Assessing Health-Related Web Sites**

Many Web sites offer helpful, legitimate health-related information. But some Web sites present myths as facts, suggest unproven methods or miraculous cures, or offer opinions rather than scientific evidence. Sometimes it can be hard to tell the difference. The National Cancer Institute offers these 10 ways to evaluate health information on Web sites:

1. **Who runs the site?** Any good health-related Web site should clearly state who is responsible for the site and its information.

2. **Who pays for the site?** The source of a site's funding should be clear. Are there advertisements on the site? If so, are they for respected products or services?

3. **What is the purpose of the site?** Check the "About This Site" link to see if it explains the goal of the site.

4. **Where does the information come from?** If the person(s) or organization in charge of the site didn't create the information, the original source should be labeled clearly.

5. **What is the basis of the information?** Medical facts and figures should have references. Opinions or advice should be set apart from information based on research results.

6. **How is the information selected?** Do people with excellent medical qualifications review the material before it is posted?

7. **How current is the information?** Medical information should be current and the site's most recent update or review date should be posted.

8. **How does the site choose links to other sites?** Some sites link only to other sites that have met certain criteria. Other Web sites link to any site that asks, or pays, for a link.

9. **What information about you does the site collect and why?** Any credible health sites asking for personal information about you should tell you exactly what they will and will not do with it. Be certain that you read and understand any privacy policy or similar language on the site.

10. **How does the site manage interactions with visitors?** There should always be a way for you to contact the site owners with problems, feedback, and questions.

research studies and clinical trials (see chapter 2). Tell your health care team that you want be involved in decision making. This will help give you a sense of autonomy as you deal with your situation.

RECOGNIZE THERE ARE SOME THINGS YOU CANNOT CONTROL

Many people are familiar with a version of the serenity prayer, which asks a higher power to "grant me the serenity to accept the things I cannot change; courage to change the things I can; and wisdom to know the difference." One essential step in coping with cancer and its progression is to acknowledge that while there are many things you can control—your attitude, for example—there are some things you cannot. Seek the wisdom to recognize the difference between the two, and don't waste your precious time or energy worrying about or trying to fix things beyond your control.

MAINTAIN YOUR PHYSICAL HEALTH AND COMFORT AS BEST YOU CAN

Sometimes, the unrelenting course of advancing cancer may make you feel out of control of your body. It's true that you can't will a tumor to spontaneously disappear or order your unruly cells to behave themselves and quit multiplying, but you can still make a conscious effort to live healthfully. Don't fall into the trap of "letting yourself go." Do all you can to make the time you have left *quality time*.

Eat a variety of healthy foods (given your appetite and what your specific treatment regimen allows), stay as active as you can (whether that means going for a slow stroll in the park or doing range-of-motion exercises in bed), and get an adequate amount of rest. Continuing to make the effort to live healthfully, even as cancer progresses, can help you combat the stress of your illness and can help boost your spirits. It can also heighten your energy level so that you have the stamina to put your affairs in order and do the things you want to do in the time you have left.

Also, don't tolerate inadequate pain relief. If you have pain or discomfort from your cancer or its treatment, talk to your health care team about pain control. Don't try to tough it out, and certainly don't let pain stop you from doing the things that bring you pleasure and happiness. Cancer pain can almost always be lessened through a variety of medications and non-medical techniques. (See chapter 8 for more information on managing pain.)

> —⁓—
>
> "You have to live in the moment. But some of the other things I do to get me through…I have my children's milestones to get me through chunks of time. You know, my son graduated from high school, and now my daughter will be graduating from high school in 2 years, and then it will be my son's turn to graduate from college, and so on. Those kinds of things have gotten me through."
>
> — Catherine

PLANNING AHEAD

Taking meaningful and purposeful action according to a well-thought-out plan can reduce uncertainty, redirect your negative emotions like anger and fear, and will also benefit both you and your loved ones. This type of advance planning can take place across many realms of your life.

Wherever you are in the continuum of cancer care, think about your next steps in terms of a conscious action plan—one that you've arrived at with input from loved ones, caregivers, and medical experts. Approach your medical treatment and care in a thoughtful, orderly fashion. Never leave a medical visit or encounter with a health care professional without an action plan or clear sense of what comes next. If there are choices available to you, or if a decision needs to be made, gather all the appropriate information and consider both the benefits and risks associated with each option before proceeding. Revisit chapter 3 for more information on how to go about this.

Focusing on those aspects of the problem that can be realistically changed or influenced and joining with your team in a clearly defined common effort can go a long way toward helping you cope with what may have originally seemed like an insurmountable challenge.

Finally, make plans for those happy events! Set goals and remind yourself of all the wonderful things you have to live for. Perhaps you want to reach a certain birthday, or live long enough to fulfill a certain dream or witness a certain special event—a marriage, a birth, or an anniversary. Let planning for and anticipating future happiness help you cope and lift your spirits in the present.

Building Your Support Network

Thinking about dying is hard, but allowing yourself to become isolated will only make the process much harder. By reaching out to others and drawing

"I've had experiences that have been so wonderful that I just can't imagine where people have all this hidden—this goodness in people. When I went through my leiomyosarcoma diagnosis and had surgery and radiation and one of the worst chemo regimens a person can have, I was in the hospital 10 times in 6 months. People from my daughter's dance school and my employer got together, and for 9 months brought meals—full meals—to our door 5 days a week."

— Catherine

your resources together, you create an environment where you and your loved ones can give and receive comfort and support. If you do not have adequate psychosocial (psychological, emotional, and practical) support from those around you, coping with a serious disease can be more difficult.

Abandonment—not dying—is the greatest fear of many people. Abandonment can be experienced on many levels. You may fear your family or friends will abandon you, or you may feel as though God or your faith has abandoned you, or you may worry about having to abandon your autonomy and independence or control over your finances as your disease progresses. *But you do not have to face the end of your life alone.* There are many places people with cancer and their loved ones and caregivers can draw support from. Support can come from other family members and friends, health professionals, support groups, and your source of spirituality or place of worship. Even if you don't have a close circle of family or friends nearby, you still have many resources that can help you face this challenge.

YOUR PARTNER

Your spouse or partner has the potential to be your greatest source of support. Communication is the key to maintaining a good relationship during this difficult time. Being honest about your emotions can help you draw support from each other. Be sure your life partner feels involved in the medical decision making, because the care and treatment options you choose have huge implications for him or her. Reaffirm your devotion to one another with loving words, hugs, and kisses.

—·ɯ·—

"My husband has been a saint through all of this. He has been my partner. The term he used was 'we.' He said at the very beginning, 'WE are going through this. Not just YOU.' He has been there through every incident that I have gone through. He has been there with me."

— Diane

Try to allow your partner room to pursue individual interests and essential life tasks. If you didn't spend 24 hours a day together prior to your illness, try to allow your spouse or domestic partner some time to engage in activities he or she enjoys. Use the time when you reconnect to learn about things that are happening beyond your world. This will give your partner more energy and an improved attitude—which translates into more support to give back!

Don't overlook the valuable services social workers and mental health professionals can offer in this realm. They can counsel you and your partner and can help couples and families talk about hard-to-discuss topics, such as end of life planning.

Physical Intimacy

You may find yourself unable to express yourself sexually as you did before because of physical changes and emotional concerns. Sexual problems may stem from feelings about your medical condition or treatment as well as from the condition or treatment itself. With patience and communication between partners, many of these problems can be solved. Understanding why sexual activity may not be the same as before can prevent unrealistic expectations and relieve feelings of self-consciousness or anxiety.

Don't be afraid or embarrassed to seek advice. Your doctor may be able to offer some guidance or provide a referral to a professional who specializes in addressing sexuality. Books that deal with sexuality or that offer people with cancer specific information on this subject may also prove helpful.

Even as your physical health deteriorates, don't give up on your needs and desires for intimacy. There are many ways to show love. Physical satisfaction can be found in a variety of ways, such as touching, kissing, stroking, and holding.

YOUR FAMILY

Your family can also be a source of support for you. During your treatment and care, daily routines around your household will probably have to change, and you may no longer be able to do the things you did before. For example, your partner may need to tackle new duties, such as cooking meals or paying bills, and your children may be required to pitch in more with duties around the house.

> "Cancer affects the whole family, and I think a family needs as much help as a patient, and too many times we forget that. We get so concerned about the patient, but we need to reach out to the family as well, to provide some of that support."
>
> — Mary Jane

Try not to feel guilty about asking others to help pick up the slack. Family members may feel powerless against your cancer, and doing concrete tasks can help them feel as though they are making a contribution to your well-being. However, be realistic about demands on your family members—especially young children and adolescents—who also may be having a difficult time.

Don't let changing roles and responsibilities build resentment. Try to allow your family to maintain a sense of routine as much as possible. If book club or poker night or 30 minutes on the treadmill every morning was a constant in your family's life prior to cancer, then try to continue with the same routine. Family members need to do familiar things they enjoy without a sense of guilt.

And as always, talk openly with one another about your fears, hopes, and concerns.

YOUR FRIENDS

Be prepared for cancer to change your relationship with your friends. You won't be able to predict how others will respond to a diagnosis of advanced cancer or your doctor's prognosis that you may only have a short time left to live. In some cases, friendships will deepen as your friends rise to the occasion to support you by visiting, keeping your spirits up, engaging you in meaningful conversations, pitching in around the house, and accompanying you to medical appointments. Letting others help is productive for both you and the other person.

In other instances, you may find that even old or familiar friends are made uncomfortable by your illness, and do not know how to act around you anymore. Try not to take this personally—some may simply be unable to cope with the emotional pain your illness causes them, and others may want to

"I had some people saying to me, 'I was afraid to call. I didn't want to say anything. I didn't want to send flowers, nothing like that.' And I said, 'Well, you know, don't be afraid. She may look a little under the weather, but she still has her great personality and she's still as friendly as she ever was. She just looks a little different now, but you know, she still has her voice, she still has her mind, and she can do anything anyone else can do. It just takes her a little while to get off the couch now, that's all.'"

— Tim

avoid confronting their own mortality. They may distance themselves from you, or say insensitive or inappropriate things. Simply let these people know how much they mean to you, and address any questions they have about your illness. If you want to try to maintain these relationships under duress, try to engage these friends in conversations about their own lives and your mutual interests, rather than your illness.

THE SUPPORT OF YOUR HEALTH CARE TEAM

Don't overlook the experts. In addition to your family and friends, your oncologist, the nurse, and social worker should be available to you to discuss your medical condition and any specific worries and concerns. In the larger health centers, access to mental health professionals such as social workers, psychologists, or psychiatrists will also be a resource you may want to consider. Actively maximize whatever professional resources are available to you.

If your oncologist does not have a team readily available to support you and your family, you should see this as an indicator that your needs may not be adequately met within this setting. Going it alone, or with inadequate psychosocial support, is a setup for unnecessary frustration and needless suffering. Don't hesitate to ask for help.

Ask to see the social worker for help and advice. Sometimes a nurse is available to be with you when you are getting medical information and to help you sort it through after the doctor leaves. Nurses and social workers are usually open to discussing your personal and family concerns. In addition to being good listeners, they know about resources that may be of help to you. This should be your first step.

"I saw that people were reluctant to come to me because they didn't know the right thing to say. And I think just letting people know that they don't have to say anything. I know there were days that, when I was in the hospital, just having a friend sit there and watch TV with me or just being in that room while I slept, made such a difference. And it doesn't have to be someone who is an expert on cancer and knows the perfect thing to say, it's just having people near you and letting people know that you need them near you and you need just their comfort and their support.

"But I think you also have to be able to tell people sometimes that, you know, I'm really uncomfortable, I feel horrible. You have to let people know that you're not there sometimes to entertain or be social. You're just struggling and you just have to tell people what really is going on in your mind and physically how you feel and just be honest with people and let them know what you need. I think that's really the most important thing."

— Michelle

If your health care team members are not readily available or able to provide you with the names of mental health professionals who are experts in helping people affected by chronic life-threatening illness and you want to find someone quickly, you have a series of other options. This is something you can do on your own. For help identifying mental health professionals (social workers, psychiatrists, psychologists, psychiatric nurses, etc.) specializing in cancer, contact the American Cancer Society, the American Psychosocial Oncology Society, and the Association of Oncology Social Work. Check the Resources section at the end of this book for contact information for these groups and descriptions of the many resources available to you. The professional groups listed can also direct you to the many patient and caregiver-led support groups available to you.

WHAT IF I AM ALONE OR
DO NOT HAVE ANYONE TO COUNT ON?

If you do not have immediate family nearby or close friends to rely on, suggestions about how to involve your loved ones in your care and coping may make you feel even more alone. It can also make you feel very lonely, abandoned, awkward, and somehow "lacking" when you see other people coming to the clinic with family and friends. Or, you may have family and friends, but they may have many other conflicting responsibilities and so cannot be there for you, even though they care for you very much. Do not despair—there are things you can do to engage others in your care. You do not have to be alone.

> "I think if anyone does some networking in their own community, they will find a counselor, a social worker, a psychologist who has had either some personal experience with cancer or has worked with other oncology patients who can be extremely helpful with dealing with some of the emotional turmoil."
>
> – Mary Jane

Asking for help and identifying yourself as someone in need of personal or emotional support is your responsibility. You should do this as early in the treatment process as possible. You may want to say to your team, "I do not have family or friends on whom I can depend for help. As experts who manage problems like this every day, can you please work with me to create a support system for myself?" A statement like this will help your health care team know that you will need their assistance and even more importantly, with their involvement, you will not feel so alone with the demands of such a serious illness.

If you are being cared for by an oncologist who does not work with a team, and you cannot rely on support from family or friends, you may need to ask your oncologist for a list of trained professionals who can help you, or be prepared to seek resources on your own. Also know that if any member of your health care team is not meeting your needs, you are free to seek out other doctors and health care professionals who may be more responsive to your concerns. You can also call the American Cancer Society at 800-ACS-2345 and refer to the Resources section at the end of this book to find sources of additional support.

SUPPORT AND EDUCATION GROUPS AND COUNSELING

Support and education programs exist in a variety of formats and include individual or group counseling, classes, and support groups. Some groups are formal and focus on learning about cancer or coping with feelings. Others are informal and social. Some groups are composed only of people with cancer or only caregivers, while others include spouses, family members, or friends. Other groups focus on specific types of cancer or stages of disease. Look for groups that are led by health professionals (a social worker, nurse, or other licensed professional) or trained facilitators. The hospital social worker, members of your palliative care team, or the American Cancer Society should be able to give you a list of groups that provide counseling, education, and support and make a referral as needed.

Cancer support groups are designed to provide a confidential atmosphere where people being treated for cancer, cancer survivors, or loved ones of those with cancer can discuss the challenges that accompany the illness with others who may have experienced the same challenges. Some people with cancer find that the mutual support of others with the disease is a source of comfort. Support groups can help people affected by cancer feel less alone and can improve their ability to deal with the uncertainties and challenges that cancer brings. Research has shown that support-group participants report an improved quality of life.

Support groups are not for everybody. Individual counseling and support is available and is worth seeking out if you are uncomfortable sharing your feelings with a group of people. Individual counseling may or may not be covered by insurance—be sure to check your policy's benefits. In addition, if you are anxious or uneasy in a public group setting, or if you have difficulty traveling, don't overlook telephone counseling and online support groups. Just be aware that chat rooms and message boards are not the best source of cancer information, especially if they are not monitored by trained professionals or experts.

> "The difficult thing for me has been learning to ask for help or learning to accept help when people offer."
>
> — Ric

> "There is an online computer site. I think it's just a stage IV cancer board, and I go in there and talk to a lot of women and see what they're experiencing…that helps me a lot."
>
> — Vickie

Seeking Meaning

Some people search for meaning as their lives draw to a close—a reason for their illness and a higher purpose for their life. For some, this challenges their beliefs; for others, the search for meaning brings comfort and solace. Seeking meaning in your life is an important coping strategy, and one that can help you come to terms with the end of your life as it nears. Many people who are facing the end of their lives develop an interest in spiritual issues. You may want to explore answers to life's big questions, like "What is the meaning of life?" "Why did this happen to me?" and "What will happen when I die?" Even if you are not a particularly religious person, you may find comfort exploring spiritual matters with someone you trust—a friend, loved one, mental health professional, or pastoral care expert.

The belief in a higher power or a divine plan can be an important source of comfort to people with advanced cancer. Others may find peace as a result of a deep connection to other people and a belief in essential human kindness and generosity. For some, individual reflection or meditation can provide peace or a sense of transcendence in times of turmoil. For others, prayer and the support of a religious community are important. See chapter 10 on spirituality for deeper discussions of these topics.

Finding a Way to Express Yourself

Tapping your creative impulses in order to express yourself is yet another powerful way not to become overwhelmed by strong emotions. For example, writing can be very therapeutic. You may want to consider writing about your emotions or experiences with cancer in a private journal. Or, you may have life stories you want to record for family members or friends. Writing letters to those you love to share your feelings for them can also help you make peace with your situation.

If you're not a writer, there are many other ways to express yourself. Listen to or play music. Sing, dance, or tell jokes. Draw or paint. Sew, knit, or whittle wood. Participate in the preparation of your favorite meal. Let loose a primal scream or have a good long cry. Go ahead and express your feelings. Do it in whatever way makes you feel better.

Talking About Advanced Cancer

Coping with advanced cancer is hard. Talking about it is hard too. Knowing how to tell a loved one you have cancer and will likely die from it isn't something many of us have experience with, yet we want to get it right. Thinking about—let alone discussing—your own mortality can be frightening and difficult to do. And finding the words to tell those we care about how we feel about them and how we want to be remembered could tongue-tie anyone.

WHY TALK ABOUT YOUR CANCER?

For many family and close friends, knowing how to best help the person with cancer is their biggest concern. It is not unusual for people to feel lost as they

"When I got cancer, me and my husband, we both wrote a journal. We wrote it together. We got a composition book out and we wrote all the do's and the don'ts—and even mad—we were mad at the cancer. We weren't mad at each other, we were mad at that cancer, you know…

"This person I read about said to do that [keep a journal]—that he and his wife did that….He lost his wife and he wrote the last paragraph of it, and it was the day that they buried her. And that made me think of me and him, and so, we did the same.

"My brother's going through cancer now. And I told my brother—for him and his wife to do that. It will make you understand your battle of cancer better. And he said, 'Sis, you're right. It does.' He said, 'Because we can talk about it.' And I said, 'Yeah, you can talk about it.'"

— Cheryl

try to guess what would be helpful. Only open communication can increase the certainty that what you are doing is wanted or helpful. Balancing the demands of facing one's own mortality, the everyday needs of the family, and other practical concerns is a challenge that is best managed through ongoing and open communication. Communicating in this way may be foreign and new for some, but there are people who can guide you through how best to talk with others at this time. The person with cancer and their concerned loved ones may initially try to protect each other by avoiding emotionally charged topics such as fear of death. Avoidance is not helpful. Although intense feelings may be initially upsetting to some, sharing emotions can make a person feel deeply understood and connected to others at a time when isolation is common. Just as important, expressing emotional concerns creates a release of physical tension and frees up invaluable psychic energy needed to confront conflicts and to overcome difficult problems together.

Even if you are a shy or quiet person, consider the many benefits of discussing your illness with the ones you care about most. Communicating openly and honestly with others about your cancer can help you in several ways. Talking about these matters allows you to communicate preferences for how you want to be treated, affirm or heal relationships, gather and give support, and seek and exchange important information. The weight of your problems

—◊◊◊—

"With Michaela, with my daughter, I tell her more than I tell anyone else. She has just come through like unbelievable for me and is one of the people that I absolutely trust in telling everything to. The support I get back from her and the love—our relationship has grown exponentially because of my diagnosis. I mean, we've had to literally cram a lifetime into, you know, just into each moment. So, I couldn't be more pleased with how our relationship has grown and where it's gone to."

– Karen

may be lightened just by talking them over with a family member, friend, spiritual advisor, or person in a similar situation. These people may even be able to think of coping strategies, resources, or ways to comfort you that you hadn't even thought of!

When you receive difficult news like a diagnosis of advanced cancer, one temptation is to bottle up your emotions and isolate yourself from others. You may find yourself thinking that no one else will understand what you are going through, or that you don't want to burden your loved ones and friends with your worries. Don't fall into this trap. Your load will be lighter if you share it with others.

Some days you may want to try to forget all that is going on and ignore your cancer and its effects on you entirely—you may *not* want to talk about it. That's okay. But most days, you'll need to accept the reality of your disease, and sharing your worries and communicating your hopes and wishes with others can provide welcome relief, comfort, and guidance.

So, how do you talk to the people who mean the most to you about your cancer? The following sections will provide you with the strategies you need—and sometimes even the words—to talk with your loved ones and caregivers about your cancer and your life. Be sure to read chapter 9 for additional strategies for talking about death and your wishes at end of life.

TALKING TO FRIENDS AND FAMILY

Try to be open in talking with friends and loved ones about your illness, your treatment, your needs, and your feelings. Many people don't understand cancer, and some may avoid you because they're afraid of your illness or worried that they will say something that will upset you. Once people know that you are

How Do I Talk to My Family and Friends About My Cancer?

- Tell friends and family what is going on. They will learn, sooner or later, that you have cancer. They will feel hurt and left out if you do not tell them.

- Find out what they feel, and try to answer their questions.

- Tell people, kindly, that you'd rather not talk at a particular time if you don't feel up to it just then. Sometimes family members can do that for you.

- It is okay to be direct with others and to express your needs and feelings.

- If you or family members usually don't like to talk about certain personal issues, it's okay not to open up completely to everyone.

- Do not set up a false front or a "happy face" when you don't feel that way. It is the other person's problem if he or she can't handle your true feelings.

- Don't hesitate to ask your nurse, social worker, clergy, or counselor to help bring together family members to talk.

receptive to discussing these things, they may be more willing to open up. By sharing your feelings, you and the people you care about most will be better able to help each other through a difficult time.

Encourage your loved ones to get their feelings out in the open so you can discuss shared hopes, fears, and worries. And for your part, speak as honestly to your family as you can (or as is appropriate, if you have younger children). You may want to tell them what you and your health care team expect in the weeks and months to come, your feelings about your diagnosis and future, and the likely effects of your illness on the family.

TALKING TO YOUNG CHILDREN AND ADOLESCENTS

Some parents or grandparents choose not to tell the children in their lives about their cancer diagnosis or their prognosis. Others choose to tell only what they feel the child needs to know, or how much they feel he or she can handle. A lot depends upon the child's age and level of maturity.

As you consider your approach, keep in mind that it is natural to want to shield children from concerns and fears about your cancer and mortality. You may feel like keeping the truth from your children or grandchildren in hopes of sparing them some pain. But even very young children are adept at sensing when something is wrong, and this secrecy can backfire. Avoiding talking to children and adolescents about cancer or even death can be especially troubling and confusing to them, and can also cause them to lose trust in what they are told by authority figures. Losing trust in the adults young people look to for guidance during what is already a scary time can be especially frightening.

Additionally, if children and adolescents don't know the truth, they may imagine that things are even worse than they are. Children—especially very

---

Figure 4-3. **How Do I Talk to Children and Adolescents About Cancer?**

-~- Before telling your children or grandchildren you have cancer, you may want to talk with your doctor, a counselor, or another expert about the best way to deliver this news. If you decide to join a support group, other members may be able to offer advice and suggestions as well.

-~- Prepare to offer the child or teen a lot of reassurance. Children's questions and concerns will probably center on how their lives might change. They will want to know who is going to take care of them and what is going to happen. Assure them that someone will be looking out for them, whether it's you or a relative or friend. Don't expect adolescents to assume too much responsibility during this tough time.

-~- Try to stay upbeat, but also be realistic and honest with the child. It's okay to say that you don't know exactly what's going to happen and promise to keep him or her informed if anything changes.

"My children were just elementary school age when I was initially diagnosed, and we didn't tell them the depth of things at the time, because nobody really knew either, initially. And as time has gone by and they have matured and grown up, we've told them more factual information. But over time, as they mature and we think that they are able to handle things, we talk about fears a little bit more, about statistics, because I think they need to know the reality of things. Because I don't want them to feel cheated that they didn't know things when they might have, and they might have changed their actions. You know, one never knows what goes on in teens' minds, but we've tempered things, because they are teens, and teens have an awful lot on their minds."

– Catherine

"I was in the hospital on a morphine drip, and it was my husband who came home and in very simple, direct language, said, 'Mommy's in the hospital. She has a sickness called cancer. She's going to be sick for a long time before she can get better, but the doctors are doing everything possible to get her better. And we'll always tell you how she is.' And the key here is that from the very first time he introduced my illness, he used the word 'cancer,' he used the word 'lymphoma,' so that these were not emotionally charged or forbidden words, but were just part of our vocabulary, so that we could talk about it."

– Wendy

young children—tend to see themselves as the center of the world, and they may think that they have done something that is causing problems in the family.

Although it is easy to understand why you might want to your protect loved ones from the truth, it is seldom possible to do so and may result in unnecessary confusion and misunderstanding. In the emotionally charged environment of life-limiting illness, not being able to openly discuss and share concerns about the impending loss of a loved one can lead to increased feelings of isolation and increased fears of abandonment that may already be part of the dying process. Talking openly about your prognosis is one way you can create an environment of caring and support.

Health professionals generally agree that telling children the truth about an illness reduces stress and guilt. The American Cancer Society has suggestions for talking with children about cancer at http://www.cancer.org/docroot/ESN/content/ESN_2_1x_Talking_with_Children_About_Cancer.asp?sitearea=ESN.

Finally, it is up to adults to teach young people how to manage crises in life. Since dying is a normal part of life, it is especially important that you model for young people how to cope with the sadness and loss that will be a part of everyone's life. If young people do not learn how to cope with dying and loss from you and this experience, then where and from whom will they learn these essential skills for living?

TALKING TO ADULT CHILDREN

The approaching loss of a parent may raise many issues for adult children. For example, it may change how adult children feel about themselves, their siblings, or their own children; it may force them to confront their own mortality; and it may affect their priorities in life. Adult children may be conflicted about juggling their multiple roles as parents, children, and professionals. They may also experience feelings of guilt if they are far away or if they are only able to spend a limited amount of time with you.

> "My most difficult thing was telling my children. They are all grown, of course, but it was very, very difficult. It's very difficult to tell children that their mother is probably going to die."
>
> – Jo Ann

One way you can initiate communication with adult children is to invite them to participate in your decision making about treatment or care. Sharing these tasks with your children can minimize conflict and fears that may arise between siblings or in-laws when other important decisions need to be made. Your ability to reach out to your adult children and openly share your feelings, goals, and wishes will help them through this time. It also will allow them to feel that they have contributed positively to making this part of your lives together the best possible.

Cancer Screening and Genetic Testing

One subject you may want to broach with your adult children is the issue of cancer screening or genetic testing. This is especially important if other members of your family have had the same type of cancer as you or if there are many family members with cancer. Ask your doctor if your type of cancer has

> —∽∞∽—
>
> "Planning ahead, finding the good in your life. Finding what I call the small miracles in your days. Making your days good rather than sitting around and thinking about the fact that there are things you can't do, that there are things that won't happen for you, that you won't be there for. That you can try, and you can't do it all the time. It's a work in progress."
>
> — Jeanne

a genetic or inherited component. If so, members of your family may be at increased risk for developing the same disease. You may want to suggest they talk to their own doctor about their personal risk for disease and the complicated subject of genetic testing.

Conclusion

A diagnosis of advanced cancer may signal that the end of your life is closer than you might have hoped. It is easy (and normal) to feel overwhelmed at first, but this may lead you to forget that many advances have been made in treatment and management of cancer symptoms and treatment side effects. You may even be able to manage your cancer as a chronic disease and be able to live a productive and fulfilling life for many more months, if not years. On the other hand, some cancers remain difficult to control and will shorten life. Given all that there is to understand and manage, it is easy to understand why people can feel overwhelmed when diagnosed with advanced cancer and forced to face the realities of their illness and their own mortality. But using the coping strategies outlined in this chapter, you and you loved ones will be better prepared to face current challenges, as well as those ahead.

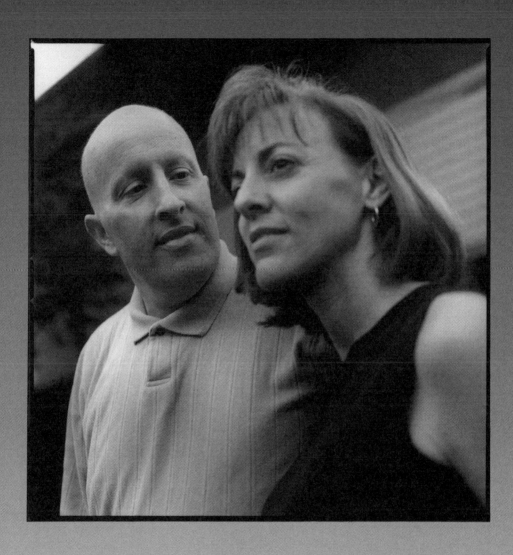

Chapter 5

Advance Decision Making

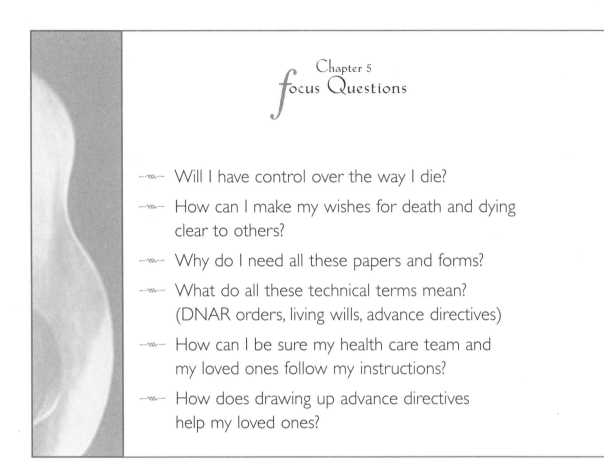

Chapter 5
*f*ocus Questions

— Will I have control over the way I die?

— How can I make my wishes for death and dying clear to others?

— Why do I need all these papers and forms?

— What do all these technical terms mean? (DNAR orders, living wills, advance directives)

— How can I be sure my health care team and my loved ones follow my instructions?

— How does drawing up advance directives help my loved ones?

"We're educated in school, we're trained in our jobs, our parents train us in living, but you know, nobody trains us to die, and real basic nuts and bolts issues like financial planning— developing your advance directives. What do you do with your body after you're dead? Making decisions about what kind of ceremony, ritual, if you want anything, and talking about that with your family. Who trains us to do that?"

— Ric

ADVANCE DECISION MAKING IS ABOUT PROTECTING YOUR AUTONOMY and ensuring you die on your own terms. It can help your family and your health care team honor what you want, but it requires that you think about these issues and discuss them with the right people before your condition declines. Advance decision making is something that most cancer patients do often when they are just diagnosed with their cancer. It is also common to do when you are writing a will (see chapter 7).

—✽—

"We had already done some of that paperwork in terms of a living will and all that, both being military when we were married. We both had wills already, and then once we got married, we updated those and had them together. With active-duty military, there's always the chance that you would have to deploy somewhere, to go to war, etc., so I think we had already dealt with some of those issues of what we wanted. And Chuck had grandparents who had strokes and things like that, so he was very much against being kept alive by machines, so we had had some of those discussions already. Which I think was probably uncommon for the age that we were at. Then once we got this diagnosis, we had some more very deep discussions from the very beginning, about what he wanted and didn't want, and we had a lot of talks then right from the very beginning about the living will, about cremation, about things like that, and we dealt with those issues honestly and openly. We realized that talking about those issues and dealing with them didn't mean that we were giving up, that we weren't going to fight, and that we were giving up hope; it was just kind of the safety net so that he knew that everything was taken care of and that I was taken care of."

– Ann I.

What Are Advance Directives?

The majority of Americans believe that decisions about the type of medical care they receive, particularly at the end of life, are personal and should be made by themselves or their loved ones. You may make casual statements about your preferences in conversation ("I don't want to be kept alive by machines" or "I want to die with dignity"), but these generalizations are not explicit enough to help doctors and loved ones make difficult technical decisions if you become too ill to communicate your preferences. *Advance directives* are legal documents—tools to help you express your wishes about end-of-life care and decision making if you become too ill to speak for yourself. Advance directives are *only* used if you are unable to speak for yourself. If you become suddenly ill or confused or delirious, your family or health care proxy can honor your preferences for care and treatment as stated in your advance directive. As long as you can speak for yourself and are competent, advance directives have no special role. There is a federal law called The Patient Self-Determination

Act, which requires that hospitals ask you if you have an advance directive when you enter the hospital for medical care.

In short, advance directives are becoming useful, commonly used documents that help health care professionals know their patients' wishes and allow these professionals to provide you with the kind of care you prefer if you are unable to tell them what you want. Advance directives were developed because of concerns of patients and their families that health care professionals did not honor families' wishes or patients' wishes.

This is your opportunity to describe what choices you would make if you were placed in a situation where you were unable to speak for yourself—even temporarily. Advance decision making is really another form of protection for you. Once you have developed your advance directives, you need to share them with your lawyer, your doctor, and your health care proxy (we'll talk more about health care proxies in a minute).

This is something you need to do when you are well. The time to make an advance directive is *before you are in a situation in which you would need one.*

The term advance directive applies to 2 basic types of legal documents we'll discuss in the next sections: the durable power of attorney for health care and the living will.

The Durable Power of Attorney for Health Care

The *durable power of attorney for health care* (DPOA) goes by several different names: sometimes it is called a *medical power of attorney*, a *health care proxy*, or an *appointment of a health care agent*. A durable power of attorney for health care is a legal document that designates someone to make medical decisions for you if you become too ill to speak for yourself. This person (called the *health care agent* or *proxy*) negotiates on your behalf with doctors and other care-givers and is required to make decisions according to your directions. In a DPOA for health care, you can indicate the specific kinds of treatments or procedures you do or do not want. If your wishes in a particular situation are not known, your agent will make decisions

> "The important thing is to have a plan, and this is what we have done. We have since retired and just a couple of years ago we went forward and we did our will because we thought that would be the intelligent thing to do, and get that behind us. We went forward and we determined who we wanted to assign our power of attorney to in the event that neither of us was in the position to make a decision for ourselves at a given time."
>
> — Esther H.

based on what he or she thinks you would want and what he or she considers to be in your best interest. Note that while you can still speak for yourself, the proxy does not have any decision-making power—the durable power of attorney for health care only takes effect when you become too sick to speak for yourself.

(There is another kind of durable power of attorney that addresses financial affairs. This power of attorney is different than the DPOA for health care, and requires a different legal form. See chapter 7 for a discussion of financial powers of attorney.)

Choosing Your Proxy

Deciding whom you will appoint as your health care proxy or agent is one of the most important decisions you will make. Choose this person carefully, and don't necessarily default to the person closest to you, such as your spouse or partner. Select someone who is reliable and trustworthy, whom you believe will be able to carry out your wishes even if they include denying life-sustaining treatments. Not everyone is willing or able to shoulder this significant responsibility and be an effective agent. It is also a good idea to name an alternate agent in case the primary agent becomes unable or unwilling to act on your behalf.

Be sure to discuss your wishes in detail with your health care proxy. Give a copy of your advance directive to your health care proxy, and discuss your advance directive periodically with that person in order to remind him or her of this important responsibility.

If you do not have an advance directive, you may receive medical care that you do not want. In the absence of an advance directive, the doctor will ask your family about your treatment. The spouse (unless legally separated) is asked first, followed by adult children, parents, and adult brothers and sisters, in that order. However, it is common for family members (especially distant family members) not to know what the patient wanted, or to disagree over what a loved one would have wanted. Occasionally, family members pressure the health care team into providing more invasive care, in part out of their own

> "It made me very sad, but just for a short period of time. And as far as how my family felt about it, they were kind of alarmed…but I want to get these things out of the way, because I can't be happy, I can't go on with my life until I can make some of these decisions. Once this is taken care of, I can be happy in my life. It just made me feel better about my total situation, period."
>
> — Vickie

feelings of guilt. If you have a life partner but are not legally married, that partner may have no legal status as a medical decision maker for you regardless of how long you have lived together or how well your partner knows you. In some situations, a court may appoint a legal guardian to make health care decisions if you do not have an advance directive. This is why it is important to express your wishes in a written advance directive ahead of time and to discuss your wishes with those close to you.

The Living Will

The other type of advance directive is a living will. Also called a *medical directive* or *health care declaration*, the *living will* gives instructions about the use of medical treatments at the end of life. Its purpose is to specify which treatments you want and which ones you refuse, and to direct your loved ones and health care team in deciding how aggressively to pursue medical treatment intended to delay death, such as life-sustaining procedures or artificial life support. As with the power of attorney, this living will only has legal status if you become too sick to speak for yourself. Also, state laws differ, so a living will may not be binding in some states. However, it can still influence decision making because it is a clear expression of intent and preference by a patient.

> "A couple of months after I was diagnosed…I made out a living will because I wanted to be in control of what was going to happen when that time did come. So once I did that, I felt better about the decisions, and who was going to be making the decisions, and what decisions would be made when that time came. And I did a lot of other things, as far as writing things down, saying how I want things to be disposed of and different little things like that."
>
> – Vickie

Considering these medical interventions and trying to understand what exactly they might mean in your case can be a little overwhelming. Ask your doctor to explain treatments or procedures that you are confused about before completing your living will.

Choosing among these hypothetical possibilities can be a little unsettling. No one wants to contemplate these scenarios. However, consider the other option: without your instructions, someone else will be forced to decide on your behalf, and family members may disagree or the physician or hospital may refuse to comply because of legal or ethical concerns.

A living will is usually more limited than a durable power of attorney for health care. It covers fewer conditions and treatments and is not as strong

Figure 5-1. **What Is a Life-Sustaining Medical Treatment?**

Each state defines life-sustaining medical treatment differently. In general, *life-sustaining medical treatment* is anything mechanical or artificial that sustains, restores, or substitutes for a vital body function and that would prolong the process for someone who is dying. Life-sustaining medical treatment *may* include the following:

- ~ cardiopulmonary resuscitation (CPR)
- ~ artificial respiration (mouth-to-mouth breathing, manual ventilation, or a ventilator)
- ~ medications to artificially alter blood pressure and heart function
- ~ artificial nutrition/hydration (including a feeding tube)
- ~ dialysis
- ~ certain surgical procedures (amputation, feeding tube placement, removal of tumor, organ transplant)

Nutrition/hydration (food and water) are not usually defined as life sustaining unless they are provided by a feeding tube or intravenous line. Medications or procedures necessary to provide comfort or ease pain are not usually considered life-sustaining procedures. In some states, tube feedings and intravenous fluids are considered comfort measures.

The decision to forego or discontinue life-sustaining treatment can be complex and difficult, and can elicit strong feelings from loved ones and health care professionals alike. Although technically there is no legal difference between withholding treatment (not starting it at all) and withdrawing treatment (removing it once it has been started), many people see the two issues differently. See the discussion on page 213 (chapter 9) for additional information, and make sure your preferences are spelled out clearly in your living will.

as a durable power of attorney for health care because it contains only written instructions. It does not name anyone to interpret the document or to ensure that your wishes will be carried out. You can have a living will and a power of attorney for health care at the same time, but if you have a power of attorney for health care, you do not need a living will. If you have both,

Figure 5-2.

Five Wishes

Five Wishes is a living will that talks about your personal, emotional, and spiritual needs as well as your medical decisions. It was developed with the help of the American Bar Association as well as many end-of-life care experts, and is supported by a grant from the Robert Wood Johnson Foundation. It has been featured on CNN, on NBC's *Today Show*, and in *Time* and *Money* magazines. The 5 wishes it covers are:

1. The person I want to make care decisions for me
2. The kind of medical treatment I want or don't want
3. How comfortable I want to be
4. How I want people to treat me
5. What I want my loved ones to know

The form is designed to be easy to complete—it is written in plain language and you simply check a box, circle a direction, or write in a few sentences. It is legally binding in all but 15 states, but residents of these 15 states can still use *Five Wishes* to put their wishes in writing and communicate their preferences to their loved ones and health care providers. To order a copy of *Five Wishes*, call 888-594-7437 or visit http://www.agingwithdignity.org. Many hospitals, doctor's or lawyer's offices, social service agencies, and houses of worship may also have copies available.

the information should be the same in both the living will and the power of attorney for health care. Some states allow you to have a single, combined advance directive.

Living wills are most commonly used to give instructions about if or when life-support treatments should be withheld or withdrawn. However, they can be used to express other wishes as well, such as a request for pain management, a preference to die at home if possible, or preferences regarding organ donation.

Other Types of Advance Directives

An *oral advance directive* is a verbal statement made by a person who is physically unable to obtain a living will or power of attorney for health care. This statement is written by someone else (for example, your doctor), and properly witnessed. Several states recognize such statements as legally binding advance directives.

A *mental health directive* defines a person's choices about treatment in the event that he or she becomes seriously mentally ill and is unable to make health care decisions.

Other Decisions to Consider

While you are making decisions about your preferences for end-of-life care, you may also want to consider making some decisions about what will happen to your body after you die. Making decisions about organ, tissue, or whole body donation and whether an autopsy should be performed, and recording these decisions and communicating them to your loved ones and health care team members can prevent stress, confusion, or their indecision later.

Organ and Tissue or Whole Body Donation

Organ, tissue, or whole body donation can enable you to help others even as your own life is coming to an end. *Organ and tissue donation* is the process of removing organs and tissues from a deceased person in order for the organs and tissues to be used for transplantation to save or enhance the life of a person in need. There are several ways you can indicate your wish to be a donor, such as specifying your preferences in your advance directives or joining a donor registry. You may also have been asked to register the last time you renewed your driver's license. By law, all hospitals must have a program to approach the families of potential organ/tissue donors and offer them the option of donation if the person is not already registered as an organ/tissue donor.

You should not assume that you cannot donate organs or tissue just because of your age or medical history. Even people with cancer may be able to donate, depending on their type and stage of cancer. While metastatic cancer may prevent you from donating your organs, if your cancer is not blood borne or has not progressed to the eye, you may be able to donate your corneas.

If your cancer is too advanced to make you eligible for organ or tissue donation, you may want to consider donating your body to a medical school or research institution. This is sometimes called *donating your body to science* or *making an anatomical gift.* Actual human bodies are helpful aids in education and research into new ways to prevent and treat diseases (including cancer) and develop innovative surgical techniques. Talk to your health care team about the options.

In both cases, be sure to make your wishes known to others.

Autopsy

An *autopsy* is a special examination of a body to determine the cause of death or the nature or extent of disease at time of death. Medical examiners may request an autopsy in the event of a sudden death, but you can also make it known ahead of time whether you want your body to undergo an autopsy. Individuals whose cancer may have a genetic component may want to request an autopsy to provide their family members with additional information about their condition. Talk with your doctor about what information an autopsy may be able to provide in your particular case.

DNAR Orders

DNAR is an abbreviation for "do not attempt resuscitation." A *DNAR order* (also called a *DNR order*, short for "do not resuscitate") is sometimes referred to as an advance directive, and while it is indeed written in advance, it differs from a durable power of attorney or a living will in one essential way: *you cannot prepare it yourself.* So technically, a DNAR order is not an advance directive. A DNAR is an order *written by a doctor* saying that a dying person will not have cardiopulmonary resuscitation (CPR) or be placed on a breathing machine before death. A DNAR order is written after the doctor talks about these issues with a patient and family. It is only valid when signed by a physician.

A patient, family member, or health care agent can ask that a DNAR order be written, but they cannot write it themselves. A person can say in a living will that cardiopulmonary resuscitation is not wanted, but this will not stop CPR until the doctor has written the order.

A DNAR order is *not* a "do not treat" order. It is narrowly confined to resuscitation. A patient can and should continue to receive any other treatments that are desired.

> "The last 3 months, Joan was in and out of the hospital quite a bit, mostly in, and at one point she had been up on the heart floor, and she had a really bad attack of something and they had to take her down to the ICU. And our doctor said, 'Joan is very, very fragile. You need to talk to her about end-of-life decisions.' And so when they got her stabilized in the ICU, we had the discussion about 'do not resuscitate' orders and stuff."
>
> — Susan T.

Ensuring Your Advance Directives Are Honored

There are several steps you can take to ensure that your wishes are followed in the event that you can no longer speak or make decisions about your health care. Talk to your loved ones and health care providers about your wishes, let them know you have specific preferences that are outlined in advance directives, and be aware of possible circumstances when your advance directives may not be honored.

Know Your Rights

There is a federal law called the Patient Self-Determination Act (PSDA), which requires all health care agencies (hospitals, long-term care facilities, and home health agencies) receiving Medicare and Medicaid reimbursement to recognize the living will and power of attorney for health care as advance directives. Under the PSDA, health care agencies must ask you whether you have advance directives and must provide you with educational materials about your rights.

Talk With Others About Your Advance Directive

No matter how thorough your written instructions, there is no way they can cover every possible circumstance. Therefore, it is critical that you talk with your agent, proxy, or trustee to ensure they know your wishes and understand your values and preferences. The more they understand about your core motivations and your desires, the better prepared they will be to make decisions that are in keeping with your wishes. For example, do you want to be at home, or is that less important? Do you want to focus on comfort? Do you want to avoid being hooked up to machines and tubes at the end? Is there any special music you would want, or people you would want to see? Is there a particular kind of funeral service you would want?

When you become too sick to speak for yourself, many family members and friends find themselves trying to help the doctors and nurses figure out what the person who is dying really wanted. When family and friends have had conversations about the end of life at an earlier time with the person who is dying, they can be very helpful advocates during this difficult time.

You can help reduce the stress on your loved ones by making sure they know what is important to you. Of course, these conversations can be difficult. You might want to have a nurse or social worker or other counselor help you get prepared for this kind of talk, or be there to help you during the talk.

Talk to your doctors and nurses about what you would want too. Your health care team should know the quality of life that is important to you to maintain. Your doctors and nurses can help you by telling you what to expect, especially for your individual situation, and they may bring up issues that are not on preprinted living will forms. So ask your doctor, "What should I expect when things get close to death? How can I make sure I'm as comfortable as possible? How can I be sure everyone on my health care team knows my preferences too?"

Ensure Your Advance Directive Is Readily Available

Your advance directive will only be useful if the doctor treating you knows that you have one. If you prepare an advance directive, tell people close to you that you have one and where it is kept. Give copies of your advance directive to your agent, family members, or friends who would be contacted should you become seriously ill. You may also want to give a copy to your attorney. Keep a copy of your advance directive in a readily accessible place so that someone else can find it if you are hospitalized, and make sure that someone close to you knows where your advance directive is kept.

It is up to you, your agent, or a family member to give a copy of your advance directive to your doctor. Federal law requires hospitals, nursing homes, and other health care agencies to ask at the time of admission whether or not you have an advance directive. However, if you are unable to answer that question or if the advance directive is not available, it may not be included in your medical record where it can help guide care according to your wishes.

"We talked early on about advance directives, and not wanting to prolong life or anything like that. Some people think that if they have told the children or whoever the responsible person might be, what they want, they've done all they need to do. But…the hospital cannot accept directives from a person unless it is documented. So according to whatever the laws in your state are, the person who is responsible should become informed in what they need to do, so that the caregiver can act for the patient. And it's important not just to have those documents. They won't do any good if they are just in a safe deposit box and the doctor doesn't know what's in them. There should probably be a copy with the will, and a copy with the primary care physician, and a copy with the caregiver, whoever the designated person is."

— Lee

Consider the Exceptions

The living will and durable power of attorney for health care are legally binding documents. The health care team should follow your wishes, but there are exceptions you ought to be aware of.

Since advance directives cannot cover every possibility, there are often situations that the health care team would want to discuss with the health care agent or proxy (remember, the documents only work when the patient is too sick to speak) so that the patient can be treated in a way that follows the spirit of what he or she wanted.

You should know that *advance directives may not be honored in emergencies,* such as when 911 is called. In general, emergency personnel are required to do whatever they can to stabilize a patient in crisis in order to transfer the person to a hospital. As a result, emergency personnel may not honor an advance directive. If you want to be sure your orders are followed, and you do not want emergency personnel to perform CPR, speak with your health care team about developing a *nonhospital DNAR* (also called a *nonhospital DNR*). This means that if you are very ill and wish to die at home, your family members and care-givers will need a clear plan about what to do if you need medical attention.

A nonhospital DNAR order is a physician's order not to attempt CPR. This order can protect seriously ill or dying individuals who are being cared for at home from unwanted resuscitation. You may need to wear a bracelet or wristband to signal to emergency crews that you have a nonhospital DNAR. While not every state has provided for such orders, many have created statutes or regulations permitting them.

Additionally, you should be aware that each state has its own laws governing advance directives. It is possible that advance directives signed in one state may not be recognized in another. Laws and regulations vary from state to state, so check with your doctor to be sure you are aware of the status of your living will in the state in which you reside.

Finally, you should always remember that advance directives are governed by state laws, which can and do vary. If a doctor or health care agency objects to your advance directive based on *reasons of conscience*, some states permit the doctor or agency to refuse to honor it. Agencies must notify you of such policies at the time of admission to the agency or delivery of the advance directive. If a refusal occurs, your advance directive is still legally binding, and the doctor and agency should help you transfer your care to a doctor who will honor the directive.

Revising Your Advance Directive

You are free to change your mind about what is written in your advance directive. Most states allow you to change or revoke it at any time, regardless of your physical or mental condition. If possible, changes should be signed, dated, and witnessed. It is also a good idea to inform your agent, family, and doctor if you change or cancel your advance directive. You should destroy the old advance directive, so there is no confusion on the part of your agent should you need it.

Why Do You Need All These Papers and Forms?

It may seem excessive to have a living will or an advance directive when you trust your doctors, nurses, family, and friends *and* have talked to them about what you want. However, if you get ill suddenly, you may be treated by doctors and nurses who you do not know, and they may not have all the information that your regular health care team has. In this case, it is very helpful to have a living will and/or advance directive, so that the new health care team knows what you would want, even before they have a chance to talk to your family or friends.

Figure 5-3. **Examples of Useful Care Plans**

The more specific you can be about your wishes for health care at the end of your life, the more likely they are to be carried out. Here are some examples of useful care plans:

- **Generally limiting aggressive care.** "I do not want to undergo more intensive care. Specifically, I direct that I have no more intubation or ventilator support. I am willing to have other treatments aimed to treat the causes of recurrences and shortness of breath. If those are inadequate, then I ask for medication to ease the struggle to breathe and allow me to pass away peaceably. I hope to be able to stay at home, and I have enrolled in a home care hospice program. Please do not call 9-1-1 in an emergency. Call xxx-yyy-zzzz for the hospice program instead. Obviously, I have an order to forgo resuscitation and the state's standard wristband to indicate that decision."

- **Wanting fully aggressive treatment but with some limits.** "I know that I have emphysema and that it will eventually take my life. However, I want to live as long as possible and I am willing to go through a great deal to stay alive. Please call 9-1-1 if I am struggling to breathe and cannot call for myself. I have a continuous positive-pressure breathing mask at home and my wife knows how to apply it. Please call her or my physician (Dr. R at sss-ttt-vvvv) if I am sick. I am willing to go through intensive care and ventilator support, so long as there is any chance that I can come home again. However, if I have permanently lost my ability to relate to others or to know myself (by a stroke or brain damage, for example), then I'd ask that you turn to my wife, who has my durable power of attorney for health care. She knows that I intend to stop life-sustaining treatment at that point."

- **Having other (unusual) priorities.** "I know that my life is coming to an end sometime soon. I have given my son John the authority to make decisions about my care and treatment, and I expect my doctors and others to let him take care of me as he sees fit. I am writing here to be sure that everyone involved understands that my view of religion requires that I die as aware as possible. I aim to seize this opportunity to gain insight and wisdom. Thus, do not aim to keep me comfortable, if doing so would blunt my experience of my body and its transition to eternity. Even if I appear to be in anguish, I believe that God does not give us anything we cannot take, and I trust that His meaning will be apparent to me at that time."

Source: Table 1 from Lynn and Goldstein. Advance Care Planning for Fatal Chronic Illness. Avoiding Commonplace Errors and Unwanted Suffering. *Ann Intern Med.* 2003; 138:812-818.

Conclusion

Many people with cancer and their loved ones want to focus on hope. Preparing advance directives is not giving up hope, nor is it being depressing or grim. If you talk about drawing up the types of documents mentioned in this chapter and someone says, "You're just being morbid," you can say, "I want to do this now so I can focus my energy on my hopes and all the positive things in my life." Preparing advance directives can also be seen as an act of love toward your family members, other loved ones, and caregivers. By clearly specifying your preferences about care and treatment in a variety of medical circumstances, you remove the burden of decision making from your loved ones' shoulders. It is an act of generosity to make your own decisions, thus preventing loved ones from having to make agonizing decisions or having to negotiate with other family members about critical issues in medical care and treatment.

Many people find that hoping for the best but preparing for the worst frees them and their loved ones and caregivers from worries and allows them to focus on what is most important in the present moment.

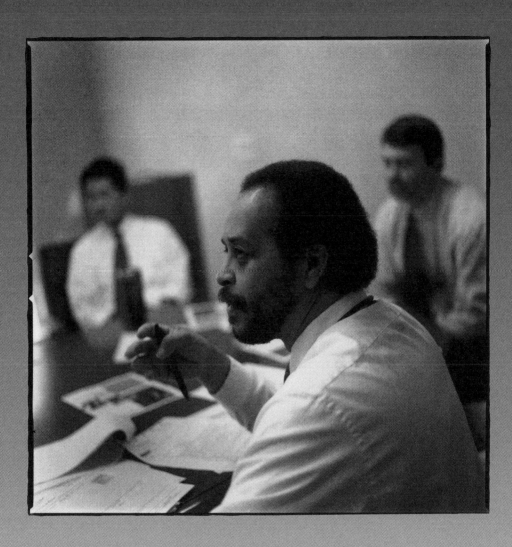

Chapter 6

Work and Insurance

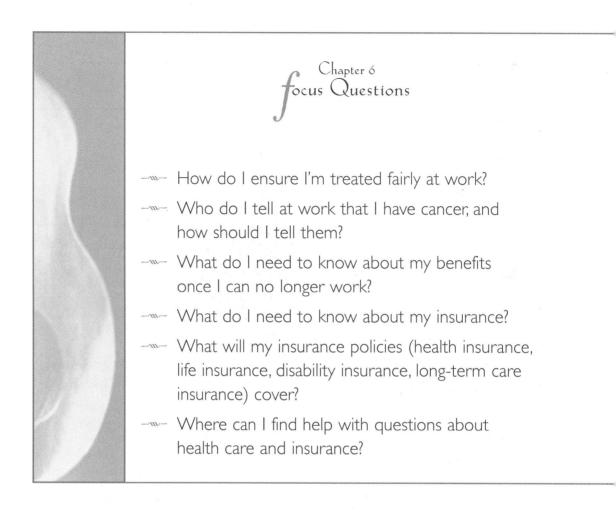

Chapter 6
focus Questions

—⚬— How do I ensure I'm treated fairly at work?

—⚬— Who do I tell at work that I have cancer, and how should I tell them?

—⚬— What do I need to know about my benefits once I can no longer work?

—⚬— What do I need to know about my insurance?

—⚬— What will my insurance policies (health insurance, life insurance, disability insurance, long-term care insurance) cover?

—⚬— Where can I find help with questions about health care and insurance?

"Insurance companies don't know what you don't know. If you don't ask them, they're not going to know what you don't know. And because they deal with so many different individuals, they're unsure what level you're at. The more questions you ask, the more informed you will be. You're going to be the individual paying the bill. You need to make sure you ask the questions, no matter how small or how large they are."

— Ron

WITH ALL OF THE PHYSICAL AND EMOTIONAL CHALLENGES that come with cancer, it may be difficult to focus on tasks as mundane as your job, your health, life and disability insurance, and what your policies cover. Yet, if you are willing to spend a little bit of time investigating these issues, you may find some useful information that can make your experience a little easier. In this chapter, we'll discuss information about your workplace, benefits, and insurance, and we'll provide resources that will help you stay on top of all three.

Work

For many people, work is an important part of their identity. For most, it is also an important part of their financial well-being. Because many people want or need to keep working as long as possible despite their progressing disease, we'll discuss work issues that will be relevant if you are still working and work-related issues that may arise after you become too ill to work.

It wasn't all that long ago that if you were diagnosed with cancer, you were on your own, subject to the whim of your employer, with no legal protections at work. Today there are both federal and state laws that protect you both during employment and after you leave work. You may also have additional rights if your job is unionized, or if your employer offers them voluntarily, which some do.

The basic law that provides employment protections for people with cancer is the federal American with Disabilities Act of 1990, generally referred to as the ADA. Although you may not think of yourself as disabled since you can work, you are "disabled" within the definition of the law if your health condition substantially limits one or more major life activities. While in general the ADA only applies to employers with 15 or more employees, other state or local laws are likely to provide similar protection. The Equal Employment Opportunity Commission (EEOC) can help you determine whether you're protected under the ADA, and point you to the correct agency in your state to learn about local laws. Call 800-514-0301 or 800-514-0383 (TTY), or visit http://www.ada.gov. Since these state laws are generally patterned on the ADA, the discussion in this chapter will be about the ADA unless another law is specified.

If You Are Still Working

If you are still able to work despite your cancer, you have special rights in the workplace. As a person with a disability, you are entitled to an accommodation at your workplace, to take time off, to have your health condition kept confidential, and to continue your health coverage even after you leave work.

JOB ACCOMMODATIONS

Employers are not required to lower standards for a disabled employee, nor are they obligated to provide personal use items such as glasses or hearing aids.

"I'm off on disability at the moment, and that has been a tremendous help. I'm sure some people would feel just exactly the opposite. They would want the distraction of working and keeping busy and so forth. With me, it didn't work that way. There was a lot of stress and it just somehow added to the problem. Since I have been out of work, I've been able to relax more. I've been able to keep up with things without being in a hurry and pressed and running around at night, and so forth. So, it's been a plus for me, but, like I say, that's not necessarily true of everybody."

— Ron

However, an employer must make a change or adjustment to a job that allows an employee with a disability to perform the "essential functions" of the job, or to enjoy the benefits and privileges of employment equal to those enjoyed by employees without disabilities. If you need time off for treatments, a reasonable accommodation may be a part-time or flexible work schedule.

Speak with your employer to clarify the benefits to which you may be entitled. To find out more about job accommodations that may work for you, contact the Job Accommodation Network at 800-526-7234 or http://www.jan.wvu.edu.

TIME OFF FROM WORK

You may be entitled to time off from your job as an accommodation. (See the above discussion.) In addition, the Family and Medical Leave Act (FMLA) requires employers with 50 or more workers to provide up to 12 weeks of *unpaid* leave. You can use this leave to receive treatment or otherwise take care of yourself. A family member also may be able to take leave to help care for you. To qualify, employees must have worked at least 1 year and 1,250 hours. To be covered by the Act, you need to tell your employer about your health condition. You may also be entitled to similar time from a smaller employer under your local state law.

TELLING PEOPLE AT WORK ABOUT YOUR ILLNESS

Under the ADA, if you tell your employer about your health condition, your employer must keep the information confidential. If you are concerned about

> ―≈―
>
> "I had tremendous, tremendous support from my family, from my friends, from my co-workers. I was really lucky on my work end that I had this great group of people who for the year and a half that I was out of work donated to me their own vacation time, and I never lost a paycheck for the whole time that I was out of work."
>
> — Michelle

losing your job because of your disability, tell your employer so you will be protected by the ADA. You always have the option *not* to tell anyone at work that you are sick. But keep in mind that if you file claims under your work-sponsored health insurance policy for cancer-related treatments and/or drugs, your employer may learn about your health condition from the insurance company. In addition, if you need time off from work or aren't working up to speed because of your condition or treatment, you can be fired. The situation changes when you notify your employer about your condition and request an accommodation.

Unlike telling an employer, there are no legal protections about telling co-workers, so think about your work environment and the people you are considering telling before you tell co-employees. Also think about how much you want to tell them.

In some work settings, people may react to your cancer diagnosis and absences due to treatment with understanding and helpfulness. In others, they may feel uncomfortable because of irrational fear, or with resentment because of additional duties they may have to take on. You may want to seek out someone in your company that you trust who has been with the company long enough to know the way the company and your co-workers respond to a person having cancer. He or she can help you determine who to tell, when, and what to say. Ultimately, though, disclosing your illness is a personal decision.

The brochure *When Someone You Work with Has Cancer* (available free from the American Cancer Society online at http://www.cancer.org/docroot/MIT/MIT_2_2x_WhenSomeoneYouWorkwithhasCancer.asp or by calling 800-ACS-2345) may also provide useful information.

IF YOU THINK YOU ARE BEING DISCRIMINATED AGAINST

Under the ADA, you cannot be discriminated against because you have cancer. However, discrimination in general, much less discrimination because of a particular reason, can be very difficult to prove. Keeping good records can help you make your case.

If you choose to tell your employer about your cancer, keep careful records of all talks with your employer or people in the benefits office. List the name of the person with whom you spoke, what you met about, the date and place you talked, and any conclusions reached.

In case you ever need to prove discrimination, a daily diary that you keep privately, at home, can be very helpful. Note in your diary each day (or as close to that day as you can), all the good things that happened to you at work, such as a pat on the back from your boss about a job well done or a good job report. Also include anything you think could indicate discrimination, such as remarks from a boss or co-worker. Write down the words that were used as best you can. Under no circumstances should you go back and change an entry. If you later remember something that occurred that you didn't include, write it down separately and note the date. If you rewrite entries you have already made in your journal, you will lose the value of the proof you were trying to create. Keeping the diary is called keeping a *contemporaneous record*.

If you feel you are being discriminated against, you must file a complaint within a short time frame, so don't hesitate to call the EEOC (800-514-0301) or the state agency that handles these issues to discuss what to do about it. The EEOC can point you in the right direction for your local agency if you don't know the right name or number.

Insurance

Your insurance is important to assure you receive appropriate treatment for your cancer. There are many types of insurance, including health insurance, life insurance, disability insurance, and long-term care insurance. Some of these policies may have been made available to you through your work, or you may have purchased them separately.

> "All of my treatments, my radiation, my chemo, my surgery, were all covered, but we did go through battles, because while I was taking my chemotherapy …one month or one week the insurance company would pay it without a problem and the next week they would send us back a statement that said I'd gone out of network, or I was doing something that wasn't covered, and it was the very same procedure we had done the week before with the chemotherapy. So, we had to go back in and, in fact, I have a bill today still sitting in my desk that we are still trying to get the codes corrected on so that the insurance company will pay for the things that they paid for during different time periods of my treatment."
>
> — Patti

Health Insurance

If you have health insurance, it is important to know how your coverage works and what it covers. For example, if you have a form of managed-care coverage, it may be that insurance company approval is needed before you can see a doctor, take a treatment, or purchase a drug. Even then, you may be limited to the doctor or treatment center of the company's choosing. Or you may have the kind of policy under which you see whatever doctor you choose and then submit the bill. The key is to learn how your coverage works. If the description from your employer or insurance company isn't clear, ask for clarification in the benefits department of the hospital or doctor's office or call the insurance company.

In looking at insurance options, be aware of differences in coverage. Ask about choices of doctors, protection against cancellations, and increases in premiums. Determine what the plan really covers, especially in the event of a catastrophic illness like cancer. What are the deductibles? (Remember, sometimes higher deductibles accompany more comprehensive coverage.) The Insurance Information Institute has a toll-free help line to answer questions about medical insurance. It also offers some free publications. Call the National Insurance Consumer HelpLine at 800-942-4242.

CLAIM DISPUTES

If you have a dispute with your insurance company, look for someone in a position of influence to help you. For example, your oncologist or primary

Figure 6-1.

Tips for Health Insurance

- Submit claims for all medical expenses even when you are uncertain about your coverage. Resubmit claims that are denied.
- Ask for help in filing a claim if you need it.
- Keep accurate and complete records of claims submitted, pending, and paid.
- Keep copies of all paperwork related to your claims, such as letters of medical necessity, bills, receipts, requests for sick leave, and correspondence with insurance companies.
- If you receive bills, submit them as you receive them. If you become overwhelmed with bills, get help. For assistance, contact local support organizations, such as your American Cancer Society or your state's government agencies.
- Do not allow your medical insurance to expire.
- Keep your insurance needs in mind when making major decisions, such as whether to stop working.
- Learn about the appeals process in case your health care plan doesn't cover what your doctor recommends. Follow the appeals process to the letter. If it gives you a time limit in which do so something, be sure to do it within the stated time limit or you may lose the right to appeal.

care physician may deal with the insurance company all the time. He or she understands what the company is looking for in accepting or denying coverage, and knows how to marshall the information necessary to change the company's thinking. Likewise, if your employer is large enough, ask the benefits department to get involved. Since they decide whether to renew the group coverage with that company each year, they can be influential.

If these methods fail, consider hiring an attorney with an expertise in health insurance. If you have trouble locating an expert, contact the state or local chapter of the American Bar Association. (A directory is available online at http://www.abanet.org/barserv/stlobar.html, or you can check your local phone directory). You can complain to the state insurance commission as a matter of last resort.

"Well, it depends on the type of plan that you have, but most groups today have an 800 number and a nurse-call type referral circumstance that you have to phone in first. So I would always encourage a person to check before they have the treatment. Now obviously, if there's an emergency, there's a provision within that to carve that out. Often, employee human resources departments can provide answers, but not always to detailed questions. If they cannot answer the question, they can at least then put you in touch with the broker or the agency that is handling the insurance for their firm…I would suggest if you have a representative that has worked with you or your family in insurance for years, that you would then lean on that person, just appeal to them to perhaps assist you in trying to identify or find out exactly what is available to you. And then, further than that, if you are in a situation maybe a little more dire…maybe don't have the coverage you need, the state or some special program could be a resource."

— Doug

WHEN YOU BECOME TOO ILL TO WORK

If you are currently employed, don't leave your job until you have explored conversion options for your insurance through your current health care plan. Many group plans have a clause for conversion to individual health care plans, although premiums may be considerably higher. These individual plans usually must be applied for within 30 days of termination.

If you leave work because of your health condition, under the federal law known as COBRA (an abbreviation for the Consolidated Omnibus Budget Reconciliation Act) you are entitled to keep your health insurance for at least the next 18 months unless you are disabled, in which event you can continue your coverage for 29 or 36 months, depending on the circumstances. No matter who paid the premium when you worked, your employer can require you to pay for the entire premium, plus up to an additional 2 percent to cover administrative costs. Your employer can help with part or all of the premium but is not under any obligation to do so.

COBRA only applies to employers with 20 or more employees. However, your state law may provide similar protection if you work for a smaller employer.

—⁂—

"After a few years, my husband's insurance abruptly changed, so that they were not going to cover ostomy supplies, which are a prosthetic device. And they didn't notify us that they were not going to be covered. So, I took it upon myself to write a letter saying basically, 'what's the story here,' and outlined the medical necessity for this and gave the rationale for it, and asked my primary care physician to write a supporting letter, which he did.

"The answer came back from the insurance company that the claim was denied, but that there was an appeal process. I went through the appeal process, again wrote a letter, also getting documentation from the original surgeon and the primary care physician. As a result of that, they gave me a timeline that they would respond. They did not respond within that timeline, so I wrote another letter saying, 'I've provided you with information, you have not responded to me within the guidelines that you set up. You have not provided me with rationale for changing your policy. This is not acceptable.'

"As soon as that letter got to the patient representative at the insurance company, I got a telephone call saying, 'If you will go with a mail order firm, we will cover your ostomy supplies forever. Will you accept that?' And I said, 'Yes, as soon as I receive it in writing.'"

— Ann F.

HEALTH CARE AND INSURANCE RESOURCES

There are many health care and insurance-related resources that can help you during this difficult time. The following is a brief list of resources you may want to explore.

Medicare

Medicare is a federal health program for people who are at least 65 years old or who have been permanently disabled for 24 months. Medicare provides basic health coverage, but it doesn't pay all of your medical expenses. Medicare benefits are subject to change, so to ensure you have the most accurate and current information about Medicare, call 800-MEDICARE.

Medicare is divided into two parts. Part A pays for hospital care, home health care, hospice care, and care in Medicare-certified nursing facilities. Part B covers outpatient services, like diagnostic studies, doctor services, durable medical equipment used at home, and ambulance transportation.

—⁂—

"My friend is a single mom with no insurance. So [I did] practical things I could think of, for instance networking people to help with child care, bringing meals to her that were freezable and that were in small portions…I had another person research Medicaid, another person research local charities, and we were able to come up with one place that paid her electric bill, another one that brought some food. We had another one take care of one of her mortgage payments. There are all sorts of things that are out there that if you have people that have background in knowing how to research these things. It can be a tremendous help."

— Dori

HMOs that have contracts with the Medicare program must provide all hospital and medical benefits covered by Medicare. However, you must usually obtain services from the HMO network of health care providers. If you have questions about Medicare, call 800-MEDICARE or contact your Social Security office.

Medicare Hospice Benefit

Recall from earlier discussions that Medicare has special provisions with regard to coverage of hospice care. The *Medicare hospice benefit* is the most common way palliative care is delivered, and this benefit covers 4 levels of required services: routine home care, continuous nursing care at home, inpatient care in a facility (acute care or hospitalization), and respite care (see pages 36–37). For a fuller discussion and the most recent information about what is covered under this benefit, see the official pamphlet online at http://www.medicare.gov/Publications/Pubs/pdf/02154.pdf or call 800-MEDICARE.

For a person with a serious illness to access this benefit, a physician must certify that his or her prognosis is 6 months or less. However, hospice care does not stop after 6 months if a person outlives their prognosis. A person with advanced cancer may receive care for as long as necessary when a physician certifies that he or she has a life expectancy of 6 months or less. Under the Medicare hospice benefit, there are two 90-day periods of care (a total of 6 months), which are followed by an unlimited number of 60-day periods.

When a person transitions to hospice care under the Medicare hospice benefit, he or she may receive palliative care but waives the standard Medicare benefits for treatments of the cancer intended to prolong life. However, the person with advanced cancer may continue to access standard Medicare benefits for treatment of conditions that are not related to the cancer, such as diseases like diabetes.

The benefit delivers comprehensive home-based supportive care designed to support primary caregivers (usually family members or other informal caregivers) and maximize the person with cancer's quality of life at the end of life. An interdisciplinary hospice team provides services including nursing care, pain and symptom management, spiritual support, grief support, and caregiver support. A hospice team includes hospice nurses and nursing aids, a social worker, a chaplain, and a physician medical director. Hospice also includes carefully trained volunteers, who provide help of all kinds.

> —m—
> "Unfortunately in this day of managed care, it may take more than one phone call and talking to more than one person, but be…persistent enough to get the answers you need."
>
> – Mary Jane

Along with home services, the benefit provides brief hospital admissions (up to 5 days per episode) for respite. This gives family caregivers a chance to rest. In addition, short periods of hospitalization (either in a freestanding hospice unit, a nursing home, or in a hospital) are covered for adjusting therapy if this has not been possible to achieve at home.

The benefit also includes a drug prescription benefit for medications and palliative procedures. It also covers bereavement support for up to a year to help people with cancer and their loved ones cope with grief and loss.

Medicare pays the hospice program approximately $120 a day to provide care to a patient at the routine home care level; most often this care is provided in the patient's own home. Because nursing homes are considered homes for certain elderly patients, hospice teams can also care for patients within nursing homes or long-term care facilities. There are more than 3,300 hospice teams in the country, and over 700,000 patients in the United States received hospice care prior to death in 2002. About half of these patients are cancer patients.

The national Medicare rates per day, effective October 1, 2003 and current at the time of publication of this book, adjusted for regional wage differences, are:

- —m— $118.08 for routine home care
- —m— $689.18 for continuous home care ($28.72/hour)
- —m— $122.15 for respite care
- —m— $525.28 for general inpatient care

For patients under the age of 65, private insurance programs support hospice care, as do a wide variety of HMOs. Although the benefits may vary, the universal focus is on supporting home-based nursing care for patients with advanced illness. When you are considering entering a hospice program, work with your insurance company to assess whether your policy provides you with the services needed. Also consider the role your family members will play in providing care.

Forced Choice: The Medicare Hospice Conundrum

The Medicare criteria for participation in hospice (that is, persons over the age of 65 or those who are currently receiving Medicare disability benefits and are expected to live fewer than 6 months) can be problematic for some individuals.

For example, the Medicare hospice benefit includes medications needed for symptom control, but people with cancer receiving treatment with life-prolonging intent are *not* eligible for hospice care. As a result, persons on Medicare who are living with advanced cancer must often choose between curative therapies and palliative care.

In addition, because of the 6-month life expectancy qualification requirement, many doctors are reluctant to refer individuals whose prognoses are uncertain to hospices, resulting in people who need critical care receiving too little care too late. The average stay in hospice is 50 days; the median is less than 4 weeks.

Medicare Home Care Benefit

The Medicare hospice benefit, which we have been discussing, is distinct from another benefit called the *Medicare home care benefit*. Under the Medicare home care benefit, if an individual is homebound, under a physician's care, and requires medically necessary skilled nursing or therapy services, he or she may be eligible for services provided by a Medicare-certified home health agency. Depending on the patient's condition, Medicare may pay for intermittent skilled nursing; physical, occupational, and speech therapies; medical social services; home care aide services; and medical equipment and supplies.

It is important for patients and families to recognize the differences between the Medicare *hospice* benefit and the Medicare *home care* benefit. In the Medicare hospice benefit, patients for the most part have to stop receiving active anticancer therapies. In contrast, under the Medicare home care benefit, patients can continue to receive cancer treatments.

Increasing attention is being given to the need to bridge palliative care teams and services within hospitals with hospice services. Some hospice programs are providing consultation teams to hospitals to help improve symptom management and provide supportive therapies. Check with your hospital to see if they have a palliative care team, or ask the hospice program if they have a consultation team available to assess patients in the hospital who require symptom management but may not be ready to receive hospice care.

Medicaid

Medicaid is another government program that covers the cost of medical care. To receive Medicaid, your income and assets must be below a certain level. These levels vary from state to state. Not all health providers take Medicaid. Some examples of groups eligible for Medicaid are low-income families with children and Supplemental Security Income (SSI) recipients. Medicare beneficiaries who have low incomes and limited resources may receive help paying for their out-of-pocket medical expenses from their state Medicaid program. Forty-five states also have a Medicaid hospice benefit. For more information, contact your state Medicaid office.

Medigap

If you are on Medicare, you may be able to add more coverage with a Medigap policy or a Medicare HMO. Currently, there are 10 Medigap policies offered in all 50 states. The plans are standardized and identified by letters A through J. Insurance carriers offer different plans, so check with them for details of coverage. Medigap policies require underwriting, which means that a person with a serious disease like cancer may not be eligible. Under the Medicare Modernization Act of 2003, Medigap policies will be changing, so contact Medicare at 800-MEDICARE or check online at http://www.medicare.gov for the most updated information.

Medical Assistance

Medical assistance programs are available for those with incomes under certain amounts. The scope of these programs varies from state to state but may provide money for expenses, such as prescription medicines. A hospital social worker or case manager should have information on these local programs. Check into the renewal requirements as you investigate this option, so that you'll be prepared if quarterly renewal is required.

Hill-Burton Program

Hospitals and other medical facilities that receive funds from the federal government must offer a minimum amount of free or low-cost services to those who are unable to pay. This is called the Hill-Burton Program. Each facility chooses which services it will provide free or at lowered cost. Those with Medicare and Medicaid services aren't eligible for Hill-Burton coverage. However, Hill-Burton may cover services not covered by other government programs. Eligibility for Hill-Burton is based on family size and income. You may apply for Hill-Burton assistance at any time, before or after you receive care. To find out more information about this program, call the Hill-Burton Toll Free Hotline at 800-638-0742 (Maryland residents call 800-492-0359) or visit http://www.hrsa.gov/osp/dfcr/obtain/freecare.pdf to view the *Hill-Burton Free Care Brochure* that describes the program and tells how to apply for services.

Veterans' Benefits

If you are a veteran, you may qualify for benefits from the government. Veterans' benefits are changing, and the number of veterans' medical facilities is declining. To get the most accurate information, contact the benefits office of the Department of Veterans Affairs at 800-827-1000 or http://www.va.gov. Veterans' benefits may also overlap with hospice benefits.

Help for Senior Citizens

For assistance, contact your local office on aging. The National Association of Area Agencies on Aging (N4A) provides the Eldercare Locator (800-677-1116 or http://www.eldercare.gov), a nationwide directory assistance service designed to help older persons and caregivers find local support resources. The Eldercare Locator Web site has links to state and local agencies on aging, where information on transportation, meals, home care, housing alternatives, legal issues, and social activities is available.

Options for the Hard-to-Insure

Health insurance options are available through some states for hard-to-insure people. A number of states currently sell comprehensive health insurance to state residents with serious medical conditions who can't find a company to insure them. These state programs, sometimes called guaranteed-access programs, or more commonly, state *risk pools*, serve people who have pre-existing health conditions and are often denied or have difficulty finding affordable coverage in the private market. They provide a safety net for the "medically uninsurable" population. To find out if your state has a risk pool, contact the state department of insurance by calling directory assistance in your state capitol.

The Health Insurance Portability and Accountability Act of 1996 (HIPAA) provides nationwide standards and a guarantee of access to health insurance coverage in the individual market. This legislation protects people from discrimination based on pre-existing medical conditions. Because of HIPAA, many employees may not lose their insurance when they change jobs or move to a different state, as long as their new employer offers health insurance as a benefit.

Options for the Uninsured

For people who are not already insured, the following are resources to consider when seeking coverage:

- **Help from independent brokers.** An independent broker may be able to help you locate a reasonable benefit package. Group insurance is usually preferable to individual insurance.
- **Health maintenance organizations (HMOs).** Health maintenance organizations (HMOs) or health care service plans in your community can provide quite comprehensive coverage. Many offer one period of open enrollment each year, where applicants are accepted regardless of health histories.
- **Help from professional organizations.** You may be able to apply for group insurance through fraternal or professional organizations (such as those for retired persons, teachers, social workers, realtors, etc.). If you are the parent of a school-age child, investigate school insurance. Look for a "guaranteed issue" plan, which means that you cannot be denied.
- **See if you can qualify under the health policy of your spouse or partner.** If your spouse or partner doesn't have such coverage, it may be worthwhile for that person to consider changing jobs to get better benefits. Larger employers (such as Fortune 500 companies or federal, state, or local

> —⁓—
>
> "Well, the financial part [of cancer], where it really hurt me in my business, was that I lost my health insurance. You know, they can't take it away from you, but in the small little firm that we are in, there's only 3 of us plus a couple of staff. They bumped the premium up so high that I couldn't afford to pay it anymore. And so consequently I lost my insurance; the whole firm lost their insurance, everybody had to go out and buy their own individual insurance."
>
> — Robert G.

governments) tend to have the best benefits. However, do your research before your spouse or domestic partner changes jobs. Some employers may make employees and their dependents wait 60 to 90 days before joining a plan, and there may be a period of up to 12 months in which pre-existing conditions are not covered. If you meet certain criteria, HIPAA (Health Insurance Portability and Accountability Act) may help protect you. Call 866-627-7748 or visit http://www.hhs.gov/ocr/hipaa for more information.

Life Insurance

Life insurance protects anyone who depends on your paycheck. What will happen to your spouse or partner, children, or other dependents if you die prematurely? Are they counting on your paycheck to cover day-to-day needs or future expenses? If so, life insurance can provide your loved ones with income to replace yours, until they can live comfortably without it. It can also provide an emergency fund for medical, legal, and funeral costs, and can help provide for longer-term expenses, like financing a child's college education or paying off a mortgage or business debts.

HOW MUCH LIFE INSURANCE IS ENOUGH?

The amount of life insurance coverage you need depends on your unique situation, such as the number of people who depend upon your income and the standard of living to which you and your family are accustomed, among other things. If you are single, or one-half of a 2-income household with no dependents, you probably won't need much life insurance. However, if you are the sole breadwinner for a large family with little savings, you are likely to need much more life insurance.

LIFE INSURANCE ISSUES TO CONSIDER
WHEN YOU HAVE CANCER

If you are still actively employed but will not be able to continue work because of advancing disease, find out whether your life insurance policy permits you to convert it from group coverage to individual coverage when you leave your employer. If there is such a right (as is generally the case), can you increase the coverage without a medical exam? Can you decrease the coverage if you can't afford the full amount you currently have?

You should also investigate whether the policy is assignable to another person or entity. This can become important if you become very ill and want to sell your policy as described in chapter 7 (see the section on viaticals on page 152). If your policy isn't assignable and your employer knows about your health condition, now is the time to speak with your employer and insurance company about allowing an assignment.

If you have life insurance and your cancer is progressing, you should update your policy to ensure the beneficiary is the person you actually want to receive the benefit. You should also find out if your insurance includes a provision that premiums are waived if you become disabled, so you can keep the coverage without having to pay additional premiums if you have to stop work.

If cancer treatment and care are putting a strain on your finances, consider asking your beneficiary to take over the policy's premium payments. This can ensure that your policy is not invalidated because of lack of payment of premiums.

OBTAINING LIFE INSURANCE IF YOU ARE ALREADY SICK

What if you don't have life insurance, but your illness is making it difficult for you to obtain life insurance—how can you get it? Here are some helpful ideas:

- Watch for periods known as "open enrollment," when you can obtain life insurance from your employer or increase the coverage you have without a medical exam.
- You may still qualify for what is known as "simplified issue" life insurance, a policy of a limited amount (say up to $50,000) that has just a few questions. A local insurance broker can let you know.
- Keep your eyes open for insurance that is guaranteed to all applicants. These policies are written for smaller amounts, but they can add up.
- You may be able to purchase life insurance for the outstanding balance on your credit cards. Contact the credit card companies. Generally, health questions aren't asked, and coverage for pre-existing conditions may be limited to a short period of time.

Disability Insurance

A disability insurance policy pays you a regular income when an illness like cancer or an accident prevents you from doing your job. You may have disability benefits from your employer and/or the government. If you have disability insurance through an employer-paid or government-sponsored program, find out what is considered to be a "disability" under the policy, so you'll know when you qualify and so you can start taking steps immediately to qualify when you need it. For instance, depression can often be considered a disability, so if you are experiencing the depression that often accompanies cancer, it can be helpful if you seek professional counseling—not only from a medical perspective but from a practical one too.

Long-term Care Insurance

Long-term care refers to the many services used by people who have disabilities or chronic illnesses like cancer. Long-term care insurance helps you pay for these services, including help in your home with daily activities like bathing and dressing, adult day care, assisted living services, meals, and health monitoring.

Quality home care or care at a residential facility can easily cost tens of thousands of dollars a year. Long-term care insurance is a way to help defray the costs associated with long-term care and to protect your assets, especially if it is purchased when you are young and/or relatively healthy. But purchasing long-term care insurance isn't always the best option, especially if you are already quite sick. Costs for a policy depend on your age and health status. If your prognosis is not optimistic, you may not qualify for a new policy. Also, if your medical bills are likely to rapidly exhaust your savings (in which case you would qualify for Medicaid), long-term care insurance may not be the wisest way to spend your money.

Conclusion

Don't make the assumption that because you have cancer you can't improve your work or insurance situation. As you've read in this chapter, that is not the case. Knowing your rights, your options, and the benefits to which you are entitled can help make the experience of your cancer treatment and care easier for both you and your loved ones.

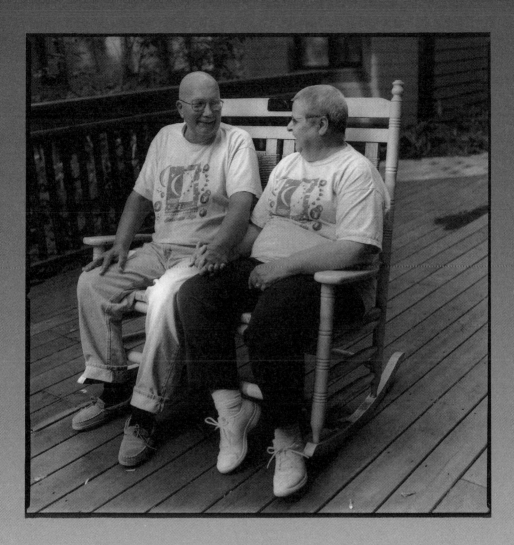

Chapter 7

Legal and Financial Matters

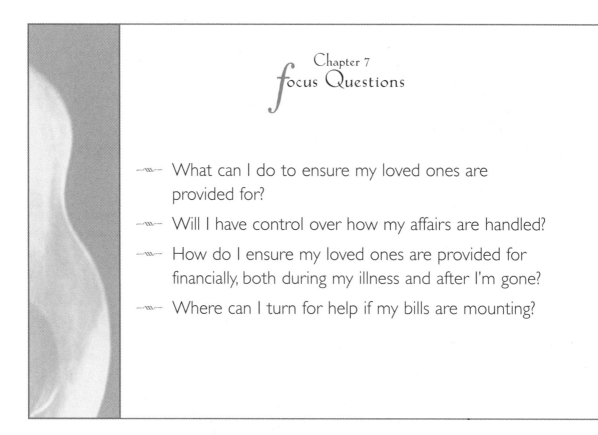

Chapter 7
*f*ocus Questions

—⚮— What can I do to ensure my loved ones are
provided for?

—⚮— Will I have control over how my affairs are handled?

—⚮— How do I ensure my loved ones are provided for
financially, both during my illness and after I'm gone?

—⚮— Where can I turn for help if my bills are mounting?

"The day after the diagnosis that the cancer had metastasized, the first thing Chuck wanted to do was go to the army base and sit down with the Judge Advocate General's office and get his will updated, get a living will done. Get all the paperwork taken care of, so that he knew that if something happened, it was all taken care of….But I think even more importantly for him and for his peace of mind was that he could go into this battle now knowing that the paperwork was taken care of, that if something did happen to him and he didn't win, that I would be taken care of financially and everything else. That I wouldn't have to deal with any of the paperwork issues, that it would be as easy for me as possible."

– Ann I.

MANY PEOPLE WITH CANCER WORRY ABOUT HOW TO PROTECT their loved ones and provide for them, both now and after they are gone. Others are worried about the distribution of their property after their death—who will inherit the well-loved baseball card collection or Grandma's quilts? Some are most concerned with the burden of pressing practical matters, like ensuring the hospital bills that are piling up get paid. These worries are very common, and the good news is, there are things you can do to manage them.

Getting your affairs in order—drawing up a will and developing a financial plan—can help ease your worries and make the time you have left less stressful for both you and your loved ones. In this chapter, we'll provide information to help you get a handle on your legal affairs, strategies to keep your financial matters in order in the short and long term, and resources to help you manage the costs of cancer care and treatment.

Will

A *will* is a legal document that describes what happens to your property after your death. Every adult should have a will—preferably one that has been prepared with the help of an attorney and is tailored to the person's unique and specific circumstances. If you have a life-limiting illness, a will is part of having a good backup plan for your loved ones, because when someone dies without a will it creates a great deal of work for the loved ones who survive them.

If you have a will, sometimes called a *last will and testament*, it will designate what will happen to your estate after you die. Your *estate* includes all your property or *assets*, which might include your house, clothes, jewelry, car, bank accounts, and retirement accounts. How this property is divided is determined by you and recorded in the will. A *letter of instruction* sometimes accompanies a will. This document includes information not covered in the will, such as how to distribute personal property with little economic value but important sentimental value, such as letters or family albums.

After your death, your debts will need to be paid, any expenses of your estate (like house payments) need to be paid, and taxes on your estate must be paid. What is left over after this is divided among the person's survivors. This process of dividing up the person's property is called *settling the estate* and may take several weeks to over a year, depending on the size and complexity of the person's estate.

If you die without a will (which is called *intestate* by lawyers), the probate court will take care of the estate until it is settled. The court will divide the property according to the laws in the state where the person lived. For example, the law in many states is that half of the remaining estate goes to the surviving spouse, and the other half is divided among children and other relatives. So if you die without a will, you will not have any control over who gets what. The way to make sure that your wishes about who gets what are followed is to make sure you have an up-to-date will.

Trust

A *trust*, like a will, is a means of transferring property from you to another person or entity—your spouse, partner, child, relatives, or other loved ones, or a charity, for example. A trust can help eliminate the probate process and minimize inheritance taxes. However, a trust is not a substitute for a will.

There are several different types of trusts. In each case, when you establish a trust, you transfer your ownership of property to that trust. Then a *trustee* (a person or a financial institution) manages that property according to your instructions. *Beneficiaries* eventually receive the assets of the trust.

Looking After Your Dependents

If you are a single parent, there is a process called permanency planning that will allow you to make arrangements for the care of your children. The laws differ from state to state, so you will need to talk to a lawyer about your particular situation. You will want to ask the lawyer about adding a *guardianship clause* in your will and about whether standby guardianship is available in your state. A standby guardian is someone you name who has legal rights to take care of your child if there is no other parent and if you become unable to do this, and a standby guardian can start to take care of the child or children prior to your death. Also, when you fill out a power of attorney document make sure it includes provisions for the care of your children.

> —⁓—
>
> "Make a will, and for middle class America, a living trust is a very fine vehicle to take care of the disposition of your estate. You can save yourself a lot of taxes, you can save yourself a lot of administrative costs, and you can decide where it goes within the limits of two generations."
>
> — Bob

Finding an Attorney

When you draw up a will, you should seek the expert advice of an attorney, so the decisions you make about taxes, beneficiaries, and how to divide up your assets are legally binding.

You will need to find a lawyer who you will feel comfortable working with and whose fees will be reasonable. You can ask friends and family for recommendations or consult your local bar association and ask for a list of lawyers who specialize in estate planning (an online directory of state and local bar associations is available at http://www.abanet.org/barserv/stlobar.html). An

"Actually, whether or not you have a diagnosis of cancer, if you have small children you should be making preparations and plans in the event that something happens to one or both parents. Part of the responsibility for a parent and planning for their children's future is to take care of the details and don't put them off!…You really need to wake yourself up and pay attention to the fact that even if you are perfectly healthy right now, tomorrow you could be hit by a car; you could have a cancer diagnosis, you could lose one or both parents at the same time. And not having a plan in place to take care of the children is a terrible tragedy for the children!"

— Susanna

attorney who specializes in elder law can also be a terrific resource. When you are trying to find such an attorney, your Area Agency on Aging or the "Experience Registry" of the National Academy of Elder Law Attorney (http://www.naela.org) are good places to start.

Your Finances: Planning Ahead

Having a life-limiting cancer affects your finances as well as your health. One estimate suggests that medical costs for people with advanced cancer are about 20 percent higher than average medical costs for people dying of other conditions. Taking stock of your financial situation and planning ahead can help you make the most of your resources and help you feel that you have some control over your situation. It can also help ensure that your cancer care and treatment don't take an undue toll on your finances, so you can ensure your loved ones are provided for after your death.

Financial Planning

Financial planning may sound like a task for only the extremely wealthy, but financial planners are for anybody who wants to make the most of their financial situation.

A financial planner can help you do a checkup on your financial status, which will give you a clear picture of your income, benefits, expenses, savings, investments, assets, and debts. A financial planner who has experience with people who are nearing the end of their lives can also help you plan for changes to your financial situation (such as lost wages) that may come as a result of severe illness and unexpected costs (such as experimental treatments not covered by your medical insurance or home health care costs). He or she can also provide advice in the event that you need to liquidate your assets and convert them to cash to pay for treatment, care, and related expenses.

> —⚏—
> "I seem to find myself worrying more about my wife and son, how they're going to do when I do go."
> – Mark

Having a good financial plan requires planning for the worst and hoping it never happens. The benefit of this is that you will know that no matter what happens, you have done your best to be prepared and to take care of your loved ones. That will help your peace of mind.

When selecting a financial planner, look for someone who is certified in financial planning (if the person is certified, the letters CFP will follow his or her name). Find someone who has experience with people like you, and who you feel you can work with. Don't forget to ask about compensation—some financial planners charge flat or hourly rates, while others charge fees and commissions.

Durable Power of Attorney for Finances

In chapter 5 we talked about durable powers of attorney (DPOA) for health care. There is also a legal document called a *durable power of attorney for financial matters*. Whether financial or medical, a power of attorney basically allows someone else to act in your name on your behalf. The purpose of a durable power of attorney for financial matters is to designate someone to handle financial matters for you if you are not able to do so because of poor health. The person you designate in the DPOA for financial affairs can do things such as pay bills and sign checks on your behalf. You can specify exactly which tasks your proxy is authorized to perform on your behalf. Assigning someone to be your power of attorney for financial affairs does not necessarily give him or her complete control over your finances. Since all powers of attorney come to an end at your death, your agent will not be authorized to make any more decisions after your life has ended.

Choose your *proxy* or *agent* (the person to whom you assign your power of attorney) very carefully. Not everyone is well suited to this task. Select someone who is honest, reliable, well organized, and trustworthy. This person will have access to private financial information, so he or she should be discreet as well. You should be confident in the person's ability to carry out your specific instructions as well as your intentions, even if family members or loved ones who have an interest in your finances have questions or criticisms. If you have any concern that people close to you will challenge your power of attorney, you may want to tell them your plans and intentions ahead of time so that your wishes will be clear to all involved.

Sources of Financial Help

Life-limiting illnesses and conditions requiring extensive medical care such as cancer often lead to a need for immediate financial resources. During treatment and long-term care, many people find themselves struggling with financial problems. Without insurance, costs can mount quickly. Even if you have insurance and your plan picks up most of your costs, out-of-pocket expenses can be a burden. If you've found gaps in your coverage, don't hesitate to discuss your needs with your doctor or hospital social worker. You may be pleasantly surprised by the number of organizations that exist to help you and other cancer patients.

You can also work directly with your creditors. Creditors will often agree to accept smaller payments or a nominal monthly amount. The Consumer Credit Counseling Service can help you make a payment plan for all your creditors. Call toll-free at 800-251-2227 to schedule a telephone or in-person session or to obtain more information. They also offer online credit counseling through their Web site (http://www.cccsatl.org).

If your financial situation is becoming problematic and mounting expenses are putting a strain on your wallet, the following resources may be helpful to you.

PAYING YOUR BILLS

You may have difficulty keeping up with the direct and indirect costs of cancer treatment and care. The easiest way to eliminate financial issues is to approach them one step at a time. You can set up payment plans with utility providers, mortgage or rental managers, doctors, and other medical providers. If you have a good history of paying your bills on time, most businesses and creditors will probably allow you to arrange a payment plan.

Because there can be many out-of-pocket expenses that aren't covered by insurance, people often use credit cards to pay for things during cancer treatment.

It isn't uncommon for people to find that their credit card bills soon become unmanageable. Try to move any credit card balances to the credit card with the lowest interest rate. Making small but consistent payments is better than making no payments at all. If you can't meet the minimum payments, call the credit card company. If you explain your situation, the company will usually try to make arrangements with you. They would rather you make some attempt to pay than not pay at all. It's also possible to negotiate for lower interest rates.

Credit counseling can help you consolidate your bills. The Consumer Credit Counseling Service is a national nonprofit service that offers free and confidential financial counseling. They help people set up budgets and make repayment plans. Their counselors are certified and often offer appointments on a same-day basis. Call toll-free at 800-251-2227 to schedule a telephone or in-person session or to obtain more information. They also offer online credit counseling through their Web site (http://www. cccsintl.org).

SOCIAL SECURITY DISABILITY INCOME OR SUPPLEMENTAL SECURITY INCOME

Check with your local Social Security Administration office to find out if you qualify for any income under the Social Security Disability Income or Supplemental Security Income programs. If you have been working for many years, you probably have contributed to Social Security. In this case, you may qualify for disability benefits. Social Security Disability Income (SSDI) typically replaces 60 to 70 percent of your income (the amount of your income has nothing to do with whether you qualify for benefits). You may also qualify for SSDI if you are currently not working but have been in the work force for many years. Eligibility for Social Security disability benefits is contingent upon your disability being expected to last for at least 12 months or lead to your death.

If you have a history of unemployment (whether by choice or not), you may be eligible for Supplemental Security Income (SSI). To qualify, your income and assets must fall below a certain level. You must be disabled, over 65 years old, and/or blind. The amount of benefits you could get varies from state to state. To locate the Social Security office near you, call 800-772-1213 or go to http://www.ssa.gov.

LIFE-INSURANCE/VIATICALS

In many states the value of an individual's life insurance policy can be realized through the acceleration of the policy's death benefit—known as living benefits. These benefits can be accessed several ways, including a *viatical* (sale of the life insurance policy) and loans from the original insurance company or a third party against the face value of the life insurance policy.

A viatical is the sale of a life insurance policy for cash. The process of selling a life insurance policy requires the person insured for a life-limiting illness to sell his or her life insurance policy to the third party. As with any sale, what is being sold and how much it is being sold for are issues both sides must agree on. A viatical insurance company is a company that buys policies from people with limited life expectancy due to illness. The viatical company pays out a lump sum—often between 60 and 80 percent of the face value of the policy—to the owner of the policy. The payment is usually tax free. After the viatical company buys a policy, the company becomes the new owner and sole beneficiary of the policy. It pays the premiums on the policy as long as the patient is alive. When the person dies, all the remaining money from the policy goes to the viatical company.

The drawbacks of a viatical are that your heirs receive no insurance money, you may not make the best trade available, and the sale is usually not reversible. Before making a decision about your life insurance, think over your options carefully and discuss the matter with a partner, trusted friend, and/or a professional.

HOME EQUITY LOANS AND CONVERSIONS

Equity is the difference between the home's fair market value and the unpaid balance of the mortgage. Equity increases as the mortgage is paid down and as the property appreciates in value. A home equity loan allows you to borrow against the value you've built up in your home.

152

You may be able to convert part of your home's equity into cash if you are at least 62 years old and own your home (or nearly own it). The most common type of equity conversion is called a reverse mortgage. This is a loan against your home that doesn't have to be repaid for as long as you live there. The loan is repaid in the future—usually when the last surviving borrower sells, dies, or moves out of the home. It can provide cash to pay medical bills and other expenses, but it is still considered a loan and includes expenses such as interest charges and service fees. A reverse mortgage can also disqualify you from some government programs. Private, public, and federally insured lenders offer many types of reverse mortgage programs. Contact a financial advisor to find out if a reverse mortgage would help you. You can also get more information about home equity conversion from nonprofit consumer groups, such as the AARP (formerly the American Association of Retired Persons).

RETIREMENT

Some people use money from their retirement plans before they retire as a source of cash. You may qualify for hardship provisions in your plan. Contact your financial advisor or speak with someone at the company that manages your retirement accounts for more information. Be aware that there may be penalties associated with early withdrawal.

FAMILY LOANS OR GIFTS

Family members can also help pay some of your cancer-related expenses or bills. If you ask for a loan from a relative, outline a repayment period and an interest rate. (Keep in mind that there are federal tax consequences if the person making the loan charges you an interest rate below the minimum federal rate.) It's important to put the agreement in writing. The tax laws in this area are complicated, so it's a good idea to consult an accountant about family loans.

If you don't think you will be able to repay the loan, consider asking for a gift. Anyone, including a relative, can give a tax-free gift of up to $11,000 per year (as of 2004). Married couples can make a joint tax-free gift of up to $22,000 per year (as of 2004). The allowable amount of tax-free gifting is increasing, so check with an expert for the latest numbers.

Also, anyone can pay the medical bills of someone else without being subject to the gift limit if the payment is made directly to the medical facility.

Other Organizations

Civic and religious organizations may offer financial help or services for people with cancer and their family members. The American Cancer Society has numerous programs that support the person with cancer. Call 800-ACS-2345 or visit http://www.cancer.org for more information. Groups such as the Salvation Army, United Way, Lutheran Social Services, and Catholic Social Services are listed in the Yellow Pages under "Social Service Organizations." Churches, synagogues, mosques, and other religious organizations may also be able to help with transportation, baby-sitting, and home care services, which may help you financially. The Federal Citizen Information Center offers information about managing debt and many other topics. You can call them toll free at 800-FED-INFO or visit their Web site at http://www.pueblo.gsa.gov.

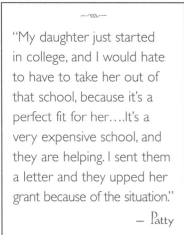

"My daughter just started in college, and I would hate to have to take her out of that school, because it's a perfect fit for her....It's a very expensive school, and they are helping. I sent them a letter and they upped her grant because of the situation."

— Patty

The National Endowment for Financial Education has collaborated with the American Cancer Society to develop a financial management program for people with cancer. For more information about the program called Taking Charge of Money Matters, call the American Cancer Society at 800-ACS-2345 or visit http://www.cancer.org for more information.

WELFARE OFFICE

Contact your county board of assistance, Aid to Families with Dependent Children (AFDC), and the Food Stamps Program for information.

BANKRUPTCY

If you try but can't make ends meet, you may have to file for bankruptcy. Bankruptcy is a complicated area of law, so consult a bankruptcy attorney if you're considering filing for bankruptcy. Legal aid clinics and other nonprofit agencies can also provide advice in this area.

ADDITIONAL HELPFUL SERVICES FOR THOSE WITH CANCER

Your hospital social worker or the American Cancer Society (800-ACS-2345 or http://www.cancer.org) can refer you to organizations who may be able to offer helpful services to you throughout your cancer treatment and care. For example, if you have to travel in order to receive cancer treatment, you may be able to take advantage of free or reduced airfare or lodging for you and your family.

You may also be able to take advantage of drug assistance programs if your insurance plan does not pay for prescription medicines used to control side effects and pain. Rather than letting this interfere with getting the supportive care you deserve, you can apply to one of the drug assistance programs listed by the Pharmaceutical Research and Manufacturers of America (PhRMA). Needy Meds (http://www.needymeds.com) is another informational resource for getting medicines from pharmaceutical companies.

You should also ask the members of your health care team for local, regional, or hospital-sponsored programs that can help defray the costs associated with cancer treatment and care.

Conclusion

The processes of drawing up a will and making a financial plan can result in many benefits. Some people find that the process of planning their estate helps them talk to their loved ones about important things. Others find that doing so gives them peace of mind. A small investment of time getting your affairs in order now can pay off later.

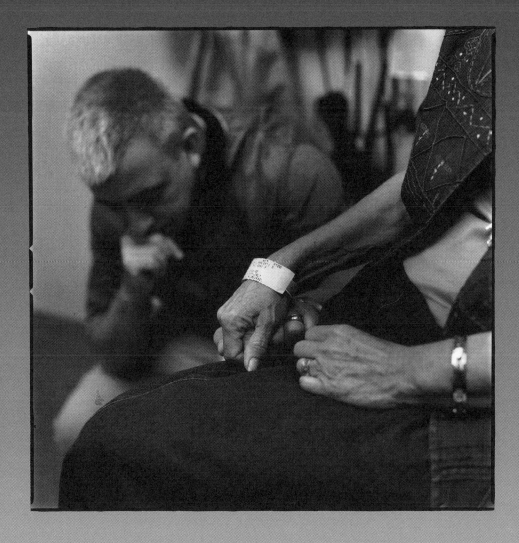

Chapter 8

Managing Your Symptoms

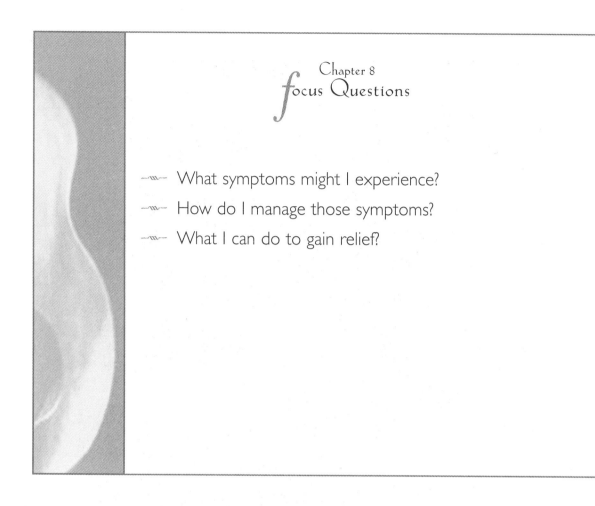

Chapter 8
*f*ocus Questions

— What symptoms might I experience?

— How do I manage those symptoms?

— What I can do to gain relief?

"I think the key is being prepared for the possibility of some of these side effects. And I emphasize 'possibility' because not all patients, even receiving the exact same treatments, experience it or experience it to the same degree. But if they're prepared for the possibility, one, they won't be shocked or surprised or try to deny to themselves that it's happening. The second part of it beyond preparation is encouraging a willingness to communicate with the health care team. Because even if something can't be done about it, having the symptom validated, knowing that if you're the patient the symptom is being watched, that anything fixable is being addressed, that any potential problems that might be related to the symptom or might be due to the symptom are being looked for, is tremendously comforting."

— Wendy

WE'VE TALKED A LOT ABOUT TREATMENT AND CARE OPTIONS, and about how to make decisions that are right for you. We've also covered coping strategies and how to talk about your illness with others. In this chapter, we'll focus on what you and your loved ones and caregivers can expect from a physical standpoint as cancer progresses through its early to most advanced stages and how your palliative care team can help alleviate the distress and discomfort associated with these conditions to ensure that you maintain the highest quality of life possible.

A detailed discussion of all of the symptoms that people with cancer may experience is beyond the scope of this book. However, there are some common symptoms that many patients experience as a result of cancer itself—we'll cover those here. There are also a wide range of treatment-related symptoms (also called side effects) that you may experience as a result of specific medical interventions. For example, if you receive radiation therapy to your head or neck, you may experience a burning sensation in the mouth or esophagus. Different chemotherapies may cause different symptoms, such as tingling in the feet, pain in your muscles, or joint pain.

> "Certainly I was briefed that there would be a lot of side effects. But it varies so much that it's difficult for them to really prepare you."
>
> — Ron

All of these symptoms (whether they are related to the cancer itself or to the cancer treatment you are receiving) should be discussed with your health care team. Many of these symptoms can be managed or eliminated. We hope that the general information in this chapter provides you with sufficient background material for you to advocate for your symptom treatment and to know what potential options are available. Further information on symptoms is available from the American Cancer Society (800-ACS-2345 or http://www.cancer.org) and from your own health care team treating your disease. Palliative care is about ensuring that you receive the best symptom management possible, and that you are as comfortable as you can be.

Talking to Your Health Care Team About Your Symptoms

Reporting your symptoms to your health care team is an essential responsibility. It helps your medical team understand your disease and your response to treatment and care interventions. In addition, treating symptoms helps you return to normal functioning.

Taking care of your symptoms is a very high priority for cancer doctors and nurses. Some patients may wonder if talking to their doctor about their symptoms will distract him from dealing with their cancer. However, doctors want to take care of your symptoms just as much as they want to try to cure your cancer or retard its growth, and it isn't an either/or choice. You can receive treatment for symptom control and cancer at the same time.

Unless you tell your health care team about your symptoms, however, they may not be aware of your discomfort. Be prepared to talk about your symptoms when you visit your doctor. Writing your symptoms down as they occur and keeping an ongoing log will help you remember to tell the doctor about them. This log might include a description of your symptom, where it occurs in your body, what its intensity is (mild, moderate, or severe), how frequently it occurs, and how it interferes with your daily tasks, sleep, appetite, and social activities. Tell your doctor or nurse which symptom is bothering you the most, so they will spend the most time on that. Most doctors find it helpful when their patients say, "there are a couple of things I want to make sure we address today—the first is pain I'm having in my leg; the second is that I have trouble sleeping at night." There are a wide range of methods to assess your symptoms and your physician may use one of these approaches in asking you about nausea, vomiting, insomnia, or other symptoms.

> —⁓—
> "Your doctors, when you've got pain, they want to make you as comfortable as they can....But the patient has to be as involved as the physician."
>
> – Jeff

Managing Treatment and Disease-Related Symptoms

As cancer progresses, you may experience a variety of physical effects from the cancer itself, or from the treatments you receive. The most common symptoms are pain, fatigue, depression, loss of appetite, and problems sleeping. As cancer advances, additional health problems like difficulty breathing and weight loss may arise. We'll discuss these symptoms and others, and will also provide tips and practical strategies for managing these health issues to minimize your discomfort.

Pain

For patients with cancer, pain is a feared consequence, but it can be effectively controlled. No one should be in pain. The goal of pain therapy is straightforward: to avoid pain that can be prevented and to control pain that cannot, while limiting medication-related side effects.

YOUR ROLE IN PAIN CONTROL

The first step in pain control is to identify your pain and tell your doctor or nurse about it. Describe your experience of pain in as much detail as possible, including the location, what it feels like, how long it lasts, when it started, and what makes it better and what makes it worse. Recording and reporting the effects of your pain and how it impacts your ability to function every day will also help. Frequently, your health care team will ask you to describe the severity of your pain on a 0 to 10 scale, with 0 being no pain and 10 being the worst pain imaginable. Presenting your doctor with specific numbers describing the intensity of your pain is a very helpful way to communicate. Your doctor will use this information to determine the best treatment options for you.

Too often, people with cancer accept pain as inevitable and do not report it to their medical team. Left untreated, cancer pain can interfere with sleep, mood, and physical and social activities.

Even though treatments exist that can significantly reduce cancer pain and improve the quality of life of people with cancer and their families, barriers persist that can prevent these treatments from being administered:

- Patients' and health professionals' lack of knowledge about the appropriate use of pain treatment is a major obstacle.
- Myths and misconceptions about pain, addiction, and tolerance may make people with cancer or other serious diseases reluctant to ask for or use pain medication and may make health professionals reluctant to prescribe pain medications.
- Health care professionals often lack knowledge about how to assess pain (that is, understand if the patient is having pain, and if so, how much pain, what type of pain, and its location or cause) and adequately treat pain.
- Health insurance companies may not adequately reimburse for pain medications, and this can restrict patients' access to needed pain control.
- People with cancer, because of societal and cultural barriers, often do not feel comfortable raising concerns about their cancer pain.

Be aware of these obstacles, and don't let them interfere with adequate pain control. Be persistent. *Everyone has a right to pain relief.*

"If you aren't getting the pain relief you think you should…be aggressive with the doctors, because there are so many different kinds of pain relief out there. Chances are there is something out there that will help your pain. I had a lot of pain. All the pills in the beginning were not working for me. Some of them were making me sicker—I was allergic to some, I was vomiting with others; but we kept trying, and then the patch, it was like a long road had finally ended. And I've been pleased as punch with it ever since, and I've been wearing it for many, many months….I thought it would make me groggy or loopy or something, but it hasn't. I can drive, I can work, I can do what I need to do in the home."

— Patty

TYPES OF PAIN

Acute pain is usually severe, begins suddenly, and lasts a relatively short time. It is often a signal that body tissue is being injured in some way, and acute pain generally disappears when the injury heals. *Chronic* pain, which can range from mild to severe, may last for a few weeks or may be ongoing. It can result from cancer itself or from cancer treatment. The most common type of pain in people with cancer is pain caused by cancer spreading to the bone. Another type of chronic pain is caused by a tumor pressing on organs or nerves. Having to cope with chronic pain on a daily basis can lead to irritability, disturbed sleep, reduced appetite, difficulty concentrating, and changes in mood, personality, lifestyle, and ability to function. Because chronic pain can make even the simplest tasks and daily activities uncomfortable or impossible, people in chronic pain may have feelings of hopelessness and depression—negative thoughts and emotions that can make pain feel worse.

Many people with chronic cancer pain have two types of pain: *persistent (continuous) pain* and *breakthrough (incident) pain.* Persistent pain is present for long periods of time—in most cases, all day long. Breakthrough pain is a brief and often severe flare of pain that occurs even though a person may be taking pain medicine regularly for persistent pain. Breakthrough pain typically comes on quickly, lasts only a few minutes or as long as an hour, and requires that you use a different pain medication, which is called a *rescue medication.*

"The pain at its worst was excruciating. I could barely go to sleep at night. I would take a lot of Motrin and try to go to sleep, and it would wake me up during the night. And if I did get to sleep, when I woke up in the morning it was horrendous just getting up. I could barely move. And I was making noise, you know, gasping for air, because the pain was just shooting through my shoulder, my breasts, my arm. And then I'd go take some pain medication and sit on the couch and weep for about 20 minutes until something started to kick in. And that was the worst. Once I got the patch, it really alleviated the pain immediately, and I was just so relieved from that. In fact, when they told me that I had cancer, it didn't bother me, because I knew there was a reason for the pain."

— Patty

There are different types of pain that occur in cancer patients as a result of cancer treatments. *Postoperative pain* due to surgery is readily managed by a wide variety of approaches. Pain management associated with a procedure is focused on preventing the pain. For example, local anesthetics are used to numb the area before a biopsy. Chemotherapy can cause a wide variety of aches and pains (such as joint pain, muscle soreness, mouth sores, and nerve pain). Before you participate in these treatments, you should discuss with your doctor the possibility of pain and how it will be managed. This is also a good opportunity to describe for your doctor what has worked or not worked for you.

TYPES OF MEDICINES USED TO CONTROL CANCER PAIN

Cancer pain can be treated in a variety of ways. One of the most effective methods of pain control is the use of medicines, or drug therapy. Pain medications are given to treat pain and to prevent new pain from occurring, and they should be adjusted as your cancer progresses. There is not one right dose for these medications, nor is there a maximum dose. The correct dose is the dose that relieves your pain. In treating your pain, your physician will likely use what is called a stepped approach (also called an analgesic ladder). This approach helps to determine what group of drugs may be helpful to you based on the intensity of your pain. For mild pain a group of nonopioid drugs (discussed later in the chapter) such as acetaminophen or aspirin and the nonsteroidal anti-inflammatory drugs are most useful. For mild to moderate pain a series of opioid drugs (discussed later in the chapter) such as codeine, oxycodone, tramadol, hydrocodone are recommended. For severe pain, a range of opioids such as morphine, hydromorphone, oxycodone, methadone, and fentanyl may be used. Your physician may use this stepped approach in tailoring the appropriate drug to your pain intensity, and she will help choose the appropriate drug based on the intensity of your pain and your experience with previous exposure to these medications. Sometimes the stepped approach is not appropriate, and your physician may decide that a drug like morphine or fentanyl is best for you.

Mild pain relievers, many of which do not require a prescription and are available "over the counter," are often used to relieve minor cancer-related pain. If pain gets worse, your doctor will most likely direct you toward specific prescription medications. Often, medications are combined to enhance pain relief or to relieve medication-related side effects. The types of pain-relief medications available are described here.

Nonsteroidal Anti-Inflammatory Drugs (NSAIDs)

Nonsteroidal anti-inflammatory drugs (NSAIDs) are the mainstay of drug therapy for those with mild pain, but they are also likely to be used for people with moderate or severe pain. NSAIDs also reduce pain and inflammation. There are about twenty different kinds of NSAIDs, including aspirin and ibuprofen. Some NSAIDs that are available over the counter require a doctor's prescription at higher dose levels.

Cyclooxygenase-2 (COX-2) inhibitors are a newer type of NSAID that can help relieve cancer pain. COX-2 inhibitors such as celecoxib (Celebrex), rofecoxib (Vioxx), and valdecoxib (Bextra) are available by prescription only and may be associated with fewer gastrointestinal side effects and bleeding problems than other NSAIDs. But beware: they are considerably more expensive, and you have to consider if they are worth the cost. Check the prescription medicine benefit of your insurance policy to figure out how much you'll need to pay for these medications. If you can tolerate the less expensive drugs, you might prefer to stick with them.

Nonsteroidal anti-inflammatory drugs are often not recommended for cancer patients receiving chemotherapy because they affect platelet function. The COX-2 inhibitors do not affect platelet function and also have less effect on your kidneys and stomach, but they have not yet been approved for cancer pain.

If you have moderate pain, opioid medication is an appropriate choice. Your doctor might first give you a trial of codeine or oxycodone (Percodan, Percocet, Endodan, Roxiprin, Oxycontin) or tramadol. Some doctors might just begin with low doses of morphine or fentanyl. (Some people still hold the misconception that morphine is a drug of last resort. Not so. In some situations, it is simply the best drug available for pain relief and one of the easiest for doctors to use.) By taking the medication on an around-the-clock basis, you will be able to prevent your pain from building up. Your doctor will then balance your dose to maximize effective pain relief and keep your side effects to a minimum.

Managing NSAID Side Effects

Stomach upset and indigestion are the most common side effects of NSAIDs. Taking your medicines immediately following a meal with food or milk may reduce or prevent these side effects. NSAIDs can also cause nausea and bleeding from the stomach. If your stools are darker than normal or if you notice blood in your stool (both signs of bleeding in the gastrointestinal tract), tell your doctor or nurse. Be careful not to mix NSAIDs with alcohol—taking NSAIDs and drinking alcohol make it more likely that you will develop stomach upset or bleeding from the lining of the stomach. Elderly people, those with bleeding disorders, or people who are receiving chemotherapy may be advised not to take NSAIDs.

Other potential side effects of NSAIDs are dizziness, headache, ringing in the ears, fluid retention, dry mouth, and increased heart rate. NSAIDs may also produce stomach ulcers. Each NSAID has a maximum dose that can be taken at one time. Higher doses produce no additional pain relief but increase the risk of side effects. Take no more than the prescribed or recommended dose.

Acetaminophen

Acetaminophen is a well-known nonopioid pain reliever that, like an NSAID, is effective against mild or moderate pain, but it does not reduce inflammation. The drug may be given alone or in a pill combined with a mild opioid (Tylenol #3 is one example). Discuss the appropriate dosage of acetaminophen with your doctor.

Managing Acetaminophen Side Effects

Side effects associated with acetaminophen are rare. However, taking large doses daily for a long period of time or regularly drinking alcohol with the usual dose may cause severe liver damage.

Figure 8-1.

Using Pain Medications

- Take the medication on a regular basis to reduce the pain.
- Use your rescue medication for breakthrough pain.
- Keep a record of your medications.
- Tell your doctor about your side effects.
- Use a laxative to prevent constipation.

Opioids

Opioids used to control pain were once made from the opium poppy or poppy juice, but today most opioid medications are synthetic and are manufactured by drug companies. Opioids are exceedingly effective in relieving cancer pain.

If pain becomes severe and does not respond to mild opioids, stronger opioids may be needed. Morphine is frequently the first choice among strong opioids for treating severe cancer-related pain. A number of brand-name drugs contain morphine or morphine-like chemicals (MS Contin, Oramorph). Other frequently used strong opioids include hydromorphone (Dilaudid), levorphanol (Levo-Dromoran), methadone (Dolophine, Methadose), and oxycodone (OxyContin). Your doctor may prescribe NSAIDs as an adjuvant medication (a treatment used in addition to the primary therapy) along with a strong opioid.

When you are first prescribed opioids, low doses are used. The dose is increased slowly (titrated) until pain is relieved. Doctors carefully adjust the doses of opioids to control the pain and reduce the side effects. Tell any doctors you deal with if you drink alcohol or take tranquilizers, sleeping aids, antidepressants, antihistamines, or any other medicines that make you sleepy. Combining opioids with these substances can cause you to become very sleepy.

There are many ways to administer opioids. They can be given by mouth, which is the easiest way to give them. If you are having difficulty swallowing, fentanyl can be given by applying a clear bandage-like patch to the skin. The drug is slowly and continuously absorbed through the skin over a 3-day period. Fentanyl can also be administered through your mouth in a "lollipop" that you suck. It goes to work immediately but doesn't last long. The "lollipop" is especially useful to treat breakthrough pain.

Figure 8-2.

Myths About Pain Medication

Unfortunately, there are many misconceptions about pain medications. Here are some of the most common myths about pain, and the facts about these mistaken beliefs.

Myth 1: Opioids cause addiction. This is an extremely rare occurrence when people take opioids for pain. Something you may find reassuring is that opioids can be decreased if the pain is adequately treated with another approach, such as radiation therapy.

Myth 2: A doctor's recommendation for morphine or a morphine-like drug means that your survival time is very, very short. This is not true. Excellent control of pain will allow you to participate in more activities of life and, in fact, may improve survival.

Myth 3: If you take morphine or opioids now, they will not work later. False—these medications have a very wide effective dose range. That is, many different doses of the drug work, and it is individualized for each person with cancer. In general, once pain is effectively controlled, the dose of the opioid does not need to be increased unless the disease progresses. An increase in the dose will then control the increased pain.

Myth 4: Opioids will make the person "high." A person's mood may improve because of pain relief, but persons with advanced cancer or near the end of life do not get high from these medications.

Myth 5: Pain-control medications cause nausea. Only about 3 in 10 people will have nausea when opioids are first started. This is almost never an allergy, as some people presume, and can be treated with antinausea drugs for a few days or weeks when the opioids are initially started. Often, the nausea will go away on its own, and the antinausea drugs can be discontinued. Sometimes switching to a different morphine-like drug will make the nausea go away. Nausea rarely occurs if you have been taking opioids for more than a few weeks.

Myth 6: Opioids cannot be used in infants and children or very frail, elderly people. False—in these 2 groups, smaller doses are usually started, but, again, the dose can slowly be increased until pain is well controlled.

If you have very severe pain or severe pain that comes and goes, you may do better with drugs that are given through a needle either under the skin (subcutaneously) or into a vein (intravenously). Whether in a vein or under the skin, you may have a pump that gives a drug continuously with a button you can push to get an extra dose of pain medication if your pain is not adequately controlled or if your pain occurs only with particular movements. This method is referred to as *patient-controlled analgesia*, or PCA. It may be used by persons at home and is very common in many cancer care facilities. For a small number of persons, about 1 in 10, pain medications may need to be delivered into the spinal fluid through a pump. This is generally recommended only if other aggressive approaches with oral and intravenous treatments have not been adequate to control the pain.

Managing Opioid Side Effects

The most common side effects from opioids are predictable and can usually be managed by either altering the dose or prescribing other medications to control the side effects. Typical side effects include sedation (drowsiness), constipation, dry mouth, nausea, and vomiting. Some people may also experience dizziness, mental effects (nightmares, confusion, or hallucinations), decreased rate and depth of breathing, difficulty in urinating, or itching. In general, the higher the dose of the drug, the more likely side effects are to occur. Treatment is available for all of these side effects. Sometimes these side effects will be decreased by changing to a different drug. However, constipation is a likely side effect no matter which opioid is prescribed.

Constipation is the most common side effect of opioids. When these pain medications are first started, doctors should prescribe a medicine to soften your stool and stimulate your bowels. The higher the dose of opioids, the more severe the constipation will be. It's important to remember that as the dose of your pain medication is increased, your dose of laxatives needs to be increased as well. We'll talk more about strategies for managing constipation later in this chapter.

When sleepiness occurs, it is usually temporary and begins shortly after the opioid has been started. Usually by 2 to 5 days, you will feel less tired. Sometimes the sleepiness results from pain relief, allowing you to finally get long-needed rest after being kept awake by unrelieved pain for many nights. If you continue to be sleepy, even after 5 days of treatment, switching to a different opioid may take care of this problem. Sometimes, however, sleepiness is a sign of progression of the cancer rather than a side effect of medication.

Confusion may occur from many causes and, especially in the elderly, may be caused or made worse by opioid drugs. If this happens, you can be switched to a different drug or take medications that are effective for treating the confusion that occurs with pain medications.

OTHER TREATMENTS FOR PAIN

Other medications are also used to treat pain. Antiseizure drugs, antidepressants, and steroids are often used to treat pain related to nerve damage. Frequently, a combination of drugs is needed to adequately control pain. In addition to medications, radiation therapy is an effective means for treating bone-related pain and may be used in combination with these drugs.

Pain is not just a physical symptom. How you think about pain affects its impact on you. If you have cancer and experience a new pain, it raises fear that the cancer has progressed or that you may lose function. These concerns make the experience of pain worse. Other symptoms, such as depression, sleeplessness, anxiety, and stress, may also make pain worse. It is important to treat the physical pain as well as address the other distressing factors that contribute to the pain experience.

Medication is not the only solution to pain or its negative effects. Nondrug therapies may also help manage pain, including applying heat or cold, massage, nerve blocks and nervous system surgery, and acupuncture. People can learn skills such as relaxation, imagery, meditation, distraction, biofeedback, hypnosis, and other techniques to increase their ability to cope with pain and remain as active as possible. These complementary nondrug methods can also help people cope with the emotional and psychological impact of pain on their quality of life and well-being, both of which can be significantly affected by pain.

> "You have to decide what you want out of your life and whether you're going to let the pain control your life or not. You wake up, maybe you can't even get to sleep, or you would get to sleep and you wake up because of the pain. Find something—whether it's medical, whether it's mental, whether it's music, whether it's a book, whether it's a ride in the country, whatever—and take your focus off that pain."
>
> — Jeff

What is most important to remember is that, though common, cancer pain can be well controlled for the great majority of persons. You have a right to good pain management, and you should not hesitate to speak up if you experience pain. *Your pain can, and should be, controlled.*

Fatigue

Fatigue is the feeling of being tired physically, mentally, and emotionally. Cancer-related fatigue is defined as an unusual and persistent sense of tiredness that can occur with cancer or cancer treatment. It can persist over time and can interfere with usual activities. Cancer-related fatigue is more severe than the fatigue of everyday life, which is usually temporary and relieved by rest. Fatigue is one of the most common symptoms for people with cancer, and many say it is the most distressing symptom of their cancer and its treatment. In persons with advanced cancer, fatigue is nearly universal.

Treatment and cancer itself can cause fatigue. The timing of the fatigue may help you sort out whether it is from the cancer or from your treatment. Radiation therapy causes cumulative fatigue, that is, it gets worse and worse as you go through the radiation therapy and is the most severe just when the radiation therapy is completed. Then it slowly but steadily improves over weeks to months. Chemotherapy-related fatigue often is the worst a few days after treatment and then slowly improves up until the time of the next treatment. Biologic therapies, like interferon and interleukin-2, may cause severe fatigue throughout the entire course of treatment.

> "I'd tell people it was almost like jet lag, because I felt totally exhausted and disoriented at times. I had a lot of people say, well, what was it like, what was it like; how can you describe it? And even now they ask me how can I describe it. And all I can say is, you know, this kind of total exhaustion."
>
> — Darcy

There are some causes of fatigue that can be easily treated. For example, anemia (a drop in red blood cell count) causes fatigue. This can be easily reversed with therapies that stimulate the production of red blood cells (erythropoietin, darbopoietin, epoetin alfa) or with blood transfusions. Hypothyroidism (decreased production of the thyroid hormone) is a less common, but reversible, cause of fatigue in persons with cancer. Some medications will produce fatigue. Difficulty with sleep, infections, or rapid weight loss will all contribute to the sense of tiredness.

"Initially, doing anything like even taking a bath was my one activity for the day. That's how exhausting the activity was. Now I have to plan my day by knowing that I have maybe 2 good hours to get things done, and then I have to go back to bed. So, it very much interferes with my ability to work, play, do anything I really want to do."

— Kathleen

MANAGING FATIGUE

What are the strategies that you can use to improve your energy? Paradoxically, getting a lot of rest actually makes fatigue worse. An exercise program, started at whatever level is appropriate for your energy level and strength, will improve both your overall quality of life and your general energy. A simple, practical prescription for exercise might include walking 20 minutes a day, 10 minutes to a place and 10 minutes back. There are additional benefits of exercise besides its effect on fatigue. These include the possibility of improved appetite, strength, self-image, and bowel habits.

If your fatigue is severe, it is worthwhile to use energy-conservation techniques. Plan your day carefully and do the activities that are most important to you and most fulfilling early in the day, when your energy is likely to be the best. Nonessential activities can be postponed. Consultation with an occupational therapist or physical therapist also may help with developing the best strategies for you as an individual for maintaining energy.

You can also ask your doctor about medications that have been tested specifically for their effect on cancer-related fatigue.

Difficulty Breathing

Difficulty breathing, also called *dyspnea* by health care professionals, is the feeling of not getting enough air, shortness of breath, or breathlessness. It is a feeling that can be more frightening than pain. This symptom is particularly common in persons with lung cancer or those who have cancer that has spread to the lung from any other primary site. Of course, difficulty breathing may be caused by noncancer-related diseases, including underlying lung disease or heart failure.

Just like pain, the feeling of not getting enough air can only be identified by you. How fast you breathe or the amount of oxygen measured in your blood does not predict how you feel.

COPING WITH DIFFICULTY BREATHING

The first step in treating this condition is often providing oxygen through a mask or little tube that goes just inside the nose. There are also a number of medications that are useful to take away the sense of air hunger. The most effective drugs for treatment of shortness of breath are opioids. Without changing how fast you breathe or how much oxygen you are getting in your bloodstream, these drugs take away the sense of not getting enough air. This is usually achieved with very low doses of morphine (2.5 to 5 mg), particularly if you have not previously been given morphine.

It is not well understood how opioids take away the sense of air hunger, but it is thought that they may alter the perception of breathing, just like opioids alter the perception of pain. These medications are safe for the relief of air hunger and will not cause you to suddenly stop breathing. A feeling of being unable to breathe is frightening and may cause significant anxiety, which may, in itself, make difficulty breathing worse. Since opioids do not treat anxiety, an anti-anxiety drug is frequently added to the morphine-like drug to control the sense of air hunger.

Oxygen does not necessarily improve the sense of air hunger. You may have a relatively normal level of oxygen in your blood but still feel significantly short of breath, perhaps because of the increased work of breathing. For example, your lungs may be stiff from cancer, not allowing you to take a deep breath. The oxygen masks used in the hospital may make you feel claustrophobic, closed in. If you do not feel that the oxygen improves your sense of air hunger, then you do not have to wear it. Cool air blowing on your face from a fan or open window may also reduce air hunger. Relaxation techniques; slow, measured breathing; and activity pacing may all help control your problems breathing.

Occasionally, severe shortness of breath is not well controlled with these approaches. In this case, you may consider taking medications to make you so sleepy that you are unaware of your discomfort. Your doctor may also suggest the aid of a ventilator. This is something you can discuss with both your family and health care team before proceeding, as it will limit your interaction with your family and friends and also has other implications.

Depression

Depression is not just sadness or feeling blue. It is a combination of symptoms that often includes a change in weight and appetite, in sleep and energy, in thinking and ability to concentrate, in your desire to participate in social activities, in your overall mood, and in your interest in both people and your surroundings. These symptoms are often accompanied by feelings of guilt, worthlessness, or helplessness that can escalate into thoughts of taking your life. *If you are experiencing pervasive feeling of guilt, worthlessness, or helplessness, or if you are thinking about taking your life, seek help immediately.* There are a bevy of approaches for dealing with depression, including medications and the help of mental health professionals.

Some degree of depression is common in people who are coping with cancer, and some cancers are more frequently associated with depression, like those that arise in the pancreas and lung. About 25 percent of all people with cancer experience clinical depression, causing distress, impaired functioning, and decreased ability to follow a treatment schedule. Not surprisingly, depression is seen more often in people with advanced stages of cancer, and in those who have more disability from their cancer and/or poor pain control.

It is not uncommon for people with advanced cancer to experience hopelessness or a sense of helplessness when they first learn that their cancer has recurred or that the treatment has failed, whether or not there are alternative treatments available for the cancer. A period of shock, disbelief, or denial is very common, often followed by a period of depression. With time, most people with cancer and their families are able to come to terms with what at first seems impossible to accept. For many, understanding what to expect and gaining more knowledge about the cancer and its progression make it easier to move forward. If the initial sense of hopelessness or helplessness persists and is accompanied by feelings of despair, guilt, and worthlessness, the possibility of significant depression should be considered. It is important that you speak with your doctor, health care team, or your family and friends about these feelings. Depression can make all of your symptoms worse.

Another reason it is important to talk to your health care team about depression is that some of the drugs used to treat cancer may make your depression worse. For example, steroids (dexamethasone, prednisone, etc.) may make depression more severe, and some biologic therapies, like interleukin-2 and interferon, can cause depression.

Both counseling and medications can make a very big difference in how you feel and improve other symptoms at the same time. There are many medications available to treat depression, some of which begin to have an effect within 2 to 4 weeks. In addition to counseling and medications, here are some other strategies to consider:

- Talk about feelings and fears that you may be having—do not keep them inside.
- Remember that it is okay to feel sad and frustrated.
- Try deep breathing and relaxation exercises several times a day.
- Don't blame yourself for feelings of fear, anxiety, or depression.
- Engage in enjoyable activities.

Depression in the setting of advanced cancer is best treated by a combination of medication, supportive therapies (such as relaxation and distraction), and counseling. Your prognosis, and therefore the time available for treatment of your depression, is an important consideration when choosing the best treatment. If you have months of survival ahead of you, you have time to wait the 2 to 4 weeks sometimes needed to see the benefit from the majority of antidepressants. If the time is very short, stimulants (which act more quickly) may be of greater benefit to you.

Many people assume that depression is inevitable if you are dying from cancer. This is not true. Treatment for depression has proven benefit for persons with cancer.

Anxiety

Anxiety is an overwhelming feeling of uneasiness, apprehension, and fear. Anxiety is very common in people with cancer and may show itself in different ways. Some people get a rapid heartbeat, palpitations, or pain in their chest. Some breathe very quickly, hyperventilate, or feel suffocated or unable to breath. Still others show their anxiety by getting sweats and chills or dizziness and lightheadedness. Some people note trembling or nausea. Many of these symptoms, particularly in combination and particularly if they cannot be explained on the basis of medical illness (i.e., a heart attack or an infection), may be caused by anxiety.

Anxiety is a very normal reaction to advanced cancer and concerns about dying. Feeling nervous, anxious, or on edge may be a reaction to the progression of your cancer, or it may be related to other things happening in your life. Anxiety is exceedingly common at the time of cancer recurrence or when anticancer therapy is no longer thought to be effective.

Anxiety also may occur because of medications you are taking. For example, some antinausea medications, like metoclopramide (Reglan), can make people feel like they are "jumping out of their skin." This is usually promptly improved with diphenhydramine (Benadryl). You may be taking medications for medical problems not related to your cancer that make your anxiety worse. Caffeine, for example, is a very common cause of feeling irritable or tremulous.

MANAGING ANXIETY

For many, anxiety is relieved by talking through their concerns. It is important to have your health care team correct any misconceptions you have about what is going to happen as your cancer gets worse, or about what to expect between the time of advanced cancer and death. The more realistic your expectations, often the easier it is to cope.

To manage your anxiety, first try to address any other symptoms that may make anxiety worse. For example, inability to sleep or poorly treated pain may worsen anxiety. Sometimes simple relaxation techniques, like focused breathing, guided imagery, or relaxation, can have a favorable effect on your overall sense of anxiety. Think about where you have found strength at other difficult times in your life. Sometimes clergy and support from your religious congregation can serve as an important means to decrease your anxiety. Social support groups are also very effective for many people.

If these methods do not work, a wide variety of medications are effective for treating anxiety. They can be given by mouth or intravenously (through your vein), or under the skin, depending on what is easiest for you and what kind of problems you have otherwise.

The most common side effect of the medicines used to treat anxiety is sleepiness. It is important to talk through with your health care team—and think through—what side effects are acceptable to you. Most anti-anxiety drugs should not be suddenly stopped. If you do suddenly stop them, it may make you feel more irritable. Frequently, antidepressants are used to treat anxiety and are very effective in improving how you feel overall emotionally.

Difficulty Sleeping

Difficulty sleeping, or *insomnia*, causes tiredness, loss of ability to concentrate, and irritability. Insomnia is a common problem in the general population but has even greater frequency in persons with cancer. Sleeplessness may make other cancer-related symptoms worse, including pain, fatigue, depression, and anxiety. Sleeplessness may disturb you as well as your family and, as a result, lessen your overall quality of life.

There are many reasons you may have difficulty sleeping. Some of the symptoms associated with cancer and its treatment interfere with sleep. For example, poor pain control will make it difficult to sleep because if you roll over the pain will awaken you. Similarly, shortness of breath, coughing, and nausea can all make it difficult to sleep.

Emotional concerns also can cause insomnia. A sign of major depression is early-morning awakening, that is, waking up early in the morning and not being able to fall back to sleep. (The opposite can be seen as well, that is, wanting to sleep too much because of depression.) Anxiety may also make it difficult to fall asleep or stay asleep. Anxiety and depression can, and should, be treated. Without adequate sleep, your other symptoms may be more difficult to tolerate.

> "I suspect that a lot of patients have sleep disturbance, and they either assume it's just part and parcel of being a cancer patient or they think that nothing can be done about it, so it's not addressed. It's not brought up as a problem."
>
> — Wendy

MANAGING INSOMNIA

If you are having trouble sleeping, stay away from stimulants like alcohol, coffee, or tobacco, particularly late in the day, as they interfere with sleep.

Unfamiliar or noisy places are difficult for everyone to sleep in, and the hospital is a particularly good example of a place where it's difficult to sleep. Talk to your doctor about what kind of problems with sleep you are having, the pattern of your sleep—that is, do you sleep too long, get up too early—or things that interrupt your sleep, to help figure out the best thing to do.

There are some symptoms that will help your doctor determine whether you have some of the sleep problems that are seen in the general population. A crawling feeling in your legs, jerking movements while you are sleeping that seem out of your control, or excessive snoring all suggest sleep problems

> "From the time of my diagnosis to the subsequent weeks and months of my intensive chemotherapy, I had a sleep disturbance. I had trouble sleeping through the night. There were times I had nightmares. Some of it was related to the stress of the new diagnosis, but as we all adjusted to the diagnosis and the routine of treatment, I continued to have sleep disturbance that clearly was related to some of my medications. And it took awhile for us to recognize that I had a sleep disturbance or to connect it with some of the medications, let alone to begin to do something about it. And the reason I bring it up is, sleep is such an important function. And I think that either inadequate sleep or poor quality sleep can make the whole cancer experience that much worse."
>
> — Wendy

that are treatable. If you are having difficulty sleeping, ask yourself whether or not you have a regular time that you go to bed and wake up, whether you are taking too many naps during the day and then are not tired enough to sleep at night, and whether you actually feel rested after you sleep. If some of these simpler tactics don't work, talk to your health care team about other options. For example, a variety of medications can help with this problem. Before starting on sleeping pills of any kind, other causes of inadequate sleep need to be ruled out and/or treated.

Things that will help your sleep in general are trying to wake up at the same time every day and limiting the amount of coffee and other caffeine and/or nicotine products that you use, particularly in the evening. Avoid alcohol use at night or heavy meals late at night, which may make you feel too full to sleep. To avoid getting up multiple times during the night to urinate, don't take in too many liquids just before bedtime. A moderate amount of exercise as tolerated will help you sleep, as long as it is not done directly before you go to bed. Be sure that you control the noise, light, and temperature in your bedroom to make it as comfortable as possible.

Setting up a bedtime ritual helps many people. For example, you can try a warm bath at bedtime to help you relax or a bedtime snack of warm milk and graham crackers. Alternatively, relaxation techniques learned from tapes or from trained health care professionals may help you. It is important to let your health care team know if you are having difficulty sleeping. They can help you figure out what the cause is and what to do about it.

Confusion and Delirium

Sometimes the thoughts of a person with cancer are disturbed and the person may have trouble thinking and acting normally. There are many reasons why someone with advanced cancer might have difficulty thinking clearly or get confused. Both cancer and its treatment can cause confusion. For example, sometimes chemotherapy causes difficulty with memory and concentration that can be long lasting. Cancer that spreads to the brain through the bloodstream can cause confusion or symptoms similar to a stroke, such as changes in the way you talk. Medications—or medication withdrawal—may cause confusion or hallucinations (seeing things that are not really there). It is important to tell your physician about any of these symptoms, so that your medications can be adjusted or these problems can be treated.

There are other reasons why persons with cancer may become confused. One important reason is an increase in the blood calcium. This happens particularly in people who have cancer that has spread to their bones and/or those who are spending a lot of time in bed, which leads to calcium leaking out of the bones and into the bloodstream. High calcium, just like a very high blood sugar, can lead to confusion. Other causes of confusion are kidney failure or liver failure, which may occur as you approach the end of your life.

It is not uncommon for a person with advancing disease to have little emotion or to become restless, anxious, depressed, irritable, or angry. These are usually symptoms of *delirium*, which is an advanced state of confusion. Delirium is similar to confusion, but is more complicated. Delirium is also very common towards the end of life.

A few of the most common symptoms of delirium are problems with memory, impaired judgment, and changing levels of wakefulness. Delirium often begins with problems sleeping, feeling on edge, and a sense of restlessness and then goes on to cause problems with thinking and attention, as well as a reversal of day and night. Sometimes delirium will cause problems with memory—making it difficult to know where you are, even who you are—and cause extremes of emotion (sadness, anger, even extreme happiness). Day/night reversal may be one of the first signs of delirium and is very difficult for families to cope with, not only because of the distress of the symptoms themselves, but because of the loss of sleep that occurs for everyone involved. These symptoms should be reported to the doctor.

"My short-term and long-term memory were significantly impaired. I had word block. I would lose my train of thought, similar sorts of intellectual dysfunction. It was emotionally very difficult because I valued my intellect. I was a physician who was used to remembering things and being in control, and cancer represented such a tremendous loss of control that here I'm an adult and I can't remember the shopping list! I can't remember to relay a telephone message! And so it was one more very significant assault on my sense of self."

— Wendy

Particularly for persons with advanced cancer, there are often multiple factors that lead to delirium. Medications can cause delirium, so if new medicines have recently been started or adjusted, it is important to consider this cause. Sometimes, particularly at the end of life, an exact cause for the delirium cannot be found. Common things that contribute to delirium in persons with advanced cancer include certain medications, particularly opioids or steroids; inadequate intake of fluids; inadequate oxygen in the bloodstream; spread of cancer to the brain; and multiple organs failing to work.

COPING WITH CONFUSION AND DELIRIUM

The ideal goal of treatment is to reverse the confusion or delirium and keep the person clear, calm, and alert. Medications given on a regular schedule can often treat these conditions effectively. There are some simple things you can do that also make a difference. For a hospitalized person, placing familiar items—a photograph or other personal things—in the room may calm the person. A well-lit room with a visible clock and/or calendar to keep the person aware of the place, date, and time may also be helpful.

When delirium occurs in the setting of very advanced cancer, it is often a hallmark of approaching death. There are medications that are effective for calming the person and taking away hallucinations, which may be frightening. If the person with cancer is very close to death and the delirium is disturbing to that person and his or her loved ones, one consideration is to make the person very sleepy. This will calm the person with cancer but may also prevent further communication between the person with cancer and family and friends. The goal of making the person with cancer sleepy is to provide comfort.

Loss of Appetite and Weight Loss

Eating a wide variety of healthy foods before, during, and after cancer treatment can help people with cancer feel better and regain their strength. However, weight loss is an exceedingly common problem in people with advanced cancer, occurring more than 80 percent of the time. Some types of cancer, particularly gastrointestinal cancers, are nearly always associated with weight loss. Others, like breast cancer, are rarely associated with severe weight loss.

The weight loss seen with cancer has many causes and generally is not simply a result of decreased appetite. The tumor itself may produce proteins, which change the way your body uses calories and cause the loss of muscle and strength. Weight loss decreases quality of life. It results in fatigue and weakness. It may cause shortness of breath and musculoskeletal pain as well as nausea. It is frequently associated with a sense of being full too fast, generalized weakness, and a change in body image. This may make you less willing to get out and about because of how thin and/or ill you look. It is typically associated with increasing problems doing your usual activities, even simple things like dusting, fixing a meal, or bathing independently.

There are many other treatment- and cancer-related symptoms that may contribute to the inability to eat. Change in taste from chemotherapy or radiation therapy, depression, difficulty swallowing, mouth sores from chemotherapy or radiation, a chronic dry mouth from radiation therapy, nausea and vomiting, and severe constipation are among a few of the symptoms that may decrease your interest in food.

It can be extremely difficult for loved ones and caregivers to see someone they love unable to eat. It is natural for them to want to provide food, to do something to help to show their care and concern. Yet, if the person with cancer has no appetite and truly *cannot* eat, it is not helpful to force food. It is easy for mealtime to become a battlefield, with you unable to eat and your family pushing you hard to eat, both in their need to *do* something for you but also, often, in the false belief that you will die from not eating.

Particularly as you get very close to the end of life, there is loss of appetite that makes food less and less appealing. There are other ways in which your family members can provide care—company, massage, reading—rather than providing food.

COPING WITH LOSS OF APPETITE AND WEIGHT LOSS

For the person with advanced cancer who would like to participate in mealtimes and would like to improve appetite, the first step is to treat other symptoms that may interfere with eating, like nausea and vomiting. Once these easily identified symptoms have been treated, then what? Many people turn to a dietitian for nutritional counseling. A dietitian can help educate you about what may be helpful to fight weight loss and poor appetite. Frequent recommendations include the following: eat as much as you want, give up old dietary limitations such as concerns about high-fat food or rich foods, start the day with breakfast, eat frequent small meals throughout the day if you find that you get full too quickly, and try to eat foods that are high in calories and protein. For example, nuts are a good source of protein and might be left in bowls around the house. If the smell of foods causes nausea, eat room-temperature or cold foods, as they have fewer aromas. Eat with other family members and friends to make eating a social activity. Drink fluids between meals, particularly high-calorie fluids, rather than with meals, so that they do not fill you up. Try to exercise before eating. If it is okay with your doctor, try a glass of wine or sherry before eating; it may stimulate your appetite. Eat what appeals to you, and eat as much of it as you want. If these strategies do not work to maintain or increase your appetite, a number of medications can help increase appetite. Ask your doctor for more information.

Dehydration

Hydration (keeping enough fluid in your body) is important for health. The loss of adequate fluid—or *dehydration*—can lead to symptoms such as dizziness, chest pain, lightheadedness, constipation, dry mouth, vomiting, drowsiness, and even confusion. Dehydration can occur as a result of cancer treatment, advanced cancer, and from noncancer-related causes. Very high blood sugar or very high calcium lead to excessive loss of fluid through the urine and then dehydration. With regard to cancer treatment, severe nausea and vomiting from chemotherapy or from radiation therapy to the upper abdomen can lead to dehydration. In these cases, dehydration is readily reversible with antinausea drugs and the provision of fluids, often intravenously if you are unable to swallow and/or keep the fluid down.

Artificial Hydration and Nutrition

The decision to begin or to withdraw the use of artificial hydration or nutrition is a complex one—one that you should thoroughly discuss with your loved ones and your medical team. The decision may have medical, ethical, legal, practical, financial, and even religious implications. We briefly cover some of these related issues in chapter 9. The following discussion covers medical information only.

The benefit of giving extra fluid (*artificial hydration*) if you have advanced cancer is not clear. Many people assume that if you aren't drinking very much and your liquid intake is not being supplemented, you could be uncomfortable, thirsty, and suffering from dry mouth. Research suggests this is not the case. A dry mouth is exceedingly common at the end of life and is caused by many different things, including medications such as pain medicines and some of the antidepressants. In studies that have looked at whether people at the end of life want fluids when given the choice, the majority of people choose not to take additional fluid. There are reasons to think that providing extra fluid at the end of life may actually worsen symptoms. For persons whose kidney function is getting worse or for those who have compromised lung function, fluid may actually increase shortness of breath or swelling of the abdomen or legs. Talk to your doctor and health care team about your feelings regarding artificial hydration at the end of life. Early discussion and planning for what you would like to happen or not happen will allow you to have more control over what happens as your cancer gets worse.

Artificial nutrition—that is, feeding through a tube in the stomach or through an intravenous line—often comes into question at the end of life. For persons who cannot swallow because of cancer blocking the swallowing tube (the esophagus) or because of problems with nerves that control swallowing, artificial feeding is frequently considered. Rather than providing a safe way to feed someone, multiple studies have shown that feeding a person through a tube in the stomach actually results in more problems with infection and no improvement in survival as compared with no artificial feeding. Although it is not uncommon to provide artificial feeding to persons with advanced cancer, not one study demonstrates improvement in survival or symptoms from artificial nutrition in persons with very advanced cancer. Loss of appetite and weight loss are to be expected, and are a natural part of severe illness and the dying process.

Constipation

Constipation refers to a decreased number of bowel movements or difficulty moving your bowels. With constipation, the stools are often abnormally hard and may be associated with discomfort with passage of the stool. Constipation is a very common problem for people with advanced cancer and occurs in 90 percent of persons, if untreated, who are receiving opioid (morphine-like) pain medications.

There are many causes of constipation, including medications (especially narcotics) used to treat cancer-related symptoms and other medical problems, eating a lot less, dehydration (getting dried out), advanced age, spending a lot of time in bed, problems with the bowel itself (such as blockage of the bowel by cancer), or neurologic problems that interfere with the movement of the muscles of the wall of the gut.

Constipation may cause you a number of different problems. It may present itself as pain in your abdomen or a feeling of fullness or bloating. It may take your appetite away or make you feel sick to your stomach or even throw up. Particularly if you are older, bad constipation can cause pressure on your urinary bladder and make it difficult to pass urine.

COPING WITH CONSTIPATION

Most of the time, constipation can be prevented. Changes in your diet can help. Drinking more fluid and adding fiber (bran flakes, etc.) or dried fruits (prunes, apricots, etc.) to your diet can be helpful, if your appetite allows. If you have the energy, increased activity also will help you move your bowels more regularly.

There are many stool softeners and laxatives available. Some drugs for constipation (products like Metamucil and Citrucel) work by making your stool bulkier and, therefore, softer. This is how increased fiber in your diet works to help your bowels move. In general, this group of drugs does not work quickly; they may take 2 to 4 days to yield results. Also, if you are spending a lot of time in bed, these medications don't work as well as they do in someone who is very active. Similarly, stool softeners alone are not very effective if you are having very infrequent bowel movements. They are most useful if the stool is hard and difficult to pass. In general, suppositories (medication placed in the rectum) work faster than pills taken by mouth. If it has been a long time since you moved your bowels or if you are having difficulty swallowing, stimulating suppositories such as bisacodyl (Dulcolax) are probably the best choice. If a suppository does not work, an enema is the next step.

It is important to keep your bowels moving, even if you are not eating. Frequently, people think that if they are not eating, they do not need to move their bowels. Being "regular" means something different for every person. Some people move their bowels every day; others every 2 or 3 days. The goal is to keep the pattern that is normal for you. If you are eating satisfactorily and are up and about, simple changes in your diet and in the amount of water and other fluids you drink may be enough to prevent constipation. If, however, you are spending a lot of time in bed and/or are unable to swallow or not very hungry, you may need daily medications to keep your bowels moving normally.

Nausea and Vomiting

Nausea—queasiness or feeling sick to your stomach—and *vomiting* (throwing up) are treatment-related symptoms that many people worry about when they are getting treatment for their cancer. There are now improved medications to prevent and treat nausea and vomiting, though overall these medications are better at preventing vomiting than controlling chemotherapy-related nausea.

It is not, however, just cancer treatment that causes nausea and vomiting. The cancer itself and other medications that you may receive may also make you sick to your stomach. For example, pain medications and some antidepressants cause nausea. In addition, you may recall having nausea after taking antibiotics in the past.

Nausea and vomiting, if left untreated, may lead to weight loss, lightheadedness, loss of appetite, or dizziness. If you feel sick to your stomach or start throwing up, it is important to let your doctor know.

Symptoms that accompany the nausea and vomiting or the timing of the symptoms may give clues to its cause. For example, nausea and vomiting associated with a severe headache, particularly a morning headache, may suggest spread of the cancer to the brain. Nausea and vomiting associated with generalized pain in your abdomen and no recent bowel movements may mean that your bowels are obstructed (blocked), especially if what you are throwing up what looks like intestinal contents. But severe constipation can cause nausea and vomiting as well. Nausea and vomiting that began shortly after starting a new medication may be drug related.

COPING WITH NAUSEA AND VOMITING

Nausea and vomiting usually can be controlled. There are many available medications that may be able to treat these problems. Often for a person with advanced disease, multiple medications are necessary for effective control of continuing nausea and vomiting. If you can't keep them down, they are usually available as suppositories, so that the medicine is absorbed through the rectum. Work with your health care team until you find an appropriate solution.

Besides asking your doctor for medications to treat and/or prevent nausea and vomiting, there are some general things that you can try. For example, you may want to consider hypnosis, distraction techniques, or relaxation therapies.

If you eat and get full very fast and this leads to feeling sick to your stomach —which is not uncommon in persons with advanced cancer—eat small meals. "Grazing" may be much more comfortable for you than sitting down to a full meal. If you have extra fluid in your abdomen (ascites), or your liver is big, or you have cancer spread throughout your abdomen—you may feel like you fill up quickly when you try to eat. There are some medications such as metoclopramide (Reglan), that are especially good for this problem.

If you feel sick to your stomach from food aromas, you are better off eating cold or room-temperature foods, as they give off fewer aromas. Stay away from greasy or fatty foods, as they are more likely to cause nausea. Stick to a bland diet, such as toast, gelatin, and clear liquids. Eat only what appeals to you, and do not eat more than feels comfortable. Often family members, out of a desire to help, may unintentionally push you to eat. This may, however, increase your nausea, particularly if you are having trouble with filling up too fast. Often, just reducing your portions and how frequently you eat will help.

> "I have to be very choosy in what I eat. Additionally, there's some foul tastes and reaction to various foods, not reactions, that's not the right word, but the taste of some of them will instantly nauseate me. I do take medication, mostly over-the-counter stuff, although there are some prescription drugs for nausea that do help."
>
> — Ron

Difficulty Swallowing

Difficulty swallowing is caused by many different things—the cancer itself, treatment for the cancer, or medical problems that have nothing to do with the cancer. It is an important symptom and may cause you significant distress because it interferes with your ability to eat and with the pleasure of eating. Mealtime is an important social event for most people. Being unable to join in celebrations and traditional holiday feasts, like Thanksgiving, can be difficult for you and your family.

The symptoms of your cancer may have begun with difficulty swallowing. For example, if your cancer originated in your tongue or your swallowing tube (the esophagus), you may have had trouble getting food out of your mouth into your stomach or feeling like it got stuck on the way down. Sometimes swallowing is not possible because the muscles that control swallowing have either been removed with surgery or damaged, and food may be swallowed into the airway instead of into your stomach. This is dangerous and can lead to life-threatening pneumonias.

Radiation therapy to the head and neck area or swallowing tube (esophagus) may cause temporary difficulty swallowing right after the treatment due to soreness of the inside surfaces. Radiation therapy can cause long-term dry mouth, which may make it difficult to swallow. Mixing significant amounts of fluid with your food can be helpful.

COPING WITH SWALLOWING DIFFICULTIES

If you are having difficulty swallowing, it is important to see an expert in swallowing who can give you pointers about how to make it easier. There are, in fact, specific exercises that you can be taught to strengthen the muscles of swallowing and make your swallowing safer. Often, thick liquids are easier to swallow than thin liquids like water. There are unflavored thickeners available that make it easier to drink things like coffee or juice.

A speech or swallowing therapist will have many recommendations, which may help you swallow more easily. For example, different ways of tilting the head or, if you had surgery for head and neck cancer, turning to the stronger side, the one not operated on, can aid swallowing. Tilting the head back allows gravity to assist with moving food toward the throat. Paying attention to the volume of food and alternating solids and liquids often will help people get solid foods down. If you have trouble getting food to the back of your mouth, which can happen if, for example, you had tongue cancer and your tongue has been removed, a long-handled teaspoon can help food get to the back of the mouth or sometimes a straw can be very effective.

A major concern with difficulty swallowing is that the food will be aspirated (go into your airway instead of into your stomach). Keeping the head of the bed straight up or sitting in a chair during eating will help prevent this. Staying upright for some period of time after you eat will also help. It is safer to eat smaller amounts of food and swallow completely before taking the next bite.

Pressure Ulcers/Bed Sores

Bedsores are a common problem for people with chronic or life-threatening diseases, who may spend a large amount of time either sitting or being in bed. These positions increase the chance that your skin will break down and you will develop a bedsore. Bedsores are also called *pressure ulcers* because they occur on the skin that overlies bony prominences (spots where you can easily feel a bone). Pressure sores begin as a small red patch on the skin at the point of pressure. If the pressure continues—that is, if you stay in one place for continued periods of time—the skin breakdown will get worse or ultimately lead to ulceration with or without drainage. The most common locations for the bedsores are the heels, lower spine, and bony areas of the buttocks.

PREVENTING AND TREATING BED SORES

Bedsores are both preventable and treatable and can be healed with good care. But preventing them is easier than healing them. If you or someone you love is unable to get out of bed, it is important to turn and change positions often so that the same bony points are not pressing against the bed all the time. Ideally, someone in bed should be moved at least every 2 hours. Pillows and foam wedges can be used to keep bony points from direct contact with the pressure of the bed. There are foam pads available for your bed that also may decrease the amount of pressure on the skin. If you are confined to a chair, like a wheelchair, it is important to shift your weight as frequently as every 15 minutes while sitting. There are special seat cushions available for wheelchairs that also decrease the chances of getting a sore because they distribute the weight over a larger area. Your health care team may recommend that you use moisturizers on your skin and try to participate in as much activity and movement as you possibly can.

How the skin and the wound look—that is, whether there is bleeding, an odor, or drainage—helps the health care team determine what local care would best lead to healing.

Spinal Cord Compression

The bones of the spine are one of the places most frequently affected by metastatic cancer. The major problem with cancer in these bones is that as it grows, it may press on nerves and cause pain much like sciatica pain from disc disease or may press on the spinal cord itself and cause both pain and nerve damage. Pressure on the spinal cord from cancer is called *spinal cord compression*. The cancers that are most commonly associated with this problem are breast cancer, lung cancer, prostate cancer, and multiple myeloma. While metastatic disease to the spine is unlikely to cause your death, it has the potential to cause very serious problems with your quality of life by causing leg paralysis and loss of control of both your urine and your bowels.

RECOGNIZING AND DIAGNOSING SPINAL CORD COMPRESSION

The sooner the diagnosis of cord compression is made, the more likely you are to keep normal neurologic function. Nine out of 10 persons with spinal cord compression experience back pain. Initially, it may stay right in the middle of your back. As the tumor grows, it will begin to irritate nerves coming out of the spinal cord, and the pain may feel like a band wrapping around from your back to your side. The pain is usually made worse by movement, coughing or sneezing, or straining to move your bowels. The majority of people have pain for a period of time, usually days to weeks, before the diagnosis is made. If you develop pain in your neck or back, tell your health care professionals immediately. After pain, the next most common symptom is weakness and loss of sensation.

You may develop numbness or tingling in your toes if the involved bone is below your neck or in your fingers and toes if the disease is in bones of the neck. One of the reasons it may take a while to make the diagnosis is that back pain can occur without the development of other symptoms (weakness, numbness, etc.) for many months even with the presence of early cord compression. Cord compression occurs most commonly in the thoracic spine (chest and mid-back). Sometimes the pain is continuous even when you are at rest but is made worse with movement. If treatment is not begun, you may develop difficulty controlling your urine or your bowels. Once this occurs, further progression is generally rapid, and the longer it goes untreated, the more likely the changes are to be irreversible.

The diagnosis of cord compression is generally made with an MRI (magnetic resonance imaging) of the spine. This is a radiologic test that provides very detailed pictures of the spinal cord and the nerves as they move between the bones of the back. An MRI examination takes about 60 to 90 minutes and requires you to lie very still in a closed, somewhat noisy space. If you are claustrophobic, you can ask to be given a medication to help you relax. Alternatively, many radiology services will allow a familiar person to stay in the room with you and even allow you to have physical contact with that person (for example, holding on to your feet while you are in the tube) to reassure you that you are not alone. If the MRI makes the diagnosis of cord compression, no other tests are necessary.

TREATING SPINAL CORD COMPRESSION

The goal of treatment is to reverse any neurologic problems, relieve pain, and maintain function and movement. Treatment begins with the initiation of steroids (dexamethasone). Steroids decrease swelling related to the presence of tumor and may take some of the pressure off of the spinal cord or nerves and improve your symptoms. This results in short-term benefit, however, and a more lasting treatment is necessary unless you have only days of life remaining.

Until very recently, radiation therapy was the standard treatment. About half of the people treated with radiation therapy for this problem were able to walk after the treatment was completed. The results of treatment are closely tied to your functional level; that is, whether or not you have weakness or numbness at the time the treatment begins. For persons who are completely bedbound, that is, unable to move their legs when first diagnosed, only about 1 in 10 will walk again. However, the sooner your health care team intervenes, the more likely you are to have a full recovery.

Some doctors feel that the results are better if the radiation is preceded by surgery to remove the tumor and stabilize the spine. There is no evidence that in someone with advanced cancer the addition of chemotherapy or other drug therapies will improve the pain and neurologic problems associated with cord compression. Cord compression is considered an emergency and warrants calling your doctor as soon as possible after the symptoms begin.

Multiple Symptoms

You may experience multiple symptoms or symptom clusters. Late in the natural course of the disease the symptoms increase and appear in groups. When this happens you may need to have a careful assessment by your health care team to develop a strategy to decrease the most bothersome symptoms. The assessment may include a measure of the severity and the frequency of each of the symptoms, and require that you report when each one appears.

Conclusion

Whatever symptoms you have, discuss them with your health care team so they can be clear with you about what you may reasonably expect. Talk about the things that frighten you, especially about being in pain, because the things you imagine may be worse than the truth.

There are many approaches to helping decrease more common symptoms like pain and fatigue and help you manage conditions like loss of appetite. Other symptoms that you develop will depend upon on where your cancer is and what kind of therapy you are receiving. Identifying your symptoms is the first step to receiving treatment and relief.

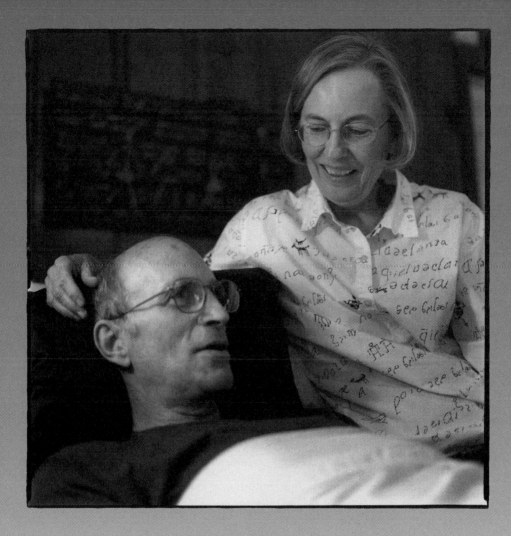

Chapter 9

Making the Most of the Last Stage of Your Life

Chapter 9
focus Questions

— How can I make the most of this last stage of my life?

— How can I prepare myself to leave this life I have built?

— How will I and those I love face my mortality?

— How do I talk about my own death?

— What if my loved ones don't want to talk about this?

— How can I die on my own terms?

— How do I say goodbye to those I care about?

— How do I make peace with myself and others?

— What will my final moments be like?

"When I look back at my life I don't have any regrets. I've lived a good life. I mean, and I continue to live a good life. It's rich and it's full, and there's not one thing I would change. Not even the diagnosis that I have would I change, because in having cancer it opened up all kinds of new adventures and new doors for me and new ways of looking at myself and looking at life and living. It's like with knowing I'm dying, I finally awoke to my life and I began to live life instead of just going through the motions."

– Karen

DEATH MAY BE A NATURAL PART OF LIFE, but that doesn't mean it's not difficult to face. This chapter is written to help you know what to expect. While no amount of information or consolation can completely erase the sorrow and anxiety that contemplating your mortality and approaching death may cause, knowing something about what to expect and how to make the most of your life in its final stage can help ease your discomfort and lessen your fear. Looking back on your life and revisiting your best moments—and even some not-so-good ones—can bring a kind of peace. Looking ahead to what life holds for your loved ones even after you are gone can foster acceptance of death as well.

"I think about how beautiful everything is and how lucky I am to be here. I count my blessings. I don't count what I don't have. I don't count what I've been through. I don't count what could have been. I just don't do that, because it would lead you back to the road that you don't want to be on."

— Lisa T.

"I just try to focus in on the things that make me happy and try to do things that I enjoy doing. There are a lot of just small things that make me happy, maybe that never made me happy before. I'm trying to enjoy my life the best I can."

— Vickie

Life Review

Although someone with a life-limiting illness generally realizes they are going to die, the actual timing of their death is always uncertain. You may be waiting for some momentous "event" to happen. More often than not, no such thing occurs at the moment of death. Momentous events occur much more frequently as you come to terms with dying and are able to put this end-of-life period within the framework of your whole life.

This may happen as you talk to a loved one about what was important in your life, what you are proud of, and what you are ashamed of. Sometimes this takes the form of a *life review*—the process of looking back on one's life and remembering what was most important to you as your life draws to a close. The life review may happen naturally as you go through old photographs with family and friends, or as you prepare your estate, or update your will, remembering when you took out a particular loan or finished paying off your mortgage, realizing that each event signified something that was happening in your life story.

The life review can also take a more formal shape. You can revisit moments in your life of great significance by yourself, in a journal, or you can set time aside for purposeful reflection. You can also do this with another person who can help you by asking you questions and perhaps writing down, tape recording, or even videotaping what you say. Many people find that the process of doing a life review helps them make peace with themselves and helps them decide what to say to the people they love.

> "I spent this past weekend looking back on a lot of aspects of my life due to a trip I made, and I think if nothing else, this whole experience of having cancer has forced me to examine things in my life and to deal with issues that I may not have dealt with….And I have looked at those issues and worked on things—bad things, dark things—and let them go, and they no longer cloud up my life. And I can look back on just absolutely wonderful times and wonderful memories, and any dark things don't hurt me anymore."
>
> — Catherine

Leaving a Legacy

In addition to looking back into your past and considering your life in review, you may want to look ahead to the future as well, to the time after you are gone. As you imagine what's ahead, you may want to consider leaving a legacy that will enable your friends and family to remember you in the ways you want to be remembered.

Leaving a legacy is not the same thing as preparing a will, or any other legal document, or about setting aside money for a person or a charity. Leaving a legacy is about communicating to the ones you love most how you feel about them and how you hope they will remember you. Leaving a legacy can give you a chance to reinforce important relationships—now and in the future.

Entering the Last Stage of Your Life

As we discussed in chapter 3, there may come a time when your doctor will tell you that further treatments to try to cure your cancer would do you more harm than good or that your cancer has advanced in a way that cannot be changed. Your doctor may have talked to you about seeing a palliative care team or entering a hospice program. Your doctor may even say that your time is very limited.

Others with advanced cancer will tell the doctor, "I know that this treatment is no longer helping me; it is time for me to stop and to focus on things that will make a difference to me and to my family after I am gone."

No matter how this conversation evolves, you will enter a stage in which you know your cancer is no longer curable, your treatments are no longer

> "What I want my children to remember about me and my life and my struggles with cancer is...that I faced it head-on. That I wasn't afraid to ask for help when I needed it. That I could recognize that I needed it. That I fought for what was important to me. That I had things that were of value to me, and I'm not talking at all about material things. That I made my decisions based on my values and was always moving forward."
>
> — Catherine

effective, your death is approaching, and your time is measured in months, weeks, or days rather than years. We refer to this time throughout this chapter as the last stage of your life.

Reacting to the News

How will you and those you love react to the realization that you have entered the last stage of your life? People react in many different ways to news of impending death. These feelings may range from acceptance to shock, anger, disbelief, fear, and grief. Frequently these feelings blur one into the other and may be very confusing. Family members and friends often have similar feelings to those you had when you realized your death was approaching. (See chapter 4 for strategies for coping with these powerful emotions.)

The way people treat you may reflect where they are along the spectrum of their own feelings and reactions—some may be drawn closer to you, while others may distance themselves from you as they come to terms with how they feel, and sort out their own grief and fear. Sometimes people just don't know what to say, and so they say nothing or stay away.

You may be fearful of what the actual dying experience will be like, not only physically (which we'll talk about later in this chapter), but emotionally and spiritually, as well. Emotionally and spiritually, it is very painful to leave this world. It is hard for many of us to leave life and to imagine the world continuing without us and our family going forward without us. But acknowledging this pain and grief helps in the healing. And allowing our family and friends to be there with us through this time can also help them in their grief and pain of loss. If you do not have family or are not close to them, close and deep emotional ties can occur with some members of your health care team.

—⚘—

"The hardest part was writing notes to my children and grandchildren. I did what I call 'I Want You to Remember,' and I wrote things that I remembered about them and about our times together that I want them to remember. I am trying to make memories to leave behind. At the present time I am trying to decide little things, not big item things, but little things that may mean something to different friends and people, to have of mine. It makes me feel better after I do it. I've done something. I think I'm doing something about it. I can't change it, but I can do something about it. I can have some control over what people remember of me, of what my memorial service will be, of what will be done with my ashes, and then after that it's all up to everybody else."

— Jeanne

On the other hand, for some who have been struggling with a long and difficult illness, death can be welcome. A comfortable death is what is desired for everyone, and that is possible with the right support.

Coming to Terms With Death

You may be thinking, "What if I'm scared to die?" This means you are totally normal. It *is* scary to think about dying. Specific fears we have may include those about pain, physical decline, inability to take care of ourselves, dependency on others for our physical needs, being an emotional or financial burden on our families, and feeling of no further use to ourselves or anyone else, to name a few of the most common.

If you are willing to think about your death, even a little at a time, you will probably discover that figuring out what part is the most scary can help you find ways to cope. For example, are you most worried about what might happen to you after death? If so, you may want to work with a pastoral care expert or the leader at your house of worship to better understand your own spiritual beliefs. If you are most worried about the process of dying and fear dying in pain, for example, you can work with a pain specialist to make sure that your pain will be controlled and that you feel confident your health care team will manage your symptoms. Or, you may be most concerned about what will happen to your children or other dependents after you're gone. You can work with a social worker, who will involve your family members and loved ones to make sure your children will be cared for after your death.

＊

"I have accepted the fact that I can't be cured. I've been told that from the beginning. That it's treatable, but it is not curable. So I have accepted the fact that barring something unforeseen, this cancer will take my life. But that has actually become just a fact for me, and I guess, it's hard to say that you've accepted it, but you do at some point. Early on it's very difficult. I was diagnosed in August, and that first Christmas, of course, I thought was going to be my last. It was a very traumatic time. Everything, at that point, I didn't know if I'd be there the next whatever. Finally, you just know that is the case and you start living more in the day."

— Jeanne

Coming to terms with your death is a process, and it may not be an easy one. Respect the way you feel, rather than denying it. Know that you and your loved ones are not alone: all of us will face death at some point. Remember there is always someone available to help you. Involve your family and friends and talk together about your eventual death and the complex emotions it raises. Seek outside help from a member of your religious community, a counselor, a social worker, or some other supportive individual. Your task is to reach out and ask for help when you need it. Reaching out for help is not a sign of weakness, but a sign of strength. Chapter 4 and the Resources section at the back of this book include additional strategies and resources for coping you may find helpful.

Seeking Support

Many people hesitate to ask for support, but when they do ask, they are pleasantly surprised by the resources that are available. It's important to think about who among your friends and family is capable of the kinds of support you might want. Different people may be capable of different kinds of support. One friend might be great for late-night phone calls; another might be able to go along with you when you see the doctor; another might be able to commiserate with your spouse or partner. You can talk at greater length to your social worker or nurse or whomever you trust most on your health care team. Psychologists, social workers, and other counselors can be very helpful when you feel like you are having a tough time with support. Support and education groups can be another useful source of support and information (see chapter

> "I wanted to live, and I wanted to be a grandmother, but I had a son that was 6 years old, and I just couldn't imagine leaving him at that age. And so my fear of dying was more the pain that he was going to have to go through."
>
> — Ana

4). Finally, spiritual counselors such as chaplains can be very valuable, as well as pastoral care counselors who are not associated with a particular religion (see chapter 10).

The most important thing is to simply ask for help if and when you need it. Don't wait, or expect others to be able to know your needs, or assume that people will react a certain way. Just starting a conversation can be the most important step you take.

Maintaining Hope

We are all born with a survival instinct. Exactly what effect this will to survive has on diseases like cancer is unknown. But what is certain is that maintaining hope, the confident desire and expectation that good things will happen (things like living the remainder of your life on your own terms), will enhance your quality of life, even if its duration has been cut short.

We're not saying that you can wish your cancer away through the power of positive thinking. But many people with dire prognoses outlive physicians' predictions. So find pleasure and happiness where you can. Emphasizing the positive aspects of your life—rather than retreating into a swirling maelstrom of anger, sadness, and self-pity—can add meaning, purpose, and comfort to your remaining days.

Living Life on Your Own Terms

Coming to terms with the fact that your life may be cut short because of an illness like cancer isn't easy to do. But some people say that accepting their prognosis freed them to say and do things they might not have done before.

Palliative care is about living life—however much of it you have left—on your own terms. Talk with your loved ones and your palliative care team about how you want to live out your days, and let them help you achieve your goals.

Talking About Death

We've spent some time covering strategies for talking to certain individuals or groups of people about your cancer (see chapter 4). But what if, now that your cancer has progressed and you are entering the last stage of your life, you don't know what to say? Confronting the possibility of death is upsetting to most people, and some may prefer to skirt the subject. Add to that the cultural taboo of talking about death and the additional fear that if you do so, people will think you are morbid or depressing.

> "Don't waste your time questioning why this is happening to me. Save your strength…to do everything you possibly can."
>
> – Jo Ann

Death—especially one's own or that of a loved one—is one of the most difficult subjects to discuss. As we have mentioned, the majority of people benefit from talking with someone about their questions and fears about death. But be forewarned, there are still some people—trained health care professionals and members of the clergy included—who are not able to openly discuss dying and death without distress and avoidance on their own part. Platitudes, superficial statements about it "is all for the best," or that "God never gives anyone more than they can handle," are seldom helpful to anyone. Avoidance of what we cannot control and neatly explain benefits no one. Some people—especially professionals—still erroneously think it is up to them to have all of the answers rather than to share an experience that leaves all concerned enriched through the struggle and honesty they have encountered together.

Do not give up if you are disappointed in the response you initially receive. Remember, their discomfort is their problem, not yours. There are many physicians, nurses, social workers, clergy, friends, and others who see the opportunity to share this difficult time with you as a gift that leads to feeling needed and deeply connected to others. Find someone who makes you feel heard and deeply understood. You will benefit from this relationship, and so will they.

By having the courage to put your concerns into words with others, you risk losing your fear but give the gift of trust, love, and intimacy. Never allow fear to keep you from engaging others in your struggle. We are all going to die, and we need to hear from and teach each other how to make meaning from the dying experience.

How Do I Talk About My Own Death?

If you are having difficulty figuring out how to talk with others about your mortality and your questions, fears, or hopes for the dying process, a helpful first step is to determine what your needs and desires are. Do you need companionship on this journey? Are you looking for chances to mend broken relationships? Do you want to celebrate and strengthen intact relationships? Do you need your friends and loved ones to help you sort out the answers to "why" questions (e.g., "Why did this happen to me?")? Do you need help finding meaning and perspective during this difficult time in your life? Do you need the comfort of your loved ones? Do they need you to be a comfort to them? The answers to questions like these can help guide you to where you need to go with important conversations.

> —\\\\\—
> "Talking about death won't kill you."
> — Karen

Next, you should seek to find trusted people who can bear to talk with you about your dying and your fears. Everyone needs at least one person to lean on in this way. You need someone with whom you can really be honest, who will listen to your thoughts and hopes and plans and fears without getting too worried or distraught themselves. You also need someone who will be able to listen without interrupting, without jumping in to try to make you feel better by simply reassuring you that "everything will be all right." Nice people do this when they're trying to be helpful but are too nervous about what they're hearing to really listen, to hear the other person out. You need someone who can stay calm enough inside themselves to really hear you out. If you have family and friends who can do this, let them give you this gift. If not, counselors and members of the clergy are trained in this kind of listening. As an alternative, ask you health care team to make a referral to someone with whom they work who is expert in this kind of care.

Ironically, you can help others you love get more comfortable talking with you by reassuring them. If you calmly initiate these important conversations, you send a powerful signal to others that you are comfortable dealing with the big questions. You may need to directly reassure some of those close to you to help them be able to talk about this. You may want to try something like, "Look, I know my time is getting short, but I want to make the most of this time we have. I'm not afraid to talk about my dying—you won't hurt me or scare me if we talk about it. In fact, there are some things I'd like to tell you that will make me feel better once I'm sure you know them."

"I have friends who dance around the issue of the fact that I'm dying. I was walking through my garden the other day and I was looking at a Japanese maple that I planted last fall, and I said to this friend of mine who's a gardener, I said, 'You know. I love this tree. I'm not going to live long enough to see it mature, but it's a beautiful tree.' And she got really angry with me. And I was surprised, and she got angry and she said, 'You know, you're always talking about dying. It's always in your conversations.' And I'm like, 'Yeah, it is in all my conversations, because I want all my friends to know that I want you to talk about how you feel. That we have to do that all the time.' And later she got back to me and said, 'You know, my problem is my denial. It's just hard. I'm grieving.'"

— Ric

What If My Loved Ones Don't Want to Talk About My Dying?

What if that doesn't work? What if the person you would choose to talk to can't tolerate being a part of that conversation? You should ask yourself if you need them to talk about it, at least right now. If there is someone else who can be your calm and trusted listening ear, talk to him or her first and give others a chance to get more comfortable with the situation (and with your reactions to it), so they will be able to bear having the conversations with you. If you feel you need to talk with someone who is uncomfortable talking about death with you, and it can't really wait, there are a few things you can do to help them be more comfortable:

- **Focus discussions on your relationship with this person, not on your dying.** "You know, you've always meant the world to me," "I am very proud of you," or "I don't want today to go by without telling you again that I love you" are good examples, but you can probably come up with just the right thing to say on your own. If you focus the conversation on your love for them, tears may come, but you'll get a conversation started. If you start out talking about dying, a worried or frightened loved one may not be able to engage in conversation. If you talk about your relationship, they're much more likely to be soothed enough to respond.

204

- **Tell stories.** Are there funny or meaningful or special stories in your family? Stories that involve your relationship with the particular person you're talking to are best. "Remember our first date?" "I'll never forget the time when...." People build meaning through stories. Families are built on shared stories. Now is a great time to take advantage of that fact.
- **Try inviting the other person to talk.** Let them choose the topic, any topic. Get a conversation started. As the other person becomes more comfortable, you can move gently toward the topics you want or need to talk about as you sense they're becoming more comfortable. They'll see you're not so fragile that you'll break down, they'll see you want to talk about things, they'll enjoy sharing stories and laughing with you. You may not need to work too hard to get them around to talking about the big questions, but if you have to take the lead, you'll know when the time is right.

Planning for Death on Your Own Terms

Although you may not be able to control all aspects of the dying process, including the timing of your death, you can certainly plan for and control many aspects of it. Having a plan helps ensure that you are cared for as you want to be cared for at the end of life and also helps ensure that those who are closest to you will be well cared for after your death.

As you begin thinking about this last phase of your life, you may want to think about what you want your death to be like. This might seem a little odd, but it can be nice to have the music you like, or the flowers you like, or a few photos of important people right by your bed, for example.

You can also plan where you want to be. At home? In a hospital or facility dedicated to providing hospice care? (See chapter 2 for more information on care options at end of life.) What do you want it to be like? For example, what "rites of transition" do you want as you are dying? These might include prayers, songs, and religious rituals, for example.

You can plan who you want to be with you and ask them ahead of time. They will need to be able to plan also.

You may want to plan things about your estate, such as financial and legal matters (see chapters 5, 6, and 7). You may want to leave a personal kind of legacy, like an album of photos, letters to the ones you love most deeply, or a book of favorite family recipes.

You can also work with your health care team to make your wishes known about your preferences for medical care. Most people want to die without excessive use of machines or tubes, and many would like to die at home. These wishes and others like them can be recorded in a living will, which we discussed in detail in chapter 5, along with other types of advance directives. Your medical team can help you make this possible if you make your wishes known to them as early as possible.

Finally, you may want to consider what happens after your death; that is, what shape your funeral or memorial services will take.

Making Arrangements for Your Funeral

Whether you participate in making plans for your own funeral or memorial service is up to you. Some people find that planning their own funeral allows them to have a say in how they want to be remembered and also allows them a way to communicate with their loved ones even after they have died.

In addition, planning a funeral can be a way to open up a conversation with your loved ones about what you want and about what you want them to remember about you. For some people, planning a funeral becomes something they do with their loved ones that helps them feel more connected. Other people find that it's too hard to think about their own funeral, and they simply want to tell their loved ones what they want or if they have any preferences. There are many variations on how much funeral planning to do, and it is an individual choice.

> "I have written my obituary. I have made notes. I have done quite a few things in preparation. I think that almost gives you a relief to have that over with; to get that out of the way."
>
> — Jeanne

Do consider that planning ahead may make things easier on your loved ones after you are gone. If you have these conversations ahead of time, or record your preferences in writing, your loved ones won't have to guess what you would have wanted and worry that what they are doing is not the right thing.

If you agree that your loved ones would benefit from knowing what sort of funeral arrangements you would like and you wish to participate in planning, here are some questions to ask yourself. Share your preferences with your loved ones:

1. How would you like your life to be celebrated or remembered?
2. Do you prefer cremation or burial?
   - If you prefer burial, is there a special outfit you would like to be buried in? Do you want to have anything with you in your casket? Is there anything special you would like engraved on your headstone? Have you chosen where you want to be interred?
   - If you prefer cremation, what would you like your loved ones to do with your ashes?
3. Are there particular songs, poems, or prayers you would like sung or read at your service? Are there particular adornments (such as a special photograph or an arrangement featuring a favorite flower) that you would like displayed?
4. If people would like to contribute in your honor to a favorite charity, where do you want those contributions to go?

Here are some steps you can take to make the logistics of your funeral easier for your loved ones:
1. Review your plans with your family and loved ones.
2. Review your plans with your clergy if appropriate.
3. Make a list of who you would want to be notified of your death, so that your loved ones can do this easily.
4. Decide what type of announcement or notification, if any, you would like to be sent to people.
5. Think about what financial arrangements need to be made for your funeral.

Of course, you may not want to think about your funeral at all; *that's okay too.* There are no hard and fast rules about how to handle this. For many people, their culture will have a way of handling funerals that is meaningful to them and that also serves as a source of guidance for this important life ritual. Religious leaders and pastoral care experts can also help with this.

Saying Goodbye

Unfortunately, many times saying goodbye happens too late—it happens at a wake when loved ones are filing past your body or at a graveside ceremony when someone drops a single rose onto your casket. Sometimes the person who

---

"My husband and I had always been really close, but whenever I went to broach subjects with him like funeral arrangements and things, when it got down to where they said he was not going to live, he wouldn't deal with it. He didn't want to talk about it. So afterwards then, I'm kind of floundering around trying to figure out what to do and what not to do. And I think that your communication has to start as soon as possible when someone is diagnosed, and it needs to be an open discussion about everything."

— Kay

---

is dying accepts their death sooner than their loved ones. So you are the one who may have to start the conversation and start saying the goodbyes.

Saying goodbye has many meanings. It may mean "I want you to know what you mean to me," or "I want you to know that I love you," or "I want you to know that I'll miss you." Depending on your religious beliefs, it might even mean "I look forward to seeing you later." Like any important message, you may want to plan to whom you want to say this and how the message gets delivered.

Don't hesitate to ask your loved ones to help you with this task—it can ease their own grief as well. For instance, consider asking a friend to write as you talk so you can remember all the things you want to put in a letter to your spouse. If you have children or grandchildren, you might want to even write several letters for them to open on special days later in their lives—when they have a birthday, a wedding, or a graduation. Or make an audiotape or video recording with the help of a media-savvy family member. You might, on the other hand, want to have a goodbye party, and ask your spouse or partner to help you pull it off. If your business or your career is an important part of your life, you may want to have a trusted co-worker help you compose a formal letter to all of your business colleagues thanking them for their support.

Making Peace With Yourself and Others

As death approaches, you may look back on your life and take stock of all the wonderful things you have done, all the gifts you have given to others. But you also probably will dwell on your mistakes and the times when you wronged others. You may be wondering, "How can I forgive myself for things that I have done?"

We are often hardest on ourselves. When faced with advancing illness, we deserve kindness and every opportunity for peace and wholeness. Forgiving ourselves helps allow that to happen. First, examine whether the thing you're having trouble forgiving yourself for involves someone else. If so, consider attempting to reconcile with them by asking for their forgiveness. Receiving the forgiveness of someone we have hurt often allows us to stop beating ourselves up for the thing we did.

If the hurt truly does not involve another person but is simply a disappointment or a shame you have within yourself, you may want to try formally forgiving yourself, as described above. For people who are religious, rituals of confession or penitence or prayers asking for God's forgiveness may lead to relief from this burden. Consulting with a trusted spiritual advisor or pastoral care counselor may be especially helpful. If you are stuck in a feeling of not being able to forgive yourself, this may be a sign of a clinical depression that would benefit from treatment.

FORGIVENESS

Perhaps in the course of your life someone else has wronged you. How can you forgive others who have hurt you? Fixing important relationships that are broken can produce tremendous benefits, including a sense of relief, satisfaction, and peace. Your illness may actually give you the opportunity you need to repair damaged relationships with those nearest to your heart. This is not always possible; sometimes the hurts are too deep. If it makes sense to try to fix things, here are some important things to remember.

First, understand the difference between *forgiveness* and *reconciliation*. You need two people for reconciliation to work, but you can forgive all by yourself— even if the other person never chooses to participate.

If you're holding hurt toward someone, you can choose to forgive that person. Forgiveness is an important part of reconciliation, but you can forgive someone even if they won't acknowledge they have hurt you, repent, or ask for your forgiveness. To do this, you simply *give up the grudge* you have held and you *forfeit the right to any kind of revenge or retaliation* for the hurt they've done to you. Ideally, you would also make an effort to *do some good toward this person* (such as praying blessings on them or showing them an act of kindness). Forgiveness is always a generous act on the part of the person who was hurt, but this is especially true when there is no repentance or chance of reconciliation. Also, it is important to recognize that it is quite possible to forgive without forgetting.

Putting your hurts aside can be very difficult to do when the person who did the hurtful thing won't admit they have hurt you or won't even deal with the subject. To make the process easier, you can view forgiveness as a way to help yourself by laying down the burden of the anger and the bitterness that the old, lingering hurt causes you. The relationship may not be fixable (through reconciliation), but you can still let the burden go through forgiveness.

RECONCILIATION

Reconciliation requires two people. The first person, the one who did the hurtful thing, has 4 tasks. First he or she *admits* to doing the hurtful thing ("I see that I hurt you two years ago when I...."). Then that person *apologizes* (here it's helpful to actually say "I'm sorry" out loud). Next the offender *repents* by stating that he or she will try not to do the hurtful thing again. Repentance involves turning away from that hurtful behavior and striving to do better in the future. Finally the offender *asks for forgiveness* ("I know I did wrong and I hurt you. I am asking if you would please forgive me."). All 4 tasks are critically important and need to be followed roughly in this order.

The second person, the one who was hurt, now has the choice to forgive or not. If he or she chooses to forgive, the forgiveness should be spoken out loud ("I forgive you."). In the interest of the relationship, both people next agree to try their best not to repeat the hurtful thing that happened, to go back to caring for one another, and to rebuild the trust in their relationship over time.

Ira Byock, in his book *Dying Well*, describes the 5 things we need to be able to say to those who mean most to us as we near the end of our lives. These things are: "please forgive me," "I forgive you," "thank you," "I love you," and "goodbye." You may not need to say all 5 of these things to everyone, but if you do, you should try to say them in the order they are listed here (for example, ask for forgiveness first if you need to, then grant forgiveness). If we can manage to say these 5 things to those who matter to us most, a great deal of healing can happen in our relationships.

Regrets and Unfinished Business

You may have regrets about your life. You may also feel as though you have important goals and dreams that will not be completed or fulfilled. If this is the case, sharing stories and thinking about your life story can be especially helpful. You are now writing the last chapter of your life's story. How does your story make sense? What does your story so far tell you about the purpose and meaning of your life? What were you able to accomplish? What can you pass on to others to do? What can you do to help them succeed in

> "It's like God jerked a knot in my tail and said, 'Hey, Jeff, open your eyes and look at your priorities, because I don't think you've got them all in line.' And things that used to be important to me prior to cancer and what's important to me now is night and day difference."
>
> — Jeff

continuing to pursue these goals? After you are gone, how will you and your accomplishments be remembered? How do you want to be remembered? What can you do now to make that happen?

Your illness may limit some of the things you can do, but try to stay aware of the gifts you *can* give now. Fix the problems you *can* fix; do what you *can* do. Don't underestimate the value of passing on wisdom and guidance to others. Determine how you can be a blessing and pass on blessings to those around you, in small ways as much as big ways. Part of being alive and connected to others is sharing the gifts we are able to give. This helps give meaning and purpose to life, even in the setting of illness. Helping others and being useful gives meaning.

If You Are Considering Hastening Your Death

During the course of advancing cancer, many people think at some point that they should just end it all. Often this is just a fleeting thought, usually at a bad moment. For a few people, the idea of hastening their death at a time of their choosing becomes a persistent, powerful idea. In either case, if you have been thinking about hastening your death, find someone on your health care team

> "I live out where I get to see the deer, the birds at the feeder, pretty clouds in the sky. My making the most of each day has more to do with finding the little things and in finding times with the people I love. You find yourself—I found myself, I should say—drawing this circle of things that were really important to me, where I maybe thought there was this whole mass of things that were important to me before."
>
> — Jeanne

that you can talk to about what you are feeling and thinking. They should be able to assess what is going on and help you process these feelings and thoughts. The most common reason for wanting to hasten death is clinical depression. Being depressed is common for people with cancer, and sometimes depression can magnify feelings about wanting to hasten death. But depression is treatable with psychotherapy, or medication, or both.

When people think about hastening their death, they are sometimes thinking about *physician-assisted suicide*, which is when a physician prescribes a lethal dose of medication that the patient can take to cause their own death. He "assists" the suicide by writing a prescription for a lethal dose for the patient, but the lethal dose of the drug is self-administered by the patient. Physician-assisted suicide is controversial. In the United States, physician-assisted suicide is legal only in the state of Oregon. The Oregon law, which is called the Death with Dignity Act, has specific criteria about who can legally have a physician-assisted suicide. (For more information about the law, visit the state of Oregon's Department of Human Services Web site at http://www.ohd.hr.state.or.us/chs/pas/pas.cfm.) Based on Oregon data, it turns out that while people may think about physician-assisted suicide at some point during their cancer, only a small number actually go through with it.

One other form of hastening death that you may have heard about is called *euthanasia*. This is when a physician injects a lethal dose of medication into a patient with the sole purpose of causing death. Euthanasia is not legal anywhere in the United States. Many people feel that euthanasia is too easy to misuse to ever become legal.

Finally, there are some people who want to take death into their own hands by stopping eating and drinking. Again, you should talk to someone on your health care team if you are thinking about this, because they will be able to assess your medical situation and also talk to you about what is going on as well as give you practical information.

WITHHOLDING AND WITHDRAWING TREATMENT

Forgoing or discontinuing treatments after they have been used for a certain period of time is an important patient right and a special circumstance that deserves additional discussion. While forgoing or discontinuing treatment are related to the topic of hastening death, it should not be confused with assisted suicide or euthanasia, which are intended to cause death.

When people discuss withholding or withdrawing treatment, they are talking about withholding (not starting) or withdrawing (stopping) *life-sustaining treatment*, not about palliative interventions designed to relieve symptoms and improve the comfort of the person with cancer. Life-sustaining medical treatment is, in general, anything mechanical or artificial that sustains, restores, or substitutes for a vital body function and that would prolong the process for someone who is dying. Examples of life-sustaining treatment include mechanical ventilation, renal dialysis, chemotherapy, antibiotics, and artificial nutrition and hydration, although state laws define life-sustaining treatment differently.

According to the American College of Physicians, court rulings and most ethicists have found no legal or ethical difference between withdrawing and withholding treatment. But from the point of view of many patients, family members, and health care workers, withdrawing a treatment after the patient has been receiving it for a while often feels harder than withholding a treatment that was never started.

The decision to withhold or withdraw treatment depends on a number of factors, such as the unique medical situation of a person with cancer, whether the person with cancer feels that the burdens of getting the treatment are worth the benefits the treatment may offer, the person's view of the quality of life that would result from the treatment, and his or her own wishes, preferences, and belief system. Refusing or discontinuing any medical treatment, including artificial hydration and nutrition and being taken off a ventilator, is not the same as physician-assisted suicide or euthanasia. The person with cancer (or his or her health care proxy, in the event the patient cannot speak on his or her own behalf) always has the right to refuse or discontinue treatment and arrange for a transfer of care to a different doctor if necessary.

Artificial Hydration and Nutrition

You may be wondering about the legal and ethical implications of *artificial hydration and nutrition* near the end of life. By artificial hydration, we mean treatments like intravenous fluids or intravenous nutrition. This term also refers to feeding tubes that go in through the nose or the stomach wall. When a person is near death, these treatments do not help comfort them, and do not help people live longer; conversely, stopping these treatments does not clearly hasten death in most cases. While people sometimes worry about starving to death if artificial hydration and nutrition are not given, the truth is that the cancer is what is causing death, and most patients in the last stage of life do not complain of hunger or thirst. In fact, people who are dying become more uncomfortable if they do receive artificial hydration and nutrition.

Ventilators

When someone has been critically ill with respiratory failure, the doctors may ask the person with cancer and his or her family whether they would like to consider the use of a ventilator (this is sometimes also called *mechanical ventilation*). A *ventilator* is a machine that pumps air and extra oxygen into a patient's lungs through a special tube (called an endotracheal tube) that goes down the patient's windpipe. When a person is on a ventilator, he or she cannot talk because of the tube, and most individuals need to be sedated, because being on a ventilator is quite uncomfortable for someone who is not medicated.

If the doctors are introducing the idea of using a ventilator, it means the person in their care is very sick. As such, there is a possibility that person will end up dying on the ventilator. If someone is put on a ventilator, it usually means that the person cannot return home to die and will stay in an intensive care unit until they die. For some people, that is not a risk they want to take. If someone is already on a ventilator and the doctors have determined that they are dying and are not going to recover, the ventilator can be disconnected and the endotracheal tube removed before death occurs. This will enable the person to die more naturally. After removal of a ventilator, death may occur very soon—sometimes within hours or even minutes.

We encourage you to ask your medical team what to expect. If a patient or the person who is that patient's legal decision maker decides that a ventilator should be withdrawn, it is generally done to avoid prolonging an uncomfortable death. While this can be seen as hastening death in the respect that it avoids prolonging the inevitable, it is definitely not the same as physician-assisted suicide or euthanasia.

PAIN MEDICATION

You may be wondering if taking pain medication is a type of assisted suicide. Many individuals (both people with cancer and their loved ones) ask questions about whether taking too much pain medicine will hasten death, and some people actually don't take the pain medicine that their doctors and nurses recommend because of this worry.

It's true that this topic is highly debated, but studies show that the use of pain medicines like morphine do not cause death and are not likely to hasten death in persons with advanced cancer. The cancer causes death, not the pain medicine. When doctors prescribe pain medicine, they are trying to treat pain to make that person's last weeks, days, or hours as comfortable as possible. Please talk to your doctor if you are worried about pain and/or the role of pain medication at the end of your life.

Signals That Death Is Approaching

Many people wonder about what might happen near the time of death. You may be curious about what to expect, and your loved ones and caregivers may want to know too, so that they can support you through your final moments. This list of signs and symptoms of approaching death may appear frightening, but for both you and your loved ones, knowing what to expect may reduce some of the anxiety about the actual process of your approaching death:

1. **Withdrawal:** Physical and emotional withdrawal, as well as increased sleep are very common occurrences as life draws to a close.
2. **Consciousness:** Some people become unconscious hours or even days before their death, while others are alert up to the last moments. Usually the dying person gradually becomes semiconscious over the period of a few minutes or hours.
3. **Reduced food and fluid intake:** This is a normal part of dying as the body starts to close down and can no longer handle or use food and water. Hunger and thirst are not usually experienced.
4. **Confusion/agitation:** This can vary in degree. This may be caused by toxins in the body as the organs start to close down and cease to function.

5. **Change in breathing pattern and noisy breathing:** The dying person may experience irregular breathing—very rapid, very slow, and/or long periods between breaths. Oral secretions may collect in the back of the throat and cause noisy breathing.

6. **Incontinence:** Loss of control of bladder and bowels may happen, and you may require a tube to drain your urine.

7. **Changes in the skin temperature and color:** These changes are a natural part of the dying process and occur as the body's circulation slows down. Skin may become cool and mottled. Sometimes, a high fever rather than cooling of the body occurs before death.

8. **Listening and Speaking:** Speech may become quiet and intermittent as a person nears death, and words or thoughts that are spoken may not relate to the people present or to current events. Hearing is generally thought to be the last sense lost.

9. **Death:** Breathing will cease, pupils will become fixed and dilated, and the person will no longer have a pulse or heart beat.

A similar list of symptoms a dying person may experience—along with information on what to do about them—is included for caregivers in chapter 12. Symptoms like pain, nausea, or shortness of breath can be controlled. The hospice team or palliative care team is specially trained to do this.

Remember that the symptoms listed above are not universal. Every person's death—like their life—is unique.

Conclusion

Although battling a life-limiting illness is undoubtedly difficult, there are also some unique opportunities for you to make the best of this tough situation. Many people have found the contemplation of their own mortality to be one of the most meaningful experiences of their lives. Being able to manage and use your emotions as important cues to identify specific concerns will help you effectively solve problems, engage others in your journey, and cope with emotions and challenges as your life enters its final stage.

Ultimately, the dying experience is about closure on life and embracing the natural cycle of living. It can be a time when every moment can be another invaluable invitation and opportunity to redefine an entire lifetime. Amazingly for some, this time in your life, despite the grief and pain of saying "goodbye," can also be a period in which can have rewards beyond the limits of any one person. For example, fear in isolation can cause unnecessary suffering, lost opportunities, and regrets; on the other hand, fear that is shared with a loved one can be a gift that leads to a sense of closeness and emotional intimacy.

For some people, the dying process and the insight and closeness with others that it may bring is one of the most meaningful experiences they will ever have. This is most likely to happen when the dying person and the people closest to them have opportunities for honest and open communication, and are able to express their love while sharing their sadness and deepest fears. By effectively working together to anticipate and manage practical problems, the person with cancer and their loved ones are often able to create, some for the first time, a series of life-affirming experiences that results in a sense of connectedness that can lead to the healing of old wounds, forgiveness, deepening respect, understanding, and love.

For some people, dying creates a sense of urgency and greater openness that makes positive change possible. Others may retreat into themselves and not be able or want to engage others in their struggle. This essential "aloneness" may be a conscious choice for some. It may be an expression of their goals and values, and family members and loved ones should respect and honor this choice.

No one can know the future, but looking back on your past (completing a life review) and assessing what is most important to you in these present and future moments (such as relationships with others and what legacy you will leave) can help you face what will come.

> "We have a fear of death, and don't really understand the process. We don't really know the shutting down process of the body and are so afraid of pain and of just not being here."
>
> – Linda E.

> "Many of us, I would include myself, have this fear of dying. When I think about the moment of death, or the minutes leading up to that, it seems very scary. I think I have to come to my own peace with that."
>
> – Andrew

—⁓—

"As far as I'm concerned, the biggest triumph for me was to live day by day. But, also to realize that by living day by day, by not letting this disease claim your spirit, even though it may be hurting your body at the time, you can win, either way. And what I mean by that is, you can win if you survive. Which I've been fortunate enough to do right now. But you can also win if you don't make it through, or the disease eventually claims your life. Because as long as it doesn't claim your spirit, you still are the same person, and you still have love and you still have laughter, still have family and friends."

— Lizette

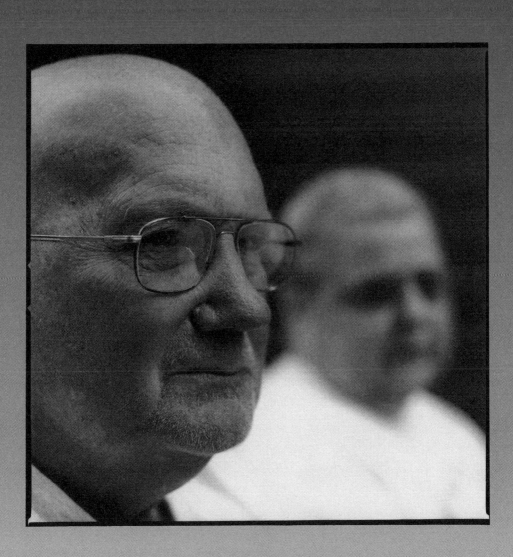

Chapter 10

Seeking Meaning, Connection, Hope, and Peace at the End of Your Life

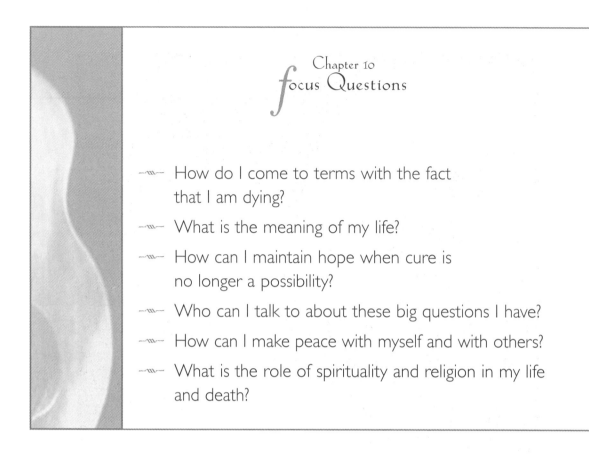

Chapter 10
focus Questions

—⚭— How do I come to terms with the fact
that I am dying?

—⚭— What is the meaning of my life?

—⚭— How can I maintain hope when cure is
no longer a possibility?

—⚭— Who can I talk to about these big questions I have?

—⚭— How can I make peace with myself and with others?

—⚭— What is the role of spirituality and religion in my life
and death?

"You know, diagnosis of cancer really has not changed anything about what my life is about. It didn't change my values. It didn't change my beliefs. You know, you hear people, that they suddenly got their priorities straight, and they were enlightened—and, you know, none of that happened for me. Cancer was just, 'Oh well, yesterday I didn't have cancer, and now today I have cancer.' And then, you wake up one morning, and 'Oh, now it's advanced cancer.' Who I am and my values haven't changed at all. Except now I really understand why it's important to live every moment, every day. I believed that before, but I didn't really understand why. Now I understand why."

— Ric

MOST OF US HAVE WONDERED AT ONE TIME OR ANOTHER, "Why am I here? What does it mean to be human? Has my life made a difference? Is there a God or some higher supernatural power, and if so, what is the nature of our relationship? What will happen to me when I die?" As humans, we tend to seek meaning beyond the physical dimensions of our existence. We are naturally curious about the big questions we don't have easy answers for.

Many people who are diagnosed with a serious illness like cancer discover that these questions have a new importance for them, and they may begin to seek answers with a renewed sense of urgency. This kind of spiritual searching can take many forms, including pursuing meaning through religious faith, through relationships with others, and through self-examination. In this chapter, we'll talk about spirituality, coming to terms with mortality, and finding meaning as the end of life approaches.

Facing Mortality

How do people come to terms with the fact that they are dying and that the time they have left is limited? How do people with chronic and severe illnesses like cancer find the strength to face their own mortality?

To come to terms with mortality, people look inside themselves and examine their thoughts and feelings across many dimensions. Here is a list of 7 of the most important aspects of life to consider as you face its close and some key questions for you to ask yourself. Seeking the answers to these questions can help you face your mortality and come to terms with death. We talked a bit about healing relationships and leaving a legacy in chapter 9, and we'll talk briefly about the other items on this list in this chapter.

1. **Relationships:** "What can I do to strengthen or repair my relationships with those I care about most? Do the people who mean the most to me know how much I care about them?" (See chapter 9.)
2. **Giving Gifts:** "What can I pass on to others? How can I share what I have and what I know to help and bless other people?" "What is the legacy I want to leave for others?" (See chapter 9.)
3. **Meaning:** "What has given my life purpose and value? What gives it purpose and value now?"
4. **Growing and Learning:** "What can I learn about myself (and about life)? What opportunities does my situation (including my illness) provide for me and for others? What do I want to do with this time?"
5. **Hope:** "What specific good things can I look forward to with confidence?"
6. **Spirituality and Religious Belief:** "What is the nature of my relationship with God or a higher spiritual being? What can I do to strengthen or repair my relationship with God or a higher spiritual being?"
7. **Peace:** "How can I feel settled in my spirit? How can I be confident that, ultimately, all will be well with me?"

Most people find strength to face challenges and bear difficult situations through their relationships. These include relationships with family members, relationships with friends, and relationships with groups or organizations. For people who are religious, a relationship with God and relationships within a community of other believers are also important. If the central relationships in your life are in good shape, you can draw on them now for strength. If your important relationships are broken, you may want to take this opportunity to work on fixing them. If this is possible, there's hardly anything else you can do that will improve the quality of your life more. You'll find a specific discussion of repairing broken relationships in chapter 9.

"I have such a new-found connection and spiritual connections that it's absolutely amazing. I've just grown spiritually leaps and bounds. I have so many more new opportunities now than I had before the cancer, which is probably odd, because you think it would limit my options. But I've actually grown, because my heart has grown."
— Lisa T.

Much like our relationships, our important stories help us cope and help us make sense of our life in times of stress. You may find it very helpful and comforting to share important stories, funny stories, or sad stories with friends and loved ones. Many people find that reviewing the story of their whole life is useful in making sense of living with an advanced illness. You may want to write some stories down or record them on video or audiotape. People who love you will not only value hearing these stories now; they will also appreciate having them later. Often, telling and hearing stories strengthens relationships, too. ("Remember when we first met?" "Let me tell you a story I remember from when you were a baby." "After that day, my life was never the same.")

Do what you can to balance your sense of independence (autonomy) with the need you may have to depend on others. When feelings of being out of control occur, they are distressing parts of dealing with diseases like cancer. Try to identify some things you can do and keep control over, even if they are little things. As your illness advances and you do need to depend more on others, try not to focus on worry about being a burden. Usually, friends and family feel really good about caring for those they love. It may help you find the grace to let others care for you to think of accepting this care as a gift—a gift your loved ones want to give you. As with all other gifts, don't forget to say "thank you." Your graceful and grateful acceptance of this gift is itself a gift you give to your family and friends in return.

—∞—

"As far as my values go, I was Christian/Catholic when I was diagnosed with cancer. But once you're actually facing the thought or the mortality, I guess that we all have, it's a lot harder to say, 'Yes, I believe in the afterlife.' Or, 'Okay, I'm confident that I'm going to be okay after this is all over.' And so I spent a lot of time dealing with that issue and trying to basically forgive myself, I guess, for whatever I had done in my lifetime. Not that I'm this terrible person, but all of a sudden you're coming to terms with all these things."

— Lizette

Fear of Death

All this talk about death may make it seem pretty matter-of-fact, and is, in fact, designed to make death a little less scary. But death can still be a frightening prospect, even if it is accepted and talked about openly. These fears are normal. You may not ever gain complete comfort with the thought of dying, but these worries and fears shouldn't ruin your ability to enjoy the life you have today. If they do, your fear of dying probably deserves specific attention.

Many people say they're more afraid of the process of dying than of death itself. Problems like pain, trouble breathing, and nausea can be complications at the end of life for people with cancer. As we discussed in chapter 8, there are many things that can be done to control these and other symptoms. If this is a worry for you, be sure to discuss these concerns with your loved ones and your health care team to ensure that a plan is in place to handle these problems.

If you're more afraid of being dead (or of what might happen to you after death), do a little thinking about these fears. Some worry about what will happen to their family once they're gone. Others worry about an afterlife. (Is there an afterlife? Is there a heaven? Is there a hell? What will happen to me after I die?) Still others worry about things they won't be able to complete, how they'll be remembered, or any number of other things. You should seek out a knowledgeable person you trust (such as a family member, a friend, a pastoral care advisor, or a spiritual or religious leader) to discuss any specific worries you may have. These conversations can help you find peace.

"One of the things I think you go through when you're in long-term care and you're experiencing pain, is you try, as a human being, try to rationalize it. And I remember that in my case, I rationalized that what I'm going through is probably what every human being will go through at some point. They may go through it when they're 10 years old, they may go through it when they're 95 years old, but the prospect of death, and in this particular case, prospect of pain associated either ultimately with death or with recovery and/or cure, it's what everyone goes through. This is all part of being a human being. There are reasons why this is happening, although with our limited intellect, we're maybe not gonna understand what those reasons are. And I think that all of that rationalization is what gets you through it."

– Dan

Seeking Meaning

How can you tell if the life you have lived has meaning? This is not a simple question with a simple answer. There are many paths to meaning, and different people will find meaning in different words, accomplishments, and events depending on their culture, values, and personal beliefs.

Consider what is meaningful to you. Look at the story of your life: What are you most proud of? What do you like about yourself? What do you admire in others—do you see those qualities in yourself? Reflect on your unique cultural or religious background: What do your traditions mean to you? Does your religion help you understand what it means to lead a meaningful life? Listen to the stories others tell you about you and about what you mean to them. Have you fixed or maintained your relationships to allow every chance to give the gifts you can give? Remember those you love or have loved. Remember those who love or have loved you. What legacy will you leave behind when you are gone? These are all reflective exercises to help you recognize what matters—what has made a difference to you—in your life.

Every life has value. If you get stuck in a feeling that your life has no meaning, this may be a sign of a clinical depression that would benefit from treatment.

—∞—

"I have cancer. And I lost a lot of things: I lost my sense of myself, I lost my body, I lost my job, I lost my income, I lost my car—I mean, lots of things. So now I fundamentally have nothing, but there is something inside of you that's intrinsically there, and that's the part that I found in myself, that there's another part of me. It has nothing to do with the body. So it was building on that faith that I didn't need all the things of life, the possessions."

— Karen

Endings and Beginnings

Death is an ending. Because of that, the last stage of your life can be a time of great sadness and upheaval. But it can also be a beginning; an opportunity for insight and personal growth. It may seem odd to think of the dying process as an opportunity, but any new experience—even a sad, tragic, or difficult one—provides the chance to learn and grow. You may want to ask yourself the following questions:

- —∞— What can I learn about myself (and about life) as a result of my illness?
- —∞— What opportunities for growth does my situation provide for me and for others?
- —∞— What can I pass on to others (knowledge, insight, experience, possessions)?
- —∞— How can I share what I have and what I know to help other people?

Finding and Maintaining Hope

Hope is the confident expectation that good things will come your way in the future. This kind of hope not only protects and buffers from suffering, worry, and distress, it adds meaning to life. This is the kind of hope that sustains.

The things we hope for have three properties in common. First, hoped-for things are *specific*—they are in this way very different from vague wishes or fantasies. We have a clear idea in mind when we hope for something. Maybe we hope to receive a visit from grandchildren or a response to a letter sent to a friend. Whatever the hoped-for thing is, the more specific and realistic it is, the more likely it is to help sustain us.

Second, hoped-for things are *reliable*. Look for good things that you can reasonably expect to have happen. Ideally, a hoped-for thing is a thing you can count on happening. Otherwise, the hoped-for thing really is a wish. Wishes can come true, and wishes are not bad things to have, but hopes are things you can look forward to with confidence. I may wish to win the lottery, but it is unreasonable for me to hope to win the lottery. It is reasonable for me to hope that the sun will return tomorrow so that I may enjoy the glorious sunrise.

Finally, hoped-for things are *things we can anticipate with pleasure*. When we hope for something, we look forward to experiencing it when it does happen. In fact, it is this property of hoped-for things (the fact that we look forward to them) that gives hope its power. The feeling we get when we think of things hoped for is the antidote to the empty, dreadful feeling that comes with losing hope. As good as hoped-for things are when they actually happen, the anticipation of good things and events is the secret of how hope helps us.

Hope involves trust. We must rely on the fact that hoped-for things will happen. We must look forward to their happening with a sense of confidence. In other words, we must trust that good things *can* and *will* happen to us and for us. Without this trust, hope cannot be—we are reduced to either wishing (at best) or losing hope altogether. One tip to help build hope is to give yourself permission to trust—to simply give trust a try if that is hard for you. You may want to think more about forgiveness (of yourself or others) if trust is really hard for you. Another tip is to initially set your sights on very realistic things, even small things, things you *know* you can count on. As these things happen and you experience the benefit of hope, trust grows, which allows more room for hope.

Don't fall into the trap of thinking about hope only in terms of hoping to have a cure. Often, doctors and nurses get stuck thinking and talking about hope only in terms of cure of a disease like cancer, but hope can help you most if you can resist putting such limits on it. Look for a variety of things to build your hope around: specific things; reliable things; things you can anticipate with pleasure.

> ⸺⁓⸺
>
> "I think that when you're facing a terminal diagnosis, I can't imagine that you can't find some spiritual relief. So in my particular case, what sounded right to me was Buddhism, and that has been like a constant source of comfort and also exploration for me spiritually in the dying process."
>
> — Karen

What Is Spirituality?

Many people use the terms religion and spirituality interchangeably, but it can be useful to distinguish between the two. The word *religion* is usually identified with adherence to a particular set of institutionalized beliefs or practices. The term *spirituality* is more neutral, and has to do with a person's sense of peace, purpose, meaning, and connection to others. Spirituality is a way to relate to the world around us and to reckon with transcendent things—things greater than ourselves and beyond our reach.

Spirituality provides a source of meaning and way to understand the significance of living. It may include habits, rituals, music, prayers, contemplation, and symbolic representations to help understand or interpret what it means to be human.

Spirituality can be expressed through organized religion, although it doesn't have to be. Spirituality can be expressed as a regard for nature or humanity in general, or can be celebrated through meditation and reflection, art, or music, for example. You do not have to be part of a church or organized religious group to be spiritual. You may be both spiritual and religious, or either one of the two.

The Effect of Spirituality on Well-being

Although scientists aren't sure exactly how spirituality affects health, a growing body of research suggests that spiritual and religious practices can indeed have a positive effect on overall health and well-being. In general, the social support provided by spirituality appears to buffer stress and enhance coping skills, and spiritual or religious beliefs or practices appear to promote a positive mental attitude that may help a person's general sense that all is well.

Spirituality and religion may be associated with improved quality of life in the following specific ways:

"My faith has a lot to do with strengthening me at my worst times….I have a strong faith that God is with me. He has always taken good care of me. And that no matter where this journey takes me…that some of the process of getting to the end is a little scary, but I do believe that whatever it is or wherever this takes me, I won't be alone, and I can make it. I can do it."

— Jeanne

"He was never very spiritual before his own cancer experience, but Dad became much more spiritual with the diagnosis and then the treatments not being helpful and all of that. It changed him immensely for the better, and at the very end he was very ready to go and felt that he would continue to live elsewhere on another plane of existence or whatever we'd like to call it, and it was a very peaceful ending because of that spirituality."

— Lu

—⁓— reduced anxiety, depression, and discomfort
—⁓— reduced sense of isolation (feeling alone)
—⁓— better adjustment to the effects of cancer and its treatment
—⁓— increased ability to enjoy life during cancer treatment
—⁓— a feeling of personal growth as a result of living with cancer
—⁓— improved health outcomes

In contrast, spiritual distress (any challenge to a person's beliefs or religious values; for example, the belief that cancer is a punishment from God) may contribute to poorer health outcomes. Therefore, seeking to resolve spiritual or religious conflicts may improve your overall health and ability to cope. A pastoral care expert can help you do this.

The Role of Pastoral Care

Pastoral care is aimed at providing spiritual care or guidance. Hospitals, hospices, and other health care agencies usually have chaplains or other clergy on staff to provide pastoral care. Hospital chaplains are people from various religious backgrounds and denominations who are ordained or consecrated for religious ministry and whose job it is to provide support and counsel to people who are very sick and their loved ones; it is *not* their job to preach or attempt to convert you. Chaplains are specially trained to provide pastoral care to people facing serious illnesses such as cancer and are typically available to see you whenever you are admitted for care. Especially if you have not established a relationship with a community of faith or with a particular religious leader or advisor, you may want to request a visit from a chaplain. Hospitals often have more than one chaplain on staff, so you may be able to state a preference for a chaplain from a particular faith tradition, request a male or female chaplain, or request another chaplain to visit you if the first one you see is not a good fit for you.

> "I called our clergy, a rabbi in this case, and the cantor in our synagogue, and we had late-evening talks with them about our feelings about what was going on, so turning to faith has been helpful for me and I think for Andrew."
>
> – Esther S.

Obviously, if you are a member of a faith congregation, your pastor, minister, priest, rabbi, imam, or other religious leader can help provide the pastoral care you need. Also, many communities of faith offer pastoral care programs staffed by laypersons trained as outreach ministers. You should contact your church, synagogue, temple, mosque, or house of worship to learn more.

When you ask for pastoral care, be clear what you want from the pastoral care expert who helps you. There are several things a pastoral care advisor can provide. Their efforts to meet your needs will be greatly enhanced if you can clearly identify what your needs are.

Among the most important parts of good pastoral care is providing what many call a "ministry of presence." One of the most distressing elements of a serious illness is the feeling of being alone and overwhelmed. Having a caring person to talk with who can really listen is a great gift. This kind of listening and presence is difficult for family and friends (who are worried themselves and may try to soothe their loved one/the person with cancer by avoiding difficult topics). Doctors, nurses, and other health care professionals often lack the time, training, or objectivity to be effective listeners. Their time and efforts are typically focused on the disease and its treatment. The pastoral care expert is able to focus on you as a person struggling with distress and spiritual concerns without having to be primarily concerned with your medical care. This "ministry of presence" is one of the most healing parts of good pastoral care.

"I'm what you call a crisis Christian. When I found out I had cancer, I thought well, my priorities, I've got to get closer to God about this, because the strength is gonna come from him, and so what I did was instead of reading *Redbook* or a novel or something, I started picking up the Bible. I think it has helped me to know that whatever happens, there's a plan for me. I don't know what it is, but obviously I'm around to fill the plan."

— Sally

"I'll never forget that he used to always tell me that, he'd say, 'When I die I'll be smiling because I'll see the angels.' And you know, I was with him when he died, and he did."

— Marilyn

A pastoral care expert can also provide other help and services to you, if you need them. Some people want to talk with a minister about religious conversion or reconciliation with their faith tradition or community of faith. An advantage of this kind of connection (or reconnection) is that a community of believers can help to provide emotional, social, and pastoral support for you. There may be a need to ask for forgiveness or participate in rituals of confession and absolution. Be careful to let your wishes be clearly known about these decisions. If you feel pressured to make a religious conversion or other decision with which you are not comfortable, or if you simply don't feel that the fit is good between you and a particular minister or chaplain, you should speak with another minister or chaplain.

You may want answers to some of the tough questions posed at the start of this chapter. You may want support and companionship at particularly stressful times (such as diagnostic tests or surgical procedures). You may want to ask others to offer prayers for you or bring elements of worship services to you if you are not able to attend services in person.

When facing serious or advanced illness, many desire a closer connection with God or a higher spiritual power. Typically, this is within the context of a faith tradition (such as Christianity, Judaism, or Islam), but not always. You may be curious how to strengthen this connection. You may desire instruction on devotional practices like prayer. You may want to work on meditation. If you desire to strengthen your connection to God, a chaplain or minister can provide help and instruction to meet your needs.

The overall goal of pastoral care is healing and whole-ness. Healing in this sense is not the same as cure but has more to do with feeling whole and at peace on the inside, in the spirit. It is quite possible to die healed. Pastoral care in advanced illness aims to achieve this goal.

FINDING THE RIGHT PERSON TO TALK WITH

Part of finding someone trustworthy to talk with about spir-itual matters is finding someone who will allow you to ask the tough questions. This trustworthy person will allow you to ask what you need to ask without making you feel bad for asking, without trying to change the subject, and with-out giving you quick, pat answers. In fact, there may not be any easy answers for your tough questions. Still, it is often very helpful to search for answers with the help and advice of someone else. If there is a pastoral care expert or religious leader you know and trust, ask him or her to help you. If you don't already know someone, ask around. Others from your faith tradition likely know a trustworthy and knowledgeable minister. Or you can ask a trusted friend or member of your health care team if there is some-one they would recommend. Paying attention to your spiritual life is an impor-tant part of your overall care. Don't be afraid to ask for help if you believe your spiritual life is not receiving the attention it deserves.

Religion

Religion is a certain kind of spirituality—one that takes place within the con-text of an organized system of beliefs and provides explanations for questions about the human condition, its origins, its purpose, and its future. Religion plays an important role in the lives of many Americans. According to a recent Gallup poll, despite the fact that Americans are generally less religious than they were a half a century ago, 95 percent of those surveyed said they believed in God, 68 percent said they belonged to a religious institution, and 58 percent said religion was "very important in life."

MAINTAINING FAITH

For believers, it is often a great challenge to maintain a trusting relationship with God when it becomes clear that an illness will not be cured. The believer may have been hoping and diligently praying for a cure. The fact that the cure may not be forthcoming may leave the believer feeling let down, deserted, or betrayed by God. He or she may think "I trusted God to heal me, and now that trust is broken." In this situation, feelings of anger toward God are very common and can be complicated by feelings of guilt for blaming God. Other believers may feel unworthy of physical healing or cure or feel that their advancing illness is evidence that their faith was not strong enough to obtain physical healing from God. Any of these situations may threaten the integrity of a believer's faith. This kind of faith crisis can be very distressing and often becomes a significant source of suffering in itself.

> "I don't care what beliefs someone has, I just hope that they have some belief. Because I really never lost faith, and I never questioned why this was happening to me. I've always just known that everything happens for a reason….That faith and trust, I don't know, is just really what keeps you going."
>
> – Jo Ann

If you feel like you have lost or might be losing your religion, first, ask yourself if keeping or regaining your faith is something important to you, something you want. If you're grappling with this issue in the first place, the answer is probably "yes." A trustworthy minister, priest, rabbi, or imam can help, whether or not you want to be connected or reconnected to a faith community or practice your faith. The key to settling this question may have largely to do with regaining the ability to trust.

CONNECTING (OR RECONNECTING) WITH A COMMUNITY OF FAITH

If you have decided to join (or rejoin) a community of faith (such as a church, synagogue, temple, mosque, or other house of worship), a member of the clergy can help guide you. You may want to participate in worship services, religious education or study, group prayer, or other activities of the faith community. You may want other members of the community to pray for you; this is called intercessory prayer. You may benefit from some of the ministries of the community—ministries aimed at helping those in all kinds of need. You may want to find ways to serve others in partnership with other members of the faith community.

"At first I was just shocked, and emotionally all I could think about was, you know, cancer—the things I was going to miss. Spiritually I was really mad at God, but then I realized, you know, God didn't do this. That He's going to help me through it and be stronger in the end to hopefully help someone else down the road. I don't understand why this happened, and I may never understand, but I think it has made me a stronger person for what I have been through this past 6 months. It's truly made me appreciate every moment I have with the ones that I love. I also know that through the prayer and support of all my friends and people that don't even know me that were praying for me, that helped me through the hard times, the dark moments when you feel like it's just never going to end."

— Carolyn H.

"I was what you might call a lapsed Catholic, and as I was going through chemotherapy, I had these days where I felt rather weak or nauseous or whatever, the side effects were actually relatively insignificant, I mean they were not anything really severe. I felt that my faith got me through those. I would start off every day by going to mass, and I felt that was just a great way of getting the strength to get through the day and at the same time, kind of saying thank you that I was still around and that I had the opportunity to even be there. So I think that it helped me. It was an incredible source of strength for me."

— Dan

There are a variety of ways to connect. You may be able to attend services and activities at the facility where the congregation meets. Alternatively, many congregations bring elements of the worship service to health care facilities or the homes of people who are not able to attend regular worship services. Clergy or other members of the congregation can suggest or provide study materials or projects that can use your talents, join you in study or prayer, or provide support and instruction for spiritual growth. Many congregations offer resources for study, growth, and worship—including recordings of worship services—via radio, television, or the Internet. Additionally, connection to a community of faith may provide new relationships with other people who can give loving, caring support to you.

"I am one of those with an inquiring and scientific mind. I think that blind faith, the faith of a child, was hard for me. And when some well-meaning individuals would say, 'God doesn't give these fights unless you're strong enough to handle it.' I'd say, 'Not my God. He didn't do this.' But it made me delve into the Bible. Gosh, I've gotten so much stronger. I'm talking about things more, and I'm learning more, and everything that I've learned just gets me stronger. But...
I still question a lot of things."

— Lisa E.

"I met Joan in a synagogue, and I didn't know that she wasn't Jewish. I'm Jewish and one of her dearest wishes was to be converted, and every time she would start to take a class for conversion then she would get sick again. So the last summer that she was still alive, a friend of ours got her rabbi certificate and she made it her job to make sure that Joan became converted, and so Joan was able to go through that, and she had a real, the whole orthodox conversion. And so she died Jewish, which was one of her dearest wishes."

— Susan T.

Conclusion

Paying attention to the spiritual and religious parts of your life can help you come to terms with the reality of your mortality, deal with your fears, and achieve a sense of inner peace that can be a great help and comfort. A number of areas may deserve attention, including finding and preserving meaning in life, holding on to the sustaining power of hope, making the most of this time as a period of growing and learning, and finding inner peace.

Establishing and strengthening connections to trusted others and—for religious believers—religious leaders, a community of faith, and God or a higher supernatural power, can facilitate spiritual growth. Your story and your journey can be enriched by attention to these matters as you search for meaning, connection, hope, and peace at the end of life.

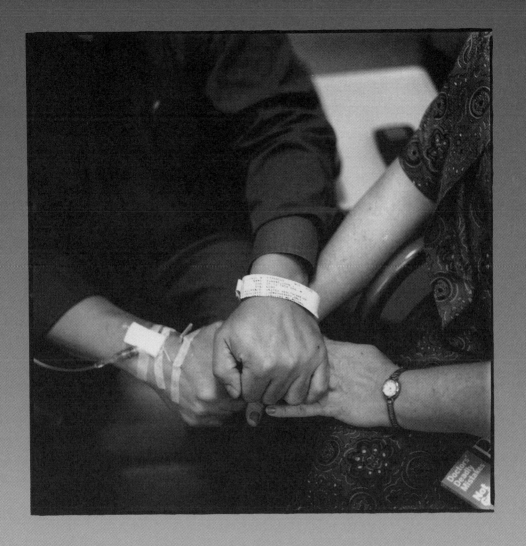

Chapter 11

Learning to Be a Caregiver

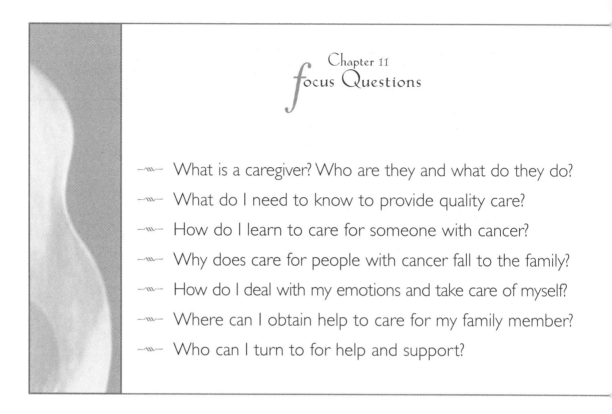

Chapter 11
*f*ocus Questions

—∽— What is a caregiver? Who are they and what do they do?

—∽— What do I need to know to provide quality care?

—∽— How do I learn to care for someone with cancer?

—∽— Why does care for people with cancer fall to the family?

—∽— How do I deal with my emotions and take care of myself?

—∽— Where can I obtain help to care for my family member?

—∽— Who can I turn to for help and support?

"The word 'caregiver' is a new word, and I never considered myself as a caregiver. I never even thought of it from that standpoint, and I'm sure these other people did not either. It's just a matter of: that's your loved one, that's your wife, or that's your son, or that's your daughter. You do what you have to do and your life goes on."

— Don

LEARNING TO PROVIDE CARE FOR SOMEONE during a serious illness or at the end of life can be complex and require entry into an unfamiliar world. Most people are very prepared through other life experiences to care for a sick or injured child, but caring for an adult, parent, spouse or partner, or sibling with advanced cancer can be a very different experience. Questions arise everyday—how to respect the wishes of the individual, how to make time in the day for all the new tasks, how to fit in time for yourself and avoid burnout, and what to do if the person resists the help you offer. In this chapter, we'll look at who caregivers are and what they do, discuss the process of learning to care for someone with advanced cancer, and address common questions and concerns caregivers often have.

Types of Caregivers—
Who They Are and What They Do

When we talk about *informal caregivers*, we generally mean family caregivers and the network of unpaid people who help with caregiving tasks on a day-to-day basis. Informal caregivers include spouses or partners, adult children, siblings, and extended family members, as well as neighbors, friends, and volunteers from the community or from your house of worship.

The professional staff members in agencies, hospice organizations, and hospitals (doctors, nurses, health aides, social workers, and allied health professionals like physical therapists) are often called *formal caregivers*. Most often, a combination of informal and formal caregivers will provide care for a person with advanced cancer.

Formal Caregivers

Formal caregivers rely on the ability and generosity of informal caregivers to perform a wide range of active caregiving tasks. They often teach specific skills to family members or loved ones who take responsibility for caring at home. Many informal caregivers learn to use medical equipment, manage medications, and even prepare and deliver special feedings through tubes after being instructed by formal caregivers. The professionals who teach informal caregivers to manage medical equipment in the home may be home care nurses, physical or occupational therapists, or physicians.

Family or Informal Caregivers

> —※—
> "For me, caring for my mom was a joy."
>
> — Delores

There are an estimated 52 million people in the United States who are engaged in caregiving within the family. One-quarter of these caregivers provide care for a person who is 50 years old or over. The majority deal with Alzheimer's disease, HIV-AIDS, debilitation and aging, and a variety of cardiovascular diseases. A smaller proportion is involved in caring for people with cancer. The actual number of people helping people with cancer is difficult to determine, since most national statistics are based on the level of disability and age rather than disease group.

An estimated 80 percent of home care services are provided by family members, usually a spouse or adult daughter. Approximately 3 out of 5 informal or family caregivers are female. The majority of family caregivers are older (ages 55 to 84), and the people they are caring for tend to be in the 55 to 84 age bracket as well. About half of those in the informal caregiver role are employed full or part time, which can cause scheduling difficulties at work or necessitate a leave of absence. These caregivers spend about 17 to 20 hours per week at their tasks and half of them have little or no outside help. The duration of caregiver activity depends on the diagnosis and the illness of the person for whom they are caring, but the average is 4.5 years. The value of these services to society has been estimated to be in excess of $196 billion.

The tasks performed by informal caregivers are quite diverse. The most common tasks include paying bills, driving to appointments, assisting with lifting and moving, dressing, bathing, toileting, and feeding.

WHY DOES CARE FOR PEOPLE WITH CANCER FALL TO THE FAMILY?

The health care system has changed a great deal over the past 20 years. Today, more medical care is delivered as an outpatient service. Also, patients stay in the hospital for a much shorter time and are discharged directly to the home even though they may not have fully recovered. In addition, cancer is a chronic disease or one that is managed over a long period of time. Some forms of cancer treatment (chemotherapy, for example) are also delivered in private doctors' offices, whereas years ago it would have been done at the hospital. These changes have all contributed to the increasing expectation that families will rise to the task of caring for members of their family when they are ill.

Caring for a family member at home still works well in some families but can be difficult when there are few family members nearby. During an earlier time in our history as a nation we tended to live closer to our roots. Families did not move so much and tended to cluster near the place where the larger family unit resided. This is no longer the case. Family members may be distributed all over a state or even in many parts of the country or the world. Home care services and hospice services may or may not be available in a specific geographic area, leaving the family to arrange for care and transportation for the patient's treatments.

"She expected from me, I think, a routine, regularity, being there, knowing that I would walk through that door, click, click down the hall, she would wait for my heels around 6 o'clock. And you know that I was to be there, not demanding, but it was a real sigh of relief when I would show up….So, I think it was more a routine and an expected reassurance….Or if she was bleeding, I knew which exact pads to get for her and she would expect me to show up with them. A certain kind of food if she could have…for instance, I would go to a certain ice cream store and get a milk shake for her, at the one hospital where she could have ice cream. And another friend offered to go get it, and she said, 'No. No. That's what Kate brings. Its fine, you know, I'll wait. Kate will show up with it at 6 o'clock.'

"These are things she expected of me. It wasn't demanding. It was more of a reassuring, a comfort level."

— Kate

Understanding Your New Role as a Caregiver

Only you can know if the effort you expend on behalf of another is a burden or an act of love and caring. Many people feel that caring for a family member during a long or difficult illness is a gift of love and part of the expectation that family members place on one another. Perhaps the person cared for you at one point in time and you consider your caring as repayment in kind. However you view this work, it will be yours to define, and the decision to be a caregiver will guide your behavior.

Preparing yourself for caregiving may seem daunting at first, but as you move into the role, you will find a pace that works for you. The repetition of tasks forms a routine, so that some of the work you perform will begin to seem quite natural. The most important challenge for many people is trying to decide which tasks they can do and which tasks they simply must give over to others. This decision also depends on the preferences of the person with cancer. For example, you may be willing to bathe your loved one, but he or she may not want you to be the one to help them with this task.

The Division of Labor

The majority of people receiving care are willing to allow immediate family members, extended family, and sometimes close friends perform certain kinds of tasks. Yet other tasks are simply too personal to allow anyone but the closest relative to perform. Life in your household will be easier if you and the person for whom you are caring make conscious decisions about who will be allowed to do certain personal tasks and who should be assigned to do more common tasks and errands. It may be helpful for you and your loved one to go through the list of potential tasks in Figure 11-1 (see page 244) and jointly consider names of people you might ask to help in those areas. Consider your role, the role of family members, friends, loved ones, neighbors, volunteers from community services or your house of worship, and paid professionals. You will still need to find out if that person is willing to perform the task, but this exercise will help you to understand the nature of the work ahead and will open up communication about the division of labor of caregiving tasks. Some of the items on the list may not be an issue at the present time, because the person with cancer may not require help with those tasks. You can always return to another version of the list later as the situation changes or as disease progresses.

The Needs of Caregivers and People With Cancer

People—both caregivers and people with cancer who are receiving care—describe their needs in various ways, sometimes in terms of services that would make life easier and at other times in terms of deficits or things that are missing. The needs of both groups overlap. The most commonly expressed needs of people receiving care include: psychological and emotional support, informational support, physical and social support, management of daily life, and help figuring out who they are once they have cancer. The most commonly expressed caregiver needs include: psychological support and information, specific skills to provide appropriate care, management of household duties, management of daily living, and respite (relief from caregiving responsibilities).

These needs fit into categories that represent aspects or dimensions of quality of life. Psychological and emotional support would represent one aspect, social support another, physical support another, and perhaps spiritual support the fourth.

Figure 11-1.

Identification of Tasks of Caregiving
and Individuals Who Could Help

Task	Effort that it requires	Persons I might allow to help
HOUSEHOLD TASKS		
Shopping – groceries	Car/driving/ money exchange	
Laundry – bed linens, towels	Carry items up and down stairs	
Laundry – personal items	Carry items up and down stairs	
PERSONAL TASKS		
Help me downstairs	No handrails/support	
Help me eat		
Prepare food, cook	Use microwave oven and kitchen appliances	
Dressing		
Changing the bed	Bending/lifting	
MEDICAL ERRANDS		
Drive to appointment	Car/driving	
Pick up pharmacy order	Car/driving/ money exchange	

People with cancer and their caregivers routinely indicate that they wish they had more help coping with their own emotional response to cancer. This help or support may come in the form of a friend offering assurance that good decisions are being made about life and health care. (See chapter 4 for more on coping strategies.) Physical support is usually seen as helping with everyday living and tasks around the house, or perhaps helping a person with cancer dress or move about. Social support can be chatting and spending time with friends and family members. Spiritual support might be a shared understanding about values and belief systems.

The way people with cancer feel about what happens around them (physically and psychologically), and their sense of whether their needs are being met affects their perception of quality of life. People who are experiencing pain or fatigue or who are feeling down in the dumps may feel as if life is not very good. This is true of caregivers too. This underscores the necessity for good support for both caregivers and the family member who receives their care.

Establishing Standards for Caregiving

It will be important to establish standards for caregiving in your home. If others are to provide part of the care or all of it during certain hours, then you should predetermine what level of quality, training, and excellence is required. Factors that will affect these standards include the family economic situation including job responsibilities; the potential toll on other family members' time and attention; and caregivers' diminished social engagement with friends and neighbors. If you use paid help, it will be important to write a simple job description listing work to be accomplished and the level of competency to which you expect the tasks will be performed. Workers in your home will appreciate your effort to help them serve the person with cancer in the most helpful manner.

Educating Yourself

Although some people seem to have naturally caring personalities, very few people have extensive knowledge about how to provide quality care for someone with advanced cancer. In this section you will learn information about the roles that caregivers often play in the life of a loved one with cancer. You will learn about the information needs of people who are caregivers, potential sources of information, how doctors use treatment goals, how you might assist the physician by paying attention to details of your loved one's condition (physical functioning, mental functioning, pain and other important symptoms), and how you could communicate your impressions to the physician.

> "They [the health care staff] did not properly prepare me for the role as care-giver other than the medical side of it. Cleaning her ports, maintaining a clean apartment, keeping things germ free, monitoring the medications, etc. So as far as the role of caregiver, I guess emotionally, no there wasn't any preparation for that….[It was] baptism by fire. It was just, when she came home, just bouncing off what she needed basically. You know, if she needed help to the bathroom, you're there for her to lean on, that kind of thing. It was almost like autopilot. You just sort of just snap into what the person needs."
>
> — Kate

Informing Yourself About the Disease

You will discover that your need for information about the type of cancer your loved one has will change over time, usually intensifying as the disease progresses. You may want to prepare yourself so that you understand the facts about cancer (the disease itself, as well as treatments and side effects), where to obtain correct information, and how the information will affect your deci-sions. You should also consider your preferred method of obtaining/receiving information. Some people prefer to receive print or electronic information while others like a verbal exchange. (See chapter 3 for more information on gathering information and making informed medical decisions. See chapter 8 for information about managing disease-related symptoms.)

Many people are still quite uncomfortable with the term "cancer," especially when the prognosis suggests that cure is no longer likely. If this is the case for you, then you will need to assess how you might become better informed and thus more helpful to your loved one. Sometimes just learning about the available palliative care options is enough to help you readjust your perspective. Your ability to gather correct medical information is essential to your own sense of control and can enable you to be more helpful and reassuring to the person for whom you are providing care.

Gathering Information About Important Topics

The information needs of primary caregivers of people with cancer vary. Some of the most critical information needs caregivers express include the following topics: prognosis, how common cancer treatments like chemotherapy work, how to manage disease-related symptoms and side effects of treatment, how to provide psychological support to the person with cancer, how to deal with an emergency, and what to expect after a particular treatment.

TERMINOLOGY

One important element in acquiring new information is to understand the definition of the terms. You will find your task of gathering information far simpler once you master some of the vocabulary relating to advanced cancer and its treatment and care. To start, you can use the glossary in this book to obtain definitions and then look up topics in the index. Other sources are also listed in the References and Resources section. Never hesitate to ask the professionals on your health care team to explain terms they use or that you have read about that you don't understand.

EQUIPMENT

Another topic that becomes important to people who provide care for a person with cancer at home is the equipment that is often used to support people who are ill. You may be assisting the person in performing daily living tasks such as bathing, dressing, and moving about in the house. If you need to learn about wheelchairs or other devices and equipment, it is important to learn how to use them safely. Training could be available through the home care nursing staff, the company representatives that deliver the equipment to your home, or a rehabilitation specialist whom you might use as a consultant. See chapter 6 for further information on home care services and reimbursement.

Treatment Goals

Another topic of great importance has to do with treatment goals. Physicians usually have different treatment goals and expectations for treatment outcomes depending on the type of disease, its stage, and its response to other treatments. (See chapter 2.)

You will need to understand how the physician views the current medical care and treatment goals of your loved one. You and the person with cancer should be clear on the goals of any treatment the health care team is recommending. For example, are they hoping to use treatments for purposes of cure or solely for comfort, or is the treatment intended to deliver a combination of objectives?

As we have discussed in other parts of this book, as disease progresses and cure seems less and less likely, the emphasis of treatment will shift from curative to palliative. The goal at the end of life is generally to diminish suffering, to decrease symptoms, and to improve quality of life through supportive care. Many caregivers are confused by this shift and fail to ask sufficient questions to identify the goals until it is obvious that the end of life is growing near. People who are unclear whether the treatment their loved one is receiving is curative or palliative (or some combination thereof) should ask for clarification.

Being a Helpful Part of the Health Care Team

The informal or family caregiver wears many hats. In addition to providing care and support for your loved one, you will be called upon to play an important role as an unofficial member of the health care team. Especially as you loved one's health deteriorates, you will be partially or fully responsible for reporting to his or her doctors about symptoms, responses to treatments, and emerging health-related problems.

Reporting Changes in Condition

Measures of health status are routinely used in medical care. Each of us is accustomed to reporting how we feel or describing changes in our physical condition. As a caregiver, you can offer assistance to the person with cancer and his or her doctor by keeping track of some simple measures of health status and the changes you observe. Changes in health status are usually meaningful and should be brought to the attention of doctors and other health care providers. When you notice changes in function or appearance, you may want to report them at the next clinic visit. Occasionally these changes are alarming and will require immediate attention.

Health status measures cover a range of topics including appearance; vital signs (temperature and blood pressure); physical health (symptoms); mental health and emotional responses; and key indicators, such as pain, of possible worsening of the condition. The following overview will provide you with basic information on some of these topics.

PHYSICAL WELL-BEING

Reporting changes in the physical health of your loved one is an important role for you to assume. There are times when your opinion of the severity of symptoms will be important to the doctor and may indicate that a treatment needs to be changed. Once the treatment has been altered you may need to report whether it is working well.

Physical Symptoms

A comprehensive description of physical symptoms that people with advanced cancer commonly experience can be found in chapter 8. These symptoms include pain, shortness of breath, difficulty urinating, and constipation or diarrhea. Fatigue is also a common problem both during curative treatment efforts and later in the course of the disease. These physical symptoms should be reported so that medical treatment can be started promptly.

Some symptoms may become obvious to the caregiver, yet the person with cancer may not complain. For example, pain is one important symptom that can be managed in 9 out of 10 cases, yet people often fail to obtain the relief that is available. People with severe illnesses may be reluctant to report these symptoms as they worry that the admission of the presence of such a problem confirms their worst fear, that the cancer has grown worse. People with severe illnesses like cancer, especially men and individuals from certain cultures, may feel that their responsibility is to remain strong and stoic and not show pain, which they may interpret as a form of frailty. But reporting the symptoms is really the only way the physician in charge may know to intervene and make everyone more comfortable. It is important to remember that palliative care is all about comfort.

Functional Capacity

One formal way that health care professionals assess the overall physical functioning of patients is to rate the person's *functional capacity* (their ability to move around and care for themselves). One scale that is frequently used in the clinical setting is called the Eastern Cooperative Oncology Group (ECOG) scale. The categories are simple to use and are displayed in Figure 11-2 on page 250.

Figure 11-2.

A Measure of Physical Functioning

Eastern Cooperative Oncology Group (ECOG) Measure of Physical Functioning

0   Able to carry out normal activities without restriction

1   Ambulatory – capable of light work, restricted with strenuous activity

2   Ambulatory – capable of self-care, but unable to work

3   Resting in bed/chair more than half waking hours, only capable of limited self-care

4   Totally confined to bed/chair, not capable of any self-care

Source: Burns CM, Dixon T, Broom D, Smith WT, Craft PS. Family caregiver knowledge of treatment intent in a longitudinal study of patients with advanced cancer. *Supportive Care in Cancer.* July 26, 2003; 11:10:629-637.

MENTAL AND EMOTIONAL FUNCTIONING

A person's mood is a reflection of their physical comfort, their general perception of quality of life, and their coping capacity. Although many people with cancer adjust and cope well with their disease, the whole cancer experience can create distress and challenge even the most optimistic person. Maintaining a positive outlook on life may not be essential to survival, but it can help you and your loved one live well for the days that remain.

People who display distress and show symptoms of altered mental functioning (such as depression, anxiety, or confusion) may require medical intervention. These signals are very important to report, and yet many people tend to ignore them or accept them as part of the disease. Refer to chapter 12 for further information on how to recognize these changes in mood and functioning in the person for whom you are caring. It is worth noting here that both people with cancer and the people who care for them are at greater risk for depression and anxiety; the important information in chapter 4 can help you cope with these conditions, whether it is you or your loved one who is experiencing them.

Keeping Good Records

Keeping track of when symptoms or problems occur is an important part of a caregiver's job. This task can be made easier if you maintain a log or journal of events in the course of your loved one's care. Designate a notebook for recording medication changes, test and clinic visit dates, and the results of treatment changes. If possible, attach dates to each of the entries and a note about who performed each procedure at the medical clinic.

You will be surprised at how helpful this record of medical care can be in the future. Our memory of events is often clouded by the pressures of more immediate tasks we must perform. Having an accurate journal entry can help enhance communication with and among the health care team, can help you track the course of your loved one's response to a certain treatment or intervention, and can even provide solid evidence for any insurance disputes or reimbursement questions in the future.

Understanding the Needs and Preferences of Your Loved One

Caring for a person with cancer is not only about observing physical signs and symptoms. It is about making a caring connection with that person and providing care in a way that reassures them that they will not be abandoned and respects their unique needs and personal preferences.

Autonomy and Independence

Retention of autonomy and control is important to most people and can become even more important to people with cancer because they may feel as though they have lost control over many aspects of their life. Discover the ways in which you as a caregiver can foster a renewed sense of your loved one's independence and control over choices. While the person with cancer may not be able to control his or her body's response to cancer, they can still exercise their autonomy in a number of ways. Each day presents opportunities to allow the individual to express personal choices, perhaps through the food chosen for a meal or for music that is played in the background in the home. These choices are the very reason that home is so comforting.

—ɯ—

"Well, I found that one of the things that's the easiest is to kind of go by the flow of the conversation with the person with cancer. You want to do everything for them, but sometimes they don't want to be hovered over. So you have to really listen and be careful as to how you approach them and do things for them. And that's a tough thing to do. But as you listen to them more closely and really pay attention to what they're saying, I think it helps you to know what's the right thing to do at the right time. It's a very difficult time."

— Patricia

Another way you can show your respect for your loved one's autonomy is to support the person's decisions about advance care directives, planning a funeral, and leaving behind a legacy.

Providing Opportunities to Do Things Your Loved One Enjoys

A person's sense of overall wellness can be directly affected by mood. You can boost your loved one's mood and contribute to his or her happiness by trying to provide opportunities for your loved one to do things he or she enjoys. For example, even if your loved one is too ill to leave the bed, he or she can still be a part of family mealtime. It is not essential to eat in the kitchen or dining room. Try placing a small table near the bedside so the entire family can gather and share stories about the way the day was spent. Another idea is to create space for favorite games or crafts that can be enjoyed by the entire family.

Consider using the newly created multipurpose table during another part of the day to help your loved one write correspondence to old friends or assemble a life-review scrapbook. Make certain the materials needed for projects he or she is interested in are stored in an easily accessible area of the room.

Balancing Work and Caregiving

If you work outside the home, maintaining your job as a wage earner may be essential to help pay for medical care for your loved one, to maintain insurance

"Wendy was a very independent person and so [providing her care] was kind of trying to learn to balance that with what she would want to do on her own. So she basically taught me what she would need help with. It was helping her with her activities of daily living, like assist with toileting, with bathing. There was a home health aide that would do some of that, but she wasn't there all the time. You would get a few hours a day, kind of thing. Helping her get dressed, helping her at night. Sometimes it was kind of being around for her 14-year-old daughter to have someone to talk to. It was definitely shared, like I said, with her mom and with friends. Cooking—which wasn't exactly my forté—and driving her places, taking her to the doctor. Her friends made a calendar and they all signed up, and so the paths were kind of rotated."

— Joanne

coverage for your loved one, and/or to ensure your own financial security in the future. Work may also be an important part of your identity and may provide success and positive reinforcement for you. For whatever reason, it is important that you find a way to balance your roles as a caregiver and a wage earner.

It may be important to keep usual schedules at work, maintain a presence at work, and keep disruptions of work schedules and routines to a minimum. Some employers are very empathic and allow workers to arrange flexible hours or split the workday. Others are not able to make these accommodations due to the nature of the work and the worksite. As many as a third of working caregivers leave their jobs to shift their responsibilities to the caregiving tasks. The majority of caregivers who work outside the home indicate that they are able to come to work late or leave early in order to take their family member to a care site. Some people reorganize career goals to care for a family member, and others arrange with employers to spend one month in the caregiving role with special accommodations for hours and then alternate to full time work the next month on the job. Most employers try to accommodate the family needs for a time. If the changes in schedule affect work productivity or the morale and work ethic of the other employees, then the employer may ask that other solutions be found.

"I tried to let my immediate supervisor know what I was going through. He wasn't the most caring, compassionate person in the world. So at one point when I had been at the hospital all night, at 9 o'clock in the morning I called him to say, 'I'm not at work. I'm still at the hospital.' He was so cold to me that I sought out someone else. I went above his head to his boss, and I said if I ever have to call out, or I'm in a situation like this, may I come to you and not deal with him. Because I just can't deal with the added stress and coldness from someone. Which was fine, and the supervisor said that's just fine with him. But it did make it harder to concentrate during the day. As soon as I would get out of a session, I would run to the phone and call Michelle and say, 'Are you okay? What's going on? How's your day?' So it was hard, it was juggling and trying to stay focused."

— Kate

Employer Support

Some corporations are beginning to develop special programs to support working caregivers. Research conducted during the 1990s demonstrated that the cost of caregiving is also borne by employers through lost productivity. At the time the study was reported, the costs per employee were estimated at $2,500. When this figure is extrapolated to a national level, it could amount to over $20 billion.

Effective programs at work might include information on local resources and counseling services in addition to flexible work hours. Specific workplace programs for caregivers of adult family members are somewhat rare; those that do exist are usually located in large corporations.

Government Support

The Family Medical Leave Act (FMLA) passed by Congress in 1993 enables many people to leave the job for a time to provide care and later return to their position. FMLA allows many (but not all) employees to take 12 weeks of unpaid leave per year if they themselves are sick or to care for an infant, newly adopted child, or immediate family member who is seriously ill. Companies must continue to provide health insurance while employees are on leave, and companies must guarantee that the employee will return to either the same job or another position with equal status, salary, and benefits.

"Caregiving kind of turned my life upside down! It was my last semester in graduate school for social work, and I was doing an internship in a hospital and I was going to classes. Here I was with my partner being very, very sick and kind of immediately paralyzed on her left side. So in addition to the cancer diagnosis, she also was pretty much in a wheelchair right after the surgery. So there was part of me that went to my advisor—I remember saying, 'I can't finish school right now. I'm just going to have to put this on hold.' I just was very overwhelmed. The academic institution that I went to and the institution I was doing my placement at, they were both very supportive, and they said, 'Let's sit down and figure out how this can work. How you could do what you want to do with Wendy and for Wendy and also continue with your life.' And so we just stretched [my coursework] out a bit….My faculty advisor talked to my professors, and my professors were great. They basically encouraged me to come to class when I could, and I turned in my papers, but I got extensions on everything. In my field placement I reduced my hours and then just did it through the summer. For instance, they would let me come in at 11 or noon and work to 7. So that gave a chance to wait for the home health aide to come before I left Wendy, because she couldn't be alone."

— Joanne

Companies with fewer than 50 employees are exempt from FMLA regulations. To be eligible, you need to have worked for the company for at least one year and have clocked 1,250 hours in the last 12 months.

Coping With the Stresses of Caregiving

The tasks of caregiving are many, and at times they may engender feelings of inadequacy, fear, frustration, and resentment. There are people who assume the role of caregiver without realizing how time consuming and difficult it can become. Often as the illness progresses, the caring demands increase in both effort and time. All of these factors can cause stress.

Stress is the response of the body and mind when we are overwhelmed by factors that are out of our control. It may be the result of daily frustrations, indecision, or simply physical exhaustion. Clues to your own response to stressful events may be found in an impaired ability to sleep well, maintain a clear train of thought, and feel cheerful. The responses to stress during the caregiving experience can be quite extreme. It is important to find out the cause of the strain in the situation and correct it if possible. Whatever the cause of the stress, the first step toward managing it is acknowledgment. The second step is to create a plan to deal with it.

Causes of Stress Responses

When attempting to identify the causes of your stress, consider the following factors:

1. Your usual coping style, or how you typically respond to feelings of stress at other times in your life.
2. The situation of your caregiving, and whether it was voluntary or you were persuaded to do it.
3. The amount of care the person with cancer in your family actually requires; sometimes it is more than you should do alone.
4. Other options open to you, such as whether there are other family members who could help if asked.
5. Your willingness to request help from others.

Exploring these factors may help you identify and acknowledge the stress response. The next step is to create a plan to decrease the stress response.

Decreasing Stress

You may be able to decrease stress by reversing the situation you identified in the acknowledgement steps. Other options are to establish some goals and realistic timetables for doing new tasks. Identify the tasks that are the least appealing and that another person might do. Ask for the help you need, and if possible, find a formal, paid helper to do some of the least appealing work. Changes in a few items on your list can change your day. The fact that you initiated the change and developed the plan will reinforce your sense of control.

People who can acknowledge their emotional response to a stressful situation may do better than others. Caregiving can generate some powerful emotions and can be a good opportunity for you to look inside yourself. For example, you may feel anger at having to deal with the care of another, frustration with the inability to do it, and/or grief that you are losing the person despite all of the care you deliver. All the feelings are legitimate; dealing with them in a forth-right manner may help you maintain your emotional equilibrium.

Taking Care of Yourself

Consider who must come first on the priority list. Try to identify why you are important. Usually people conclude that they must care for themselves in order to stay healthy and manage the care of another. It is not a selfish act to care for yourself when you are caring for another. It is imperative! You need to renew your health, sleep, and adjust your thinking in order to face another day and fulfill your role. Failure to address your own needs can lead to added frustration, stress, and inability to function at your best.

Making Time for You

Carve out some hours or minutes each day to attend to some of your own needs. This may mean simply going grocery shopping or sitting quietly to read, listen to music, or perhaps do some task such as paying the household bills.

Staying healthy depends on retention of some degree of focus on self. You still need to interact with friends and family, go to a movie if possible, and continue to enjoy even brief respites away from the planning and caregiving tasks. Your social engagement with other people helps you to stay focused in the present. Maintain contact with people. Isolation will not serve you well in the long term, since you will need all of your friends and acquaintances later, when you could be alone. Picking up on lost connections and relationships later is much more difficult than maintaining friendships. Make time to initiate phone calls as well as to return them. People will appreciate your efforts to keep them apprised of the events in your household, and you will alleviate their need to ask "How is everything?" when they fear that things are not going well. You may also want to appoint one person to be a contact individual that everyone can call for information when you are particularly busy. This strategy has worked well for people who work full time and still manage a household with a seriously ill family member.

Sometimes you will have to acknowledge that you cannot do it all. When you need to get away and take time for yourself, consider the possibility of respite care (someone who can help with caregiving responsibilities). We'll talk more about respite care later in this chapter.

—⁂—

"When I had my cancers, everybody was worried about me. I had church groups praying for me….And one day my wife had to go to the doctor because she was very sick. She came home from the doctor, and I asked her, 'Well, what was it? What did Doc say?' And she said, 'I don't know. We never got to me. All they ever did was talk about you.'

"And I've thought this over the years….I had the doctors and nurses, specialists, God, you know, all the prayers working for me, but my family—my wife and my children—didn't have anybody working for them. And it finally dawned on me that when somebody goes, 'Hey, Jeff, how are you doing?' I go, 'Hey, I'm doing fine, but ask my wife and my kids how they're doing, and honestly ask them, 'Hey, do you need anything? How are you feeling?' Because they're going through more than you are, because most of the time, when you're going through cancer—a major cancer—you know, they've got you so messed up on different medicines you don't know what's going on all the time. But the family is the one that's dealing with it 24 hours a day."

— Jeff

Eating Well

Another issue you must attend to is your diet. There is no question that you will be under stress if you are a caregiver. It will be critical to watch your weight and be certain you are eating a well balanced diet. You may have to prepare special food for the person with cancer and other food for yourself. Remember that the household runs well when you are healthy, so eating well is just as critical for you as it is for the person with cancer. If you are unable to prepare all of the food yourself due to time constraints, consider asking a friend or relative to make special food for you as well as for the person with cancer.

Exercise

Exercise and physical activity should not be ignored. Go for a walk or ride your bike several times each week, perhaps once a day. The time is well spent, as you need to stay healthy and fit. You may think that you are already getting plenty of exercise as you take care of the needs of your loved one, but most of these activities are probably not aerobic.

—⁊⁊⁊—

"Take care of yourself first. You have to be healthy in mind and physically to be a good caregiver. I think that is the most important thing, because you don't want to give your loved one something to worry about. They already have enough worries without worrying about their caregivers. And I can't stress that enough: don't feel guilty when the time comes and you need space. You deserve it and you need it."

— Arlene

"I think that in order to be a good caregiver you have to take care of yourself, because you have to be strong, and emotionally if you're not upbeat, and with it, and capable of just rising to the occasion, then you're really a drag on the person who's ill. And so I think that you need to be shored-up in terms of getting enough sleep; in terms of eating properly; in terms of surrounding yourself with people who are good and positive for you."

— Mary Ann

Certain types of exercise—such a going for a walk, swim, or bicycle ride also give you an opportunity to get outside the house and enjoy a change of scene.

Finally, don't pass up exercise because you are too tired from caregiving to engage in it. On the contrary, regular exercise can energize you and provides numerous psychological benefits, including improved mood and relief from mild depression. Regular exercise can also help you sleep more soundly at night.

Sleep

Personal fatigue and overwhelming exhaustion near the end of life of a loved one can be a real problem. The tasks of caring for a very sick person can gradually increase in intensity and there may be little opportunity for a good night's sleep. Interrupted sleep patterns over many nights generally lead to feelings of exhaustion. Some people go through weeks being sleep deprived, and it can impact their ability to make good decisions and deliver good care. The feeling of exhaustion may even be a sign that the family caregiver needs professional help. Again, seeking respite help may be one way to diminish your stress, make the person for whom you are caring and the family comfortable, and ease the burden for all members of the informal caregiving network.

"It was like a 24-hour, 7-day-a-week marathon that I was running, with Nancy being the focus about 90 percent of the time. And people would come up to me and say, 'Oh, how are you doing?' 'I'm just fine, I'm just fine.' I sort of like pushed people away, and I didn't really allow myself to get in conversations about how I was personally doing, because I was more concerned about how Nancy was doing.

"And looking back on that, it was probably wrong for me to do that, because I think I could have used some help every now and then, you know. I'd get a little short tempered, but I would never do it in front of Nancy. I'd keep it to myself and then when I was on my way driving into work, I would like yell for no reason at all, just to get the anger out."

— Tim

Supportive Services

You may need support for the immense tasks that you assume as a caregiver, and you will likely need to turn to others for your own support at times. Sometimes people are surrounded by a large supportive family, but other caregivers with very small or distant families may be in need of finding support within the community. Since caregiving is a 24-hour job, even if you assume the lion's share of responsibility, you will probably need some additional help.

Most communities have many resources that are not apparent until you suddenly require them and begin your search. Revisit chapter 2 for a more detailed discussion of care options and places that deliver care to people with advanced cancer at end of life, including hospice programs, home care, and private personal care agencies.

You may also find that you need help not only delivering caregiving services, but that you also need psychological or emotional support for your caregiving. There are many potential sources of help where you can gather information and emotional support from other people and agencies. We'll cover some options here, but you can also ask the health care staff caring for your loved one with cancer; they can provide a referral to a psychiatrist, medical social worker, or psychologist.

Asking for Help

The decision to share caregiving tasks or shift responsibilities to others may be difficult. It can seem like an admission of defeat, but it is actually a demonstration of personal strength to identify those tasks you do best. Your loved one will get better care if you focus on the things you do best and have the energy to do and delegate other responsibilities to those who can help in specific areas. The sharing of tasks and coordination of caregiving work is essential for both patient and caregiver well-being, and grows more important toward the end of the life of the person with cancer.

Respite Care

As we've mentioned, caregiving can be a stressful responsibility, even while it provides reasons for happiness and satisfaction. Because the demands on caregivers can be so great, it is a good idea to become familiar with agencies and other resources that offer home care services, respite care, and even interval admission care for people who are very ill. Using formal services with professional staff or relying on friends or volunteers may enable you to take a few days off and renew your personal strength.

Respite help can provide you with a brief reprieve from your caregiving responsibilities. Whether for an hour, a day, a weekend, or a regularly scheduled visit, a trained professional can take over in your absence.

Agencies that place staff as personal assistants or caregivers often charge by the day, hour, or sometimes by the week, so you should request financial information before making any commitment to hire one of their staff. Check to see if your policy covers respite care before you proceed. You may also explore other care options to help spread around the caregiving responsibilities, so that you are not the only one providing care. For example, you may want to consider adult day care centers or live-in caregivers. Sometimes live-in helpers will accept a place to live in your home as a partial form of payment for their services.

It is not only important to explore the cost of this type of care, but also the training of the staff. Sometimes home health aides are extensively trained and sometimes they receive little or no training. They may have a minimal understanding of the type of cancer your loved one is facing or the tasks involved in meeting their needs. It is also vital to secure a background check, since you may leave the person in the company of your loved one and all your household possessions. Your local Office on Aging is one source that can help you find someone to assist.

Once you select a respite care worker or home health aide, it is important to determine the tasks you want to be accomplished. Establish a routine for the person to follow and write down telephone numbers to call in an emergency or in case of questions.

THE MEDICARE HOSPICE BENEFIT AND RESPITE CARE

If the person with cancer has qualified for and is receiving care under the Medicare hospice benefit, respite care may be provided in a Medicare-approved facility such as a freestanding hospice facility, a hospital, a nursing home, or some other long-term care facility. Under these circumstances, respite care is covered by Medicare for up to 5 days at a time.

Support or Education Groups

You can also find comfort, support, and information through groups designed for caregivers. Look for a group where members are dealing with problems similar to your own and where the leader is trained and well prepared. Look for resources within this book, or consult your health care providers and local hospital social work department for names and contacts. See the section on support groups in chapter 4 for more information on finding a support or education group that is right for you.

Since everyone reacts differently to speaking about his or her life in front of others, the support group experience is not for everyone. The support group concept is about sharing ideas, experiences, and feelings. Some people find it is safer and more comfortable to talk to people who do not know them well, while others may prefer the comfort of confiding in old friends.

Self-help Through Use of the Internet

Some caregivers are uncomfortable seeking support from a support group; others may not be able to attend a group meeting due to the demands of care. For these caregivers, the Resources section at the end of this book offers Internet sites that can be good sources of support and information for you and your family. You can find support through online chat rooms and message boards, and you can also use the Web to seek information about your loved one's disease, treatment and care options, and additional resources for you. Just be warned that all the information you read on the Web is not necessarily accurate or trustworthy information. Refer to page 86 of chapter 4 for tips on evaluating a Web site for credibility.

Spiritual/Religious Support

Spirituality refers to your individual belief system and interpretation of the meaning of life. As we discussed in chapter 10, you need not practice a religion to be spiritual. Many people consciously decide not to participate in a religious affiliation, yet have profound personal beliefs and internal strengths that enable them to lead a philosophical and spiritual life.

Spirituality is one method people use to come to clearer self-understanding; it can also be part of a helpful coping strategy. Just as people who know they have advanced cancer often call upon spirituality as a means of support, caregivers can benefit from spiritual reflections.

Religion and spirituality may provide feelings of hope, peacefulness, and meaning and may also provide a way for caregivers to deal with loss, to forgive themselves and others for not living up to former, perhaps unrealistic, expectations, and to continue life in the face of grief.

Religious guidance and spiritual support are also available through formal affiliations with clergy members or other religious leaders. Consult the hospital for a referral if you are not a member of a local house of worship. Cancer centers usually have pastoral care available for their patients and their loved ones and caregivers.

On a more pragmatic level, members or your local congregation or community of faith can be a source of support, providing meals and opportunities for respite care, helping with errands and household tasks, and even offering intercessory prayer.

Informal Sources of Support

Most people have extensive networks of friends and acquaintances that could be potential sources of support. If you are well connected in your building, neighborhood, or community, you are very fortunate—many of these friends will likely step forward to provide assistance and needed care. Refer to Figure

"I was very fortunate that one of the local hospitals has a very fine caregivers' support group, which meets every week. And I found that a godsend, because I could go there and I could be with people who were experiencing similar emotions, some of which we tend to feel guilty about. There's nothing calm about one's emotions when we're going through this. Sadness is certainly there, but along with that, there's guilt, there's anger, there's fear. Fear and sadness are socially acceptable. Anger is something that perhaps we don't expect in that kind of situation and we're a little concerned about expressing it, and I was able to go to the support group and find that others felt the same way. I could talk about my anger at being in this situation, at being extraordinarily weary, at being fearful, at being sorrowful…just the whole unruly, unfair ball of wax.

"And to be able to express that, and to find that it was very normal and was perfectly acceptable, and indeed, to be expected."

— Janet

11-1 on page 244 for some ideas of tasks you may want to delegate to friends and neighbors. Remember to give them the option of selecting the task they are most comfortable providing.

Don't forget to think about the other family members, friends, or acquaintances who have also been caregivers at some point in their life. They can be wonderful sources of support, because they can sympathize with what you're going through, and they may also be able to offer caregiving tips, strategies, or coping techniques that helped them during their caregiving experience.

Conclusion

People who serve in the caregiver capacity for someone they love frequently reflect on the experience with mixed emotions. The experience differs for each person who undertakes this act of loving care. There is a sense of relief once the task is over, but there is also a sense of joy at having the opportunity to make the days of a person's life more comfortable, more pleasurable, and happier. Perhaps there is some satisfaction in helping the person achieve their aspirations and realize their dreams or complete their life with dignity. There

> "Even when you feel so incredibly alone and like there is nowhere to go, you're not alone. There is someone else who is going through something or has gone through something similar. There are people out there who want to listen, and that can assure you that you will get through it. It's okay not to know how you're going to get through it....I think that one of the things for me was as a caregiver—especially the same-sex caregiver—sometimes you can feel very invisible, and just because you might feel that way, know that everything you're doing counts just so much and is just so valuable."
>
> — Joanne

may also be a sense of admiration for the person's strength and final sense of resolution. You may be surprised by the number of people who later tell you how much they admire your courage, generosity, and strength of caring.

Many former caregivers report that they have grown through the experience. Sometimes the growth seems to be spiritual, while others report a sort of growing up and becoming more responsible. You definitely learn things about yourself through the experience. It may be that this is the time you really grasp the full picture of your financial situation. Perhaps the caregiving enabled you to explore your beliefs and values, leading you to a more solid philosophy about life. Even if you learn to appreciate each day and value the lives and perspectives of others, you will probably agree that you learned through caring.

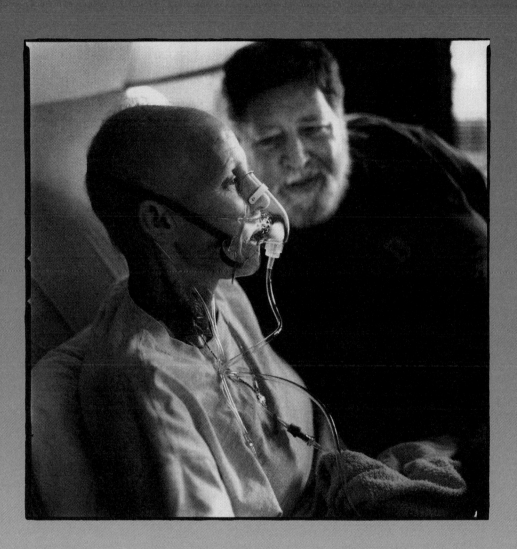

Chapter 12

Caregiving in the Final Days

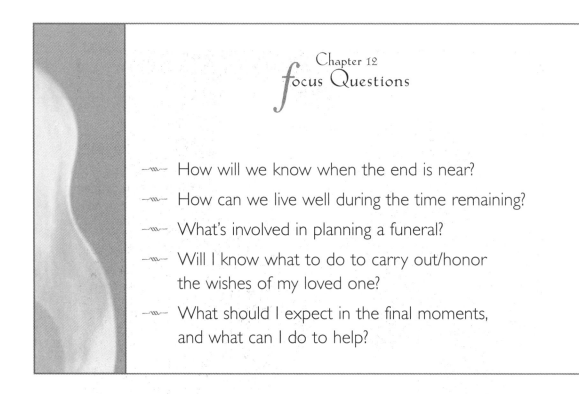

Chapter 12
*f*ocus Questions

—⫴— How will we know when the end is near?

—⫴— How can we live well during the time remaining?

—⫴— What's involved in planning a funeral?

—⫴— Will I know what to do to carry out/honor
the wishes of my loved one?

—⫴— What should I expect in the final moments,
and what can I do to help?

"As difficult as it sometimes can be emotionally to try to be part of a support system for someone who is dying…we all come away from these experiences having gained something and having grown and found our own lives enriched in some way. Even in the dying process. And perhaps going through that process with someone else takes some of that fear and mystery and sting out of the end of life."

— Dick

AS CANCER ADVANCES, THE FOCUS OF CARE SHIFTS toward making the person with cancer comfortable for the time that remains. There is rarely a clear demarcation or a single transition point between curative treatment and palliative care. Curative treatment is intended to alter the course of the disease, whereas palliative treatment alters the symptoms and disease manifestations. Sometimes one phase merges into the other and sometimes they coexist. When comfort becomes the primary focus of care, the transition is moving toward palliation.

How Will We Know
How Much Time Is Left?

Physicians may not raise the topic of the transition to end-of-life palliative care or openly discuss the amount of time a person with cancer has left unless the patient or caregiver asks directly about the prognosis. Asking specific questions helps, because it encourages openness and may facilitate planning for the remaining time. As we discussed in chapter 3 in the section on prognosis, doctors are rarely able to accurately predict the length of time remaining in a person's life. There are always some people who survive longer than predicted and some who survive for less time.

How Can We Live Well During
the Time That Remains?

Your role as a giver of care, love, and support will be increasingly important throughout this last phase of your loved one's illness. As you move through these remaining months, days, and hours, the number of tasks you take on may become greater or the tasks themselves may become more difficult. As you contemplate these challenges, know that there are many things you can do to ensure that you and the person you love live well and make the most of the time that remains. We'll discuss these things that you can do to improve both physical comfort and emotional well-being.

Physical Comfort

Providing for your loved one's physical comfort means controlling and managing symptoms from treatment and from the cancer itself and monitoring your loved one's ability to perform daily tasks and functions.

SYMPTOM MANAGEMENT

First, take care of the symptoms that appear. They not only diminish the overall sense of well-being but they can lead to psychological changes such as depression. Symptom management means reporting changes to the health care team and paying attention to things like pain, fatigue, and loss of

"I suddenly was doing things for her that she had done for me when I was a baby and always; showers—everything and trying to get her to eat. Three days before she died, we had a conversation, and I just looked at her and I said, 'Do you know who I am?' Because I wasn't sure she was understanding anything and she looked at me and she said, 'You're my mother.' That broke my heart. And then I said, 'Well, who are you?' And she said, 'I'm your daughter.' I waited a few minutes and I asked her again, and she said the same thing… it still kind of haunts me a little bit."

— Suhaila

appetite. These problems need to be reported promptly so that your health care team can provide appropriate care. Refer to chapter 8 for further detailed information about how symptoms are managed and what to look for in the person with cancer.

Functional Capacity

Second, pay attention and report any changes in the ability of the person with cancer to perform everyday activities. Most people nearing the end of life begin to focus attention on comfort rather than function. Following diagnosis, especially if the cancer is in an early stage, the person will probably be very functional and able to do most self-care or daily living activities and even go to work. Over time, subtle changes may occur: diminished appetite, gradual weight changes, or a decrease in energy and diminished interest in social engagement. Some cancers lead to rapid functional decline and death, whereas other cancers are slowly progressive and the person may remain functional for long periods. Later, toward the end of life, people with advancing cancer may become more introspective and sleep with greater frequency or for longer periods. This final period can also be marked by loss of function, acute weight loss, decreased ability to eat and drink, drowsiness, and in some cases confusion and delusional behavior. (See the section on What to Expect in the Final Moments and What You Can Do to Help beginning on page 278.)

—⁓—

"The cancer is definitely having an effect on me now, and a lot of times I need to lie down. And it doesn't mean that I don't want company around me or people around me, but it's like if I'm lying down it doesn't mean you need to go out grocery shopping or go and fix something or, you know—it means that you could sit there on the bed with me or just lie on the bed with me and be there, and sometimes to me that would be the most comforting thing, and it's one of those things I don't get. People have a tendency to, you know, like, 'Oh, she's not feeling well. Let me go do something. Let me go cook dinner.' Even though they know I won't eat it. Or, 'Let me go this place or that place,' or, 'Let me fix this.' And it's like, 'No! You don't have any idea how much comfort it would give for you to just be in the room with me.'"

— Karen

Emotional Well-being

Your loved one's declining physical health may be an opportunity for him or her (and for you) to strengthen emotional bonds. Attending to the emotional needs and psychological well-being of the person with cancer and listening to your own body's cues about the same things are important parts of being a good caregiver to someone nearing the end of his or her life. This might include providing opportunities for self-expression, reminiscing, planning for end of life, confirming social connections, and grieving.

Self-expression

Allow yourself and your loved one to express and experience a full range of feelings and encourage open discussion of topics you need to plan together. Sharing feelings and ideas will help you, the person with cancer, and others to feel freedom of expression. You will no doubt experience a broad range of emotions. It is healthy to experience laughter and sadness, and to reflect on the past and the value of long-term relationships. You may even begin conversations about your sense of loss and other feelings that arise as your loved one nears the end of his or her life. Stay active and verbally engage with other people. Caregivers who isolate themselves physically and emotionally

---㎅---

"My problem was that John was in denial from day one, and I did not get much help…I played the role of, 'John, we have to talk about this,' and I kind of put him on the spot by saying you know, 'We need to make arrangements. Your brother is out of state, your parents are out of state. What do you want me to do?' And he'd say, 'Do whatever you want to do.'"

— Arlene

are at greater risk for personal illness and unresolved grief that lasts for long periods. Revisit chapter 4 for additional discussion of the importance of self-expression as a coping mechanism.

Planning

Encourage your loved one to discuss plans for his or her final days, and begin the process of saying goodbye. Some people are very fortunate to have time to plan and say thanks and farewell to friends and family. Ask your loved one how he or she would like to be remembered or if there are special things to acknowledge about his or her life in a memorial service or funeral eulogy (see chapter 9).

Some important conversations should involve decision making around the topic of medical emergencies, life-saving interventions, and the desire to use resuscitation (see chapter 5). These are not easy topics to discuss or broach, but they are essential for any family facing the final months, weeks, or days of life.

Social Connections

Maintain as many connections with your friends, family, and neighbors as possible during this time. This will ensure that you distribute information about the progression of the illness to these people and it is an effective way to alert others to the needs of the family. Social interaction also provides affirmation for you as a caregiver, making it easier for you to carry the weight of your caring tasks. It is wise to remember that not all people act alike and some cannot visit or interact with you during this period. They may pull away due to their own inability to deal with the disease, the situation, or because they do not know exactly what to say or how to help.

"It was very hard. I had no help and she didn't want help from other people. And it was really—it was really hard on me to watch her day by day just slowly slip away. I have 2 brothers. One is in the South, but when he was here, he was with my other brother. Neither one of them liked to be around her. They would see her, but just for very short periods of time. Five minutes. At first everybody offered to help. Then there was just nobody. Other than her doctors and her nurses, nobody. Nobody wanted to see her with no hair. They really didn't like being around her. Then after chemo, she just basically slept all the time. So there was just—around the middle of July, she didn't even want me to leave the house. She just wanted me to stay with her."

— Suhaila

Reminiscing

Use the time you have together to think about life, remember what has always been of value to you, and share those values with one another. For example, you may want to look through old photographs together as a way to encourage reflection on important moments in your loved one's life. Or you may have videos that record family gatherings—perhaps you can use this time to review them. Encourage the person with cancer to revisit his or her high school or college yearbook to renew acquaintances with people from the past. Reflecting on a life well lived can be an important part of coming to terms with death—for both the caregiver and the person with cancer.

Grieving

Finally, allow yourself to grieve. Don't feel as though you need to postpone grieving until after your loved one's death. Grieving now can help acknowledge the reality of the situation and provide a healthy outlet for the many complex emotions you and your loved one are likely to experience at this time.

You and your loved one may even have begun the process of grieving as early as when cancer was first diagnosed. As death approaches, you are likely to experience something called *anticipatory grief*. During this grief process, which precedes the actual death, you begin to recognize the inevitability of the loss of your loved one and begin to anticipate how your life will change after his or her passing. You should not be surprised by this response; it is natural and acceptable to express these feelings. In fact, you can learn a great deal about grief during this time. The behaviors you demonstrate during a period of anticipatory grief may be good predictors of your responses following the death of the family member. (See chapter 13 for more information on grief and bereavement.)

Leaving a Legacy

One of the greatest gifts a loved one can give a person with advanced cancer is support that will enable the dying person to come to terms with the loss of his/her life and leave the desired legacy. A legacy is often thought of as "leaving a mark" on the family and the world. It doesn't have to be a financial legacy, although it might be. The opportunity to collect important objects, photos, letters, or other memorabilia can be very meaningful in the creation of an individual legacy. Some people leave a box of items for young children to open at a later date. Others leave written messages, either in the form of letters to loved ones or notes hidden in strategic locations to be found by a specific person. Notes left in favorite books or hidden within favorite items could be at risk of never being found, so the location should be carefully considered.

A measure of peace and acceptance of approaching death is required to be able to be reflective, transcend physical problems, and contemplate the legacy of a life. Everyone brings different life experiences, strengths, and capacity for coping with stress as they enter the final passage of the life course. For some people, the passage through the end of life is rapid with little time for preparation and reflection. For many people with cancer, there is time to prepare and consider the legacy one wishes to leave behind. Caregivers should do all they can to assist in this process.

Denial and Acceptance

The end of life represents significant loss—loss of life, loss of important relationships, and loss of opportunity. These losses can generate strong emotions, including grief, anger, and frustration. As you, your family members, or the person with cancer experience such emotions, you should all be allowed to express your feelings. Family members may want to repress their own feelings,

"My father died very early in the morning, around 4 a.m., and I left there around midnight that night, and he was begging my mother, 'Please let me go. I don't feel I can let go and leave until you let me, and everything will be okay. I'll still be there somewhere, so it's not like an end.' Finally, in addition to convincing his other children, he finally conveyed to my mother, his wife, that everything was going to be okay and it was okay to move on. I knew as soon as Dad started with this conversation with Mom about 'Please let me go, everything will be okay,' I knew he wouldn't last the rest of the night; he was ready. They had given him 6 months to live. He lived 9 months, and I think it was because Mom and my siblings couldn't let him go. He knew or felt he couldn't leave without their permission or without their acceptance of him leaving, and it was very good to finally see that he had that understanding with them and for them to accept it, and for them to let it be okay that he was going to leave us."

— Lu

or shield the person with cancer from their personal emotions, yet openness often accomplishes more than denial. Avoiding the topic of impending death can isolate each person with his or her own feelings.

Denial and disbelief may be common emotions for both people with advanced cancer and their families, but lasting denial has been shown to diminish the capacity to deal with treatment, financial and legal plans, and even discussion of preferences for funeral arrangements. Not surprisingly, as many as 1 in 4 people with advanced cancer demonstrate moderate to severe denial. Grief and other emotions are a natural part of the process of coming to terms with impending death. Denial may delay coming to terms with the death.

On the other hand, denial can be a protective coping mechanism, and in that regard it can be helpful to an extent. Also, just because a person who is seriously ill does not want to dwell upon or talk about their impending death does not mean they are in denial.

Accepting the inevitable death can bring a peacefulness and comfort to all who are involved in the end of life. Sometimes it is a relief to know that your loved one will be released from further discomfort or decline in health.

Planning Funeral and Memorial Services

Talk to the dying person in advance of impending death to ask for preferences. Some people want only a simple memorial and are happy to let a loved one or caregiver make plans, while others may become actively involved in planning by specifying who should read a eulogy, where the memorial should be held, and at what time of day. Some people are specific about preferences for music to use in the service and the atmosphere within the room. A few people use the funeral service as an opportunity to celebrate a life while others use the time to simply share the mourning process. (See chapter 9 for more on planning a funeral.)

The caregiver or loved one can play an important role in this process by encouraging the person with cancer to talk about his or her preferences (if he or she is comfortable doing so), recording these wishes, and ensuring they are acted upon after the loved one's death.

In addition to planning memorial services and celebrations, you'll need to consider the practical topic of final disposition of bodily remains. If the religious affiliation of the person with cancer mandates certain rituals be followed, then they should be respected and followed as meticulously as possible. Make certain that you or someone close to you knows what the dying person's preferences are. They may be specified on paper through a will, but many people simply relate this information verbally. It is a relief for you to know ahead of time how these details should be handled. You can carry out final requests and feel satisfied that you fulfilled all of the requirements of the dying person.

Acknowledging the Person Who Died

Funeral and memorial services are used to acknowledge the attributes of the individual through public statements such as a eulogy and by displays of objects that are reflective of the person's interests. The displays may reflect personal values, accomplishments, or perhaps items from a military career. Some people use photographs to depict the life of the individual. These can be displayed for visitors at the funeral home or during a service in a house of worship. The verbal statements read by one person who knew the deceased well may be compiled from a collection of statements, or a series of speakers may address different aspects of the person's life. These statements usually portray the values of the deceased, their special interests, their passions, their personality, their favorite pastime and music, and their professional and personal accomplishments.

Memorial services are often used especially in the circumstance of a person who wished to be cremated. The final disposition of cremains (the cremated ashes) can be discussed in advance or decided by family members following the services. Many people bury the cremains, which are returned to the family in a sealed container. Others elect to scatter the ashes in a location that has special meaning for the deceased. There is rarely a required time period during which the memorial must be scheduled; some people prefer to delay the memorial service for a date that is convenient for the family. These decisions are personal preferences and do not require that you follow any set procedure. Just be sure you respect the wishes of the dying person.

Families handle death, bereavement, and religious rituals in very unique and personal ways. Only you and your loved one can decide the best way for your family and community. Trust that with a little thought you will do an excellent job of closing this chapter in your loved one's life.

What to Expect in the Final Moments and What You Can Do to Help

Many people wonder about what happens near the time of death. Knowing what to expect will ensure you are prepared to support and care for your loved one in the best way possible. In addition to the following descriptions, see also Figure 12-1 on page 280, for a list of possible changes in body function and what the caregiver or loved one can do about them.

> "I had never been around anybody with cancer. I have never taken care of anyone who was dying. I didn't know what to do."
>
> — Suhaila

Consciousness and Sensory Perception

Some people become unconscious for hours or even days before death, while others remain clear and alert up to the last few moments. Usually people who are dying gradually become confused and semiconscious over a few minutes or hours. In addition, speech may become quiet before death, and the thoughts expressed may be quite unrelated to the events or people present.

Often the semiconscious person can still hear, although he or she is unable to respond. Words of endearment and support may still be understood and appreciated. Touching, caressing, holding, and rocking are all appropriate and comforting.

Pain

Pain is one of the first senses to decline just before death. Still, even though people with cancer may no longer be able to express their pain, it is important to continue providing pain medication up to the end of life.

Fluids

Ice chips, water, or juice may be given as requested but should be stopped if the dying person has difficulty swallowing. Because the person no longer needs nourishment, solid food should not be given unless the person requests it.

Care of the person's mouth is important. Apply petroleum jelly or some other lubricant to the lips to prevent drying. Remove mouth secretions with the tip of a towel after turning the person to his or her side.

Temperature

As the circulation of blood begins to decline, the dying person's hands and feet become cooler, darker, or sometimes more pale than usual. Later, the same changes occur in the face. Although the skin is cool to the touch and either dry or damp, the dying person is usually not conscious of feeling cold, and light bed coverings provide enough warmth.

Breathing

Often breathing becomes irregular, alternating gradually between rapid and slow. Breathing may be easier when the person is lying on his or her back or slightly to one side with a pillow under the head. Of course, any position that makes breathing easier is acceptable, including sitting up with good support. Whatever position the person is in should be relaxed and comfortable.

While oxygen may help some people, it offers little for others. Medications can be given if breathing becomes uncomfortable for the person with cancer.

Figure 12-1.   **Signs and Symptoms of Approaching Death**

	Possible Changes	What the Loved One or Caregiver Can Do
Body Function	• Increased periods of sleep during the day • Difficulty waking from sleep • Confusion about time, place, or people • Restlessness or picking or pulling at bed linen • Increased anxiety, restlessness, fear, and loneliness at night • Less desire for food and drink	• Plan to spend time with your loved one when he or she is most alert, or during the night, when your presence may be comforting • Remind your loved one who you are and what day and time it is • Use a calm, confident voice to reduce chances of startling or frightening a confused person • Apply cool, moist washcloths to the person's head, face, and body for comfort
Secretions	• More mucus in the mouth that collects in the back of the throat causing a distressing sound sometimes called a "death rattle" • More thick secretions due to less fluid intake and the inability to cough	• Keep oral secretions loose by adding humidity to the room with a cool mist humidifier • Provide ice chips or sips of liquid through a straw if the person with cancer is able to swallow; this will thin secretions and relieve thirst and dry mouth • Change the person's position—turning the person to his or her side may help drain mouth secretions
Circulation	• Cooling of arms and legs • Deepening of color and mottling of skin of arms, legs, hands, and feet • Dusky, pale skin in other areas of the body	• Provide blankets if needed or requested • Avoid use of electric blankets and heating pads
Sensory Perception	• Blurred or dimmed vision • Decreased hearing, though most people are able to hear you even after they can no longer speak	• Leave indirect lights on as vision decreases • Never assume your loved one cannot hear you • Continue to speak with and touch your loved one to reassure him or her of your presence
Breathing	• Irregular breathing caused by poor blood circulation and the build-up of waste products in the body • Periods of no breathing (10–30 seconds)	• Raise person's head and chest with pillows or by raising the hospital bed
Elimination	• Decreased urine output • Darkened urine • Loss of bladder and bowel control	• Pad bedding with layers of disposable pads • Learn how to care for the person's catheter, if necessary
Death	• Breathing stops • Pulse stops	• Call appropriate authorities in accordance with local regulations

Source: *Advanced Cancer and Palliative Care Treatment Guidelines for Patients*, Version I/December 2003.
Courtesy of the American Cancer Society (ACS) and the National Comprehensive Cancer Network (NCCN). p. 18-19.

> "I was with her when she died….She had had a real bad day. The oncologist had come in and had told me that she wasn't going to make it, and they came in and gave her a dose of morphine….They put her on a morphine drip and she lasted a day and a half. The Friday that she died we had a huge number of people at the hospital and finally right around 10 o'clock or 10:30 everyone left and went home except for a core group of people that stayed with me. They insisted on staying, and I lay down with her on the bed and told her that she could go. She died about 15 minutes later….I told her it was okay to go, you know, that she could go if she needed to. It was pretty amazing that she took me up on it."
>
> — Rebeca

Rattling or gurgling with each breath results from secretions in the back of the throat. Although these sounds may be distressing to listen to, typically these sounds do not indicate that the person with cancer is uncomfortable. Medications can be given to dry up excessive secretions if this becomes a problem.

Involuntary Movements

Some people may have involuntary or reflex movements as they are dying. These movements, while rare, may involve any muscles. They most commonly occur in an arm, leg, or face muscle. In addition, the person may lose control of the bladder or the bowels as these muscles relax.

Death

When breathing and the heartbeat have stopped, the eyes become fixed in position and the pupils dilate. After death, you may sit with your loved one as long as you wish. Many families find comfort praying or talking together at this time. The family may reconfirm their love for each other as well as for the person who has passed away.

Once the person with cancer dies, if he or she passed away at home, the family is responsible for calling a physician or coroner to pronounce death. Regulations concerning proper notifications and removal of the body differ from one community to another. The doctor or cancer care team can provide this information for you in advance. If funeral arrangements have been completed, the funeral director and doctor will need to be notified.

Conclusion

Families face intense emotional feelings and potential stressors when confronted with the impending loss of a loved one. Good care at the end of life requires continuity of care, a good care plan, and lots of help. Knowing what to expect in these final months, days, and hours and knowing what you can do to provide good care for your loved one can help lessen the burden.

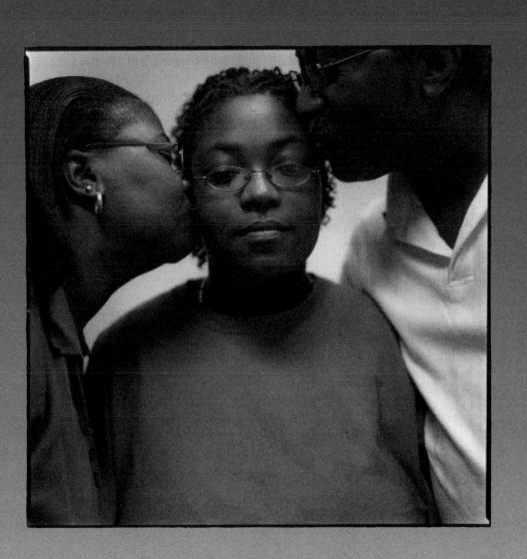

Chapter 13

Redefining Life
After a Loved One Dies

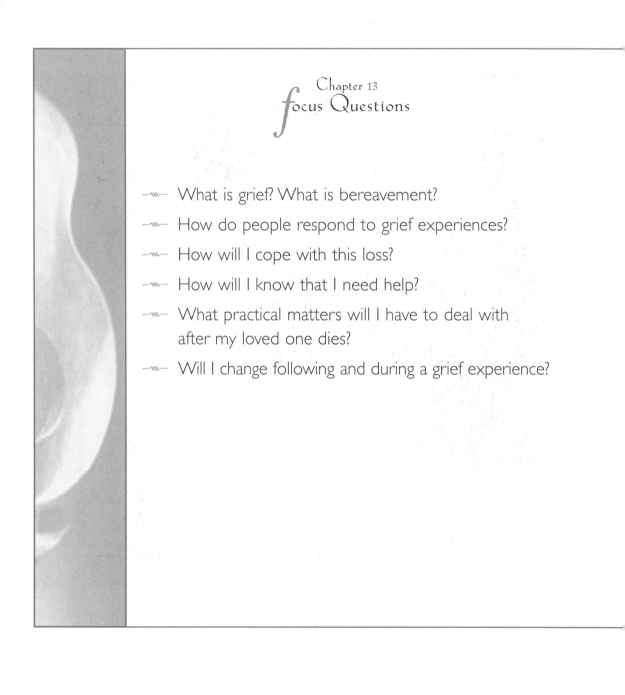

Chapter 13
focus Questions

—⚏— What is grief? What is bereavement?

—⚏— How do people respond to grief experiences?

—⚏— How will I cope with this loss?

—⚏— How will I know that I need help?

—⚏— What practical matters will I have to deal with after my loved one dies?

—⚏— Will I change following and during a grief experience?

"After we went to the neurologist and he gave Wendy the prognosis of 3 months…she asked me in the parking garage of the hospital, 'Would you go to a therapist to do grief counseling with me?' Together, we went, until the last few weeks of her life, when she was too ill to go, and I remember the day before she died, I was on the phone with the therapist. I was sitting with Wendy all day, and we had an appointment and I had to cancel it, and I was talking to the therapist and I was crying and she said, 'Joanne, it's time to let go. You need to give Wendy permission to go. You need to give her permission so that she can move on with her journey, and you need to let her know that it's okay.' And I said, 'I don't think I can do that.' And she said, 'Yes. You can do it, and you need to do it and you can do it.'

"And it was just excruciatingly painful. On the other hand, it sort of felt like this one last gift that I just really needed to give Wendy, and so I told her…that everything was okay, that her daughter was going to be okay and that I loved her and that she didn't need to hold on for anyone any more. And she died the next morning."

— Joanne

THE GRIEF EXPERIENCE CAN BE VERY PAINFUL and can open up old wounds or call attention to unresolved difficulties. The process can take a long time and may not be easy to reckon with. Coping with grief over the loss of a loved one can be one of life's most difficult challenges.

But the death of someone we love often sets in motion a series of changes in our lives. Although it sounds unusual, people who have experienced grief often note that the grief experience also has the potential to expand your understanding, provide you with a new outlook for the future, and help you to understand more about the range of human emotions, despite (or perhaps because of?) the enormous challenge it presents. You may even discover personal strength you didn't know you had.

However your life changes, the grief experience can teach you important things about yourself. In this chapter, we'll talk about coping with and responding to grief.

What Is Grief?

Grief describes the emotional distress we feel when we are confronted with great loss, such as the death of a person we love. Almost everyone experiences grief at some time. Children may confront grief and feel sadness when they lose a beloved pet or a friend. Adults may experience loss and grief after learning of the death of a distant relative or parent. Even health care professionals struggle to deal with the loss of patients with whom they have grown close. Grief is a common experience that brings everyone to similar sorts of emotional responses. The differences are in how we cope with the loss and in how we apply the experience in the context of our belief systems. Some people rely on their religious beliefs to organize their thinking and their response, while others rely on personal philosophy to guide their conduct.

Bereavement is the state that a grieving person enters upon the loss of the loved one. Bereavement is more general and nonspecific; it does not reflect the emotional reaction. It is a period of time that society recognizes, during which the grieving person may require additional support and consideration. We refer to the bereaved family or the bereaved spouse or partner and acknowledge that they may require time to reflect on their loss before they can return to their daily routine. *Mourning*

> —m—
>
> "I still am in shock. It's been 16 months and I'm still in shock. I really didn't expect it. Even though I knew that she was really sick and she didn't have very many bounces left in her, I just didn't expect it, so that's hard. Maybe I would have done something different, although I don't know what I might have done."
>
> — Susan T.

is the process by which a person adapts to the loss. The mourning process may be influenced by cultural customs, rituals, and societal expectations.

Responding to Grief Experiences

The grief experience can vary in intensity, from mild sadness to inconsolable anguish to melancholic depression. There is not a standard for the grief a person should feel. Everyone will experience grief in their own unique way, and the way a person responds to the loss of a loved one will depend upon his or her own personality and relationship with the person who has died. Your cultural or religious background, your satisfaction with the care and treatment your loved one received during his or her illness, and your coping skills may also influence the grief experience. The grief response may also depend upon other external factors, like the experience the person with cancer had as he or she was dying, the way the disease progressed, or the support the person with cancer received from his or her health care providers.

For example, health professionals recognize that grief may be very pronounced among young people, women, and people with very limited social support networks. Although the reality of the death of a loved one is a shock even when it is anticipated, people who experience an unexpected death may have more profound grief reactions.

Grief frequently triggers an emotional response that is expressed through tears. Some people cry profusely, while others save these responses for more private moments. Still other people say that they cried so much in anticipation of the death that when death came there was a sense of relief. Grief may also make you feel tired, because the grieving process may demand intense amounts of physical and emotional energy. Grief can bring about a range of emotions: it might make you feel frustrated at the doctors who couldn't cure the disease, angry with your loved one for leaving you, helpless that you couldn't stop the cancer from taking the life of your loved one, or even guilty if you are relieved that death ended the suffering of a loved one.

All of these emotions and responses are appropriate. There is no *right way* to grieve for the loss of a loved one. Grief requires gradual adaptation and changes in one's expectations. In other words, we should all expect that the experience of grief will change us and alter our lives.

For Loved Ones and Caregivers

Stages of Grief

Grief is a gradual process of change that helps us adjust to a new condition in life. This process includes:

1. **Separating from the person who died.** To separate from the person who died, the mourner must find a way to say goodbye and to accept his or her loss. This may involve coming to terms not only with the loss of a loved one, but with the unfulfilled wishes and plans for the relationship with that person, or with the things that were left unsaid or undone. Separating from the person who died does not mean that he or she should be forgotten—it simply means that the person experiencing the loss must begin to find emotional satisfaction from other sources.

2. **Readjusting to a world without that person.** The grieving person may need to reexamine or adjust their roles, their identity, or their self-perception in order to go on living in a world without the person who dies.

3. **Forming new relationships.** The mourner must redirect the emotional energy that was given to the loved one to other people or activities.

How Long Does Grief Last?

How long you mourn depends on your family, religious, and cultural traditions and your own interpretation of when it is appropriate to resume your life and establish a new normal. Mourning, a process that may take several years to complete, may begin its expression through some form of ritual such as a religious ceremony. Some families spend a specific length of time following the death using the time to perform rituals and extend support through togetherness. The Jewish tradition of "sitting Shiva" is an example of the family spending time mourning together. Other families go through the rituals of death with the religious leader of their house of worship and/or a funeral director assisting them in decisions about the sequence of events.

Grief in Special Populations

As we have mentioned, different people understand death and cope with grief in different ways. These different approaches and understandings can be a function of many things, including age and ethnic and cultural contexts.

—⁓—

"With me, having a 3-year-old child…of course, the questions that a 3 year old asks, 'Where's Papaw?' I think that was the hardest thing. And her not really saying so, but not understanding that we meant that Papaw wasn't here anymore, that he went to heaven."

— Lu

Children and Grief

Unlike adults, children do not experience continual and intense emotional and behavioral grief reactions. A grieving child may appear sad one minute and playful the next. Children may seem to show grief only occasionally and briefly, but in reality a child's grief usually lasts longer than that of an adult. The child's mourning is a process that continues over time, and will likely need to be revisited as the child grows. (See Figure 13-1 on page 290 for information on how children understand death and express grief at different ages.)

In addition, grieving children may not show their feelings as openly as adults. This is because children cannot think through their thoughts and feelings like adults and have trouble putting their feelings about grief into words. Instead, a child's behavior may reveal his or her response to the loss of a loved one, and feelings of anger or fears of abandonment or death may show up in their behavior. They may also play games that take death as their subject as a way of working out their feelings and anxieties. These games provide safe opportunities for grieving children to express their feelings.

Children who are grieving may express some or all of the following common concerns: Did I cause the death to happen? Is it going to happen to me? Who is going to take care of me? You can help children cope with their grief by explaining to them in words they understand the answers to these questions. Explanations should be simple and direct, and should be tailored to a child's age and level of understanding. Finally, you should provide every reassurance to children that they are loved and will be well cared for.

Not talking about death does not help children learn to cope with loss. In fact, allowing children to participate in discussions about the loved one ("I remember Grandma used to sit me on her lap and sing to me") can be very helpful. If children seem interested, you should also include them in memorial ceremonies. If you do, be sure to tell them what they will see and hear at the funeral. You can use the suggestions in Figure 13-2 on page 291 as a guide when talking to a child about death.

Figure 13-1.

Children and Grief

Age	Understanding of Death	Expressions of Grief
Infancy to 2 years	• Is not yet able to understand death. • Separation from mother causes changes.	• Quietness, crankiness, decreased activity, poor sleep, and weight loss.
2–6 years	• Death is like sleeping.	• Asks many questions (How does she go to the bathroom? How does she eat?). • Problems in eating, sleeping, and bladder and bowel control. • Fear of abandonment. • Tantrums.
	• Dead person continues to live and function in some ways. • Death is temporary, not final. • Dead person can come back to life.	• Magical thinking (Did I think something or do something that caused the death? Like when I said I hate you and I wish you would die?).
6–9 years	• Death is thought of as a person or spirit (skeleton, ghost, bogeyman).	• Curious about death. • Asks specific questions. • May have exaggerated fears about school.
	• Death is final and frightening.	• May have aggressive behaviors (especially boys). • Some concerns about imaginary illnesses.
	• Death happens to others, it won't happen to ME.	• May feel abandoned.
9 and older	• Everyone will die.	• Heightened emotions, guilt, anger, shame. • Increased anxiety over own death. • Mood swings.
	• Death is final and cannot be changed.	• Fear of rejection; not wanting to be different from peers.
	• Even I will die.	• Changes in eating habits. • Sleeping problems. • Regressive behaviors (loss of interest in outside activities). • Impulsive behaviors. • Feels guilty about being alive (especially related to death of a brother, sister, or peer).

Source: National Cancer Institute. Loss, Grief, and Bereavement (PDQ®).
Available at: http://www.nci.nih.gov/cancerinfo/pdq/supportivecare/bereavement/patient/.
Accessed February 25, 2004.

Figure 13-2.

Talking to Children About Death

- Explain what happened in a way they can understand. Children know when you are hiding something, so be open and honest.

- Encourage communication. Listen and accept their feelings, no matter how difficult it may be.

- Answer their questions in brief and simple terms. Telling them they are too young to understand only avoids dealing with the problem. It is okay to not have all the answers.

- Reassure them that they will still be loved and taken care of.

- Show affection, support, and consistency. Let them know that you will be there to help as much as possible.

- Share your feelings in terms they will understand, and in a way that won't be overwhelming. For example, it is okay to let them know that you hurt too. If you try to hide your feelings, they may think they shouldn't share theirs.

Grief and Bereavement Across Ethnic and Cultural Groups

Culture influences everyone's experiences of death, grief, and bereavement. Out of respect for the wide variety of traditions surrounding death and grieving across ethnic and cultural groups, we will not attempt to describe any specific practices or traditions, but we suggest that you do as much as you can to understand your own grieving experience within the context of your culture. This self-understanding can be an important coping mechanism, and it can also help you define and communicate your preferences to your health care providers.

Your health care providers should be sensitive and respectful of your unique world view, family, and cultural characteristics and should tailor their responses to your loved one's death and your grief accordingly. You play an important role too, because without your direct input, others around you are left to make assumptions about how you prefer to be treated. Once you help them understand more about your culture, background, and personal preferences, they should be responsive to these unique circumstances.

"Toward the end of her life, my mother decided that she did not want to pass in the hospital, that she wanted to go home….And during that period of time there were a lot of tribal people that came and family members that came, and a lot of people were there to kind of help with the family who was going through the dying process with my mother….

"One of the ladies had told us that at the time that my mother passed that we were to make sure and stay away from her feet, and at the time that she passed that her spirit would be going through her feet and leaving through her feet. So when that did happen, at the time that she did pass, we made sure that no one was at her feet, and the ladies also told us to open up all the doors and to make sure and allow her to go out so that her spirit could leave her without having to have any impediment.

"And at the time that happened, my sister, my second sister, was very upset and very sad and having a hard time because Mom had just died, and she was out with one of the traditional ladies at that time outside, and she was crying real hard, and the traditional lady said, 'Look up there.' And circling above our house at that time was an eagle, and it seemed as though the eagle was talking and saying, 'Well, what's going on?' It was as if it was my mother saying, 'Where are the boys? Where is my husband? Where is such-and-such people?' And so we told the eagle that her sons had gone to go hunt for the meal at the funeral and that her husband had gone to town to take care of some business and that a traditional man was to be coming from our local community, and it's as though the eagle heard us and it took off towards the mountain to where my brothers were hunting. And as time was going on, within about half an hour people seemed to know already that my mother had passed. My stepfather said that as he was coming back from the local community there was an eagle that was following him up the grade. When our traditional person came from another small community, he also saw the eagle, as the eagle was coming towards our house.

"So I truly believe that my mother, with the help of the eagles, was telling people of her passing. And in a lot of ways it was very comforting for me to have my mother pass by having the eagles take her, just because of what I've learned as my own traditional beliefs that I've been taught."

— CeCe

Efforts to better educate health care professionals about how to provide culturally competent care (not only for patients with cancer but for their loved ones as well) are underway. The importance of this topic—a cornerstone of quality palliative care—cannot be overstated.

Managing Grief and Coping With Your Loved One's Death

Loss of a child, spouse, or another family member is known to be a source of considerable stress. Although the loss registers high on the list of events that could constitute a family crisis, most of the stress is based on how you interpret the event. What is difficult for one person may not be so difficult for another. We are all unique individuals, and we interpret these life events in the context of our own personal experience.

As we discussed in chapter 4, coping refers to the behaviors people use to manage stressful situations or events. In this next section, we'll review some coping strategies that you can use to make the grieving process less painful and decrease the emotional impact of your loss. The coping strategies listed in chapter 4 can also be adapted to coping with grief over the loss of a loved one.

1. **Be patient with yourself and others.** A loss due to the death of a loved one inflicts much pain that is difficult to heal.
2. **Express yourself.** Many people keep a diary or journal with their reflections about the events and the changes that occur. You may also consider other forms of expression, such as singing songs or creating art.
3. **Talk about your loved one with family and friends.** Other people will also welcome the opportunity to talk and remember the person, their personality, and interests. Sharing personal stories can be very healing.
4. **Recognize that holidays and special events can be especially difficult after the recent loss of a loved one.** Discuss and try to decide how you want to handle the situation; you may want to incorporate some prayer, remembrance, or new tradition in acknowledgement of your loved one.
5. **Allow yourself to experience the pain of loss.** It is unlikely that you would feel such pain if deep affection was not present in the relationship. Cherish the time you had together and value your memories, which can never be taken away from you.

"People said that to me, it's easier at first. It gets harder later. And they're right, because now Sherry's life is over and essentially all the loose ends are wrapped up. People miss her, but they have adjusted to life without her…and I'm left here having to figure out what to do with the rest of my life, and it doesn't feel very good or very fair. You don't want to be the one that's left behind, but yet so many of us are, and we manage somehow. But it's not easy."

— Rebeca

6. **Reach out to others.** Take the focus off yourself and your pain by volunteering to help others.
7. **Avoid isolating yourself in grief.** Stay in touch with other people. Keep communication open with family, friends and colleagues. Accept invitations for social events, even if you do not feel like going to the event.

Meeting the Challenge of Adversity and Loss

Coping with the loss of a loved one is a very important challenge. A death can inspire you to reassess your own skills, look back at how much you changed through the experience, and begin to plan for the future. Many people learn a great deal about themselves during the course of the serious illness of a loved one. They take on new responsibilities and begin to discover new talents and abilities that were not previously obvious. Some people discover a new inner resolve to change the way they live or they discover that they are very strong. The human capacity for growth and change is remarkable and many people are surprised by their own resilience.

What might you consider adversity? Sometimes the tremendous physical and emotional toll of caregiving can be considered adversity. Some people may think of the disease experience as the adverse condition that triggers change in their lives. Others may think that they learned so much about themselves and the connectedness to friends and family that the adversity of the illness experience can be overcome because of the close-knit group behaviors. Whatever the adverse condition was for you, it is important to put

> *―₩―*
>
> "I was very bitter and angry for a while. I felt so robbed…I remember at her memorial service. There was like over 300 people, and these people would give stories and say, I've known her for 15 years, and I've known her for 10 years, and she was all this, and I just felt so envious of them, you know? I just felt so ripped off, and so what did I do to take care of myself? I'm not sure I did a whole lot at that time. It took me a while to figure that out. I was just trying to get through the day."
>
> — Joanne

it behind you. Do not ignore it or erase it, but try to view it as a growth experience. Consider how you want to live the rest of your life keeping memories alive but honoring the person you lost by creating new opportunities for yourself and your loved ones. For example, you may want to turn your grief into action for others by entering volunteer work.

Professional Help and Support for the Grieving

Some grieving—even intense sadness and feelings of depression—after the loss of a loved one is normal. However, these feeling are generally temporary, and eventually most people are able to resume their daily activities. People who find themselves unable to move on with the daily tasks of life may want to obtain professional help.

How do you know if your grief reaction requires professional help? Signals include profound sadness, changes in eating habits and sleep patterns, suicidal thoughts, inability to converse with others in your support circle (friends and family), and inability to confide in others.

Grief and depression are known to occur together following the death of a loved one. A quarter of people who are grieving suffer from depression while grieving, and about half of those people have suicidal thoughts within a 6-month period after the death. When grieving people think they are depressed, they should seek medical care, because depression can make the grief symptoms worse. When profound feelings of great sadness persist, the situation should be

"She was the kind of person that other people gravitated to. She was very dynamic, and she had been a massage therapist and she just had that special touch about her. Before I knew her, when she had her cancer surgery, she had a whole circle of friends that was her care circle. Many of the people didn't really know her very well but were recruited to help with her care. I still run into some of those people who were so impressed with her. She was just a very special person."

— Susan T.

discussed with a health professional. *If you are considering taking your own life, seek the help of a health care professional immediately.*

The Medicare Hospice Benefit

People who have recently lost a loved one should know that the Medicare hospice benefit provides grief and bereavement support to patients and families at the end of life and for up to a year after a loved one's death. Members of the hospice team are available to provide support, information, and counseling and to help family members make the transition to life without their loved one.

Additional Bereavement Interventions and Sources of Support

Most of the support people receive after a loss comes from friends, family members, and other loved ones. There are also several types of support available within the community. Supervised interventions often include discussion groups, educational programs, behavioral modification and training, and individual psychotherapy.

The AARP can put you in touch with local grief and loss support groups, for example (http://www.aarp.org/griefandloss/). You can also find support on Web sites with discussion boards. One example is the Cancer Survivors Network offered on the Web site of the American Cancer Society (http://www.acscsn.org). These discussion groups offer the opportunity to share your feelings and experiences with other people in similar situations.

—⁓—

"I faced grieving and Chuck's dying the same way we faced the cancer. And look, there's a lot of options out there. There are support groups, there are a lot of very good books out there, there's information on the Internet, there are such things as guided imagery, there are so many options out there…you don't have to go through fighting the cancer alone. The same thing is true with the grief process. You don't have to go through that alone.

"We're not going to be perfect at it. We're human, and for a lot of us it's the first time we're going through something like this. And even if it's not, every time is going to be different because of the relationship you had with the person that you just lost.

"So there's no right or wrong way, there's no perfect way to do it, but there's a lot of things out there from hospice grief support classes to counselors to a variety of books to journaling. There are so many things out there that you can try, and you can see, and you can get help from, as well as other people, family, and friends. I think you need to know that it's okay to seek help and to look at what's out there and gain knowledge of the grief process and understand that anger can be a part of that. Guilt can be a part of that. And so when you understand those kinds of things and understand the grief process, I think it's easier to deal with those if they do come up. That's the main point that is made to you over and over, is that there's no way out but through."

– Ann I.

Sometimes you may need additional support—the kind that can be provided by a professional. Doctors, nurses, and other members of the palliative care team are excellent sources of support. Social workers, psychologists and psychiatrists, and pastoral care experts or members of the clergy are also available to help. Organizations such as the American Cancer Society (800-ACS-2345 or http://www.cancer.org) or Growth House (http://www.growthhouse.org) are good resources for potential referrals. Finding a person you are comfortable talking with about your feelings is the key to moving forward.

The Satisfaction of Carrying Out Last Requests

One of the ways you can honor the person who died is by carrying out his or her final requests. Dying people often designate someone special to care for their children, maintain a garden or other property in perpetuity, or scatter their ashes in a designated place. Completing these tasks can be very satisfying and can help to bring closure.

People sometimes leave funds through their will to enable others to carry out final requests. If you are asked to complete a final request, you should check with the executor of the will to be certain there is funding available for the task.

Wills may contain guardianship agreements and trust funds to provide for the care of children. If you are part of such an agreement, you are obligated to honor the agreement and make all necessary arrangements for surviving children. This may require that you make plans for the education of underage children, possibly administer the financial agreements, or arrange for the children to live with you. See chapter 7 for more information about legal matters.

Survivors' Tasks: Taking Care of Business and Other Practical Matters

There are some business and practical matters that must be taken care of immediately after the death of the family member.

Bank Accounts

Banks should be notified as quickly as possible, since they usually freeze the account and await instruction from the estate as to the final disposition of funds held by the deceased in a sole owner account. (Joint accounts are not frozen.) The same thing happens to safe deposit boxes. If the will is in the safe deposit box, it may require a letter from the attorney to retrieve it. These actions are really safeguards for the family: since deaths are routinely announced in the newspaper, the bank attempts to shield the family from unauthorized entry into the accounts.

> ——∿——
>
> "After someone died and you're the executor of their will and also their last partner, you get to be in widow mode for a while. You've got to take care of all the details of wrapping up someone's life, and so that sustained me for a while. It gave me focus. I kind of had a script. I've got to take care of this and I've got to take care of that. Do this, do the other, and so that helped."
>
> — Rebeca

Outstanding credit card balances should be settled and accounts should be closed to avoid the possibility of fraud.

Wills and Other Documents

The family needs to determine if the deceased person wrote a will prior to dying. Ideally, a loved one will have drawn up a will and left it in a secure place that is easily accessible. A will is a written, legal document that at the very least names a person to settle the estate and usually directs the efforts of that individual to distribute remaining property to family and friends. It is necessary for someone to be able to manage the affairs of the deceased, which may mean paying bills and researching life insurance policies. If there is no will, someone in the family will have to go to the county courthouse to obtain instruction in how to name an individual to be the executor. The executor reports to the court all the transactions needed to close out the person's business.

In the event that there is substantial wealth involved in an estate, there is probably a will in existence. The family should know in advance of the death where the original copy is stored. When considerable funds or a home is left to a spouse, tax laws are fairly lenient. If wealth is left to others, however, taxes may be substantial. Family members and the executor may need to rely on the services of an attorney who specializes in estates for final disposition of the funds and material goods. Learning about the will and planning for the distribution of the estate prior to the death can be a source of relief and consolation to the entire family.

Redefining Your Life Following a Grief Experience

The process of accepting the death of the loved one and redefining your life through a grief experience may be a very slow process. Perceiving yourself in a new context is an important transition. If you lost a spouse, you are no longer a wife or husband. Are you now single, or are you a widow(er)? How will you define yourself to new people you may meet? The death changes your definition of self.

Death of a loved one may also affect your social relationships. You may discover that some friends may step up their efforts to include you in their social events and activities, while others stop inviting you to join them for dinner or special occasions. Sometimes people reflect their discomfort with your (and their) loss by withdrawing from you. Although this rejection may hurt you, you will heal more quickly if you make an effort to accept it as part of the other person's own adjustment to a new relationship. You must move on. Make new friends who may share some life experience with you and share your new status as an individual.

If you were a primary caregiver, it takes time to stop the routines you used to provide care. If caregiving tasks were a major part of your life, you could find yourself going through the motions of the tasks even after the death. You must gradually instruct yourself to sleep all night, eat alone, and entertain yourself with constructive new activity. Explore your talents, travel, and develop new relationships as soon as possible.

> "All you want is to just get through this situation the very best you can. And there is no wrong way to grieve. Whatever works for you, that's the way it's good for you."
>
> — Lee

> "Many people naively think that after such a devastating event you can go back to your old normal way of living. Instead, you have to create a new normal that includes the loss of a loved one."
>
> — Glenda

How Do You Know When You Are Recovering?

You will know that your recovery has started and that you are successful with recreating a life for yourself when you can look at the following situations and see that they no longer upset you or cause you to respond emotionally.

- You begin to sleep in a normal pattern, regain your usual appetite, and no longer feel fatigued all the time.

—҂—

"When my mom first died, it was a physical pain. The nights were horrible. I mean, I actually still—now I've grown to where it's not as often—but when I do get that, it's in your chest. I can't describe it. It's a physical pain. This year, when I was Christmas shopping with my daughter, was the first I had felt it for a long time. I was almost glad that I did because I thought, I don't want to lose that intensity of the feelings that I had for her.

"And it almost can become a good thing. Maybe that's weird, but it's like I said. I was Christmas shopping last week and I just thought back for a moment, 36 years ago. What a different place the world is. What would she think of it now? What would she think of my children? Then I got that feeling. And I thought, 'Well, you know, I still have that intense feeling, so that's good!'"

— Diane

— You can look at old photographs or read books and materials written by the deceased without crying.
— When some days pass and you do not think about the deceased. Although at first this may make you feel guilty, it is a good sign.
— You get up in the morning actually looking forward to the tasks at hand, whether that is going to work or going shopping.
— You begin to form new relationships with other people with some joy in your heart.
— You can drive the car without crying.
— You can participate fully in religious services and listen to prayers, readings, or songs without crying.
— You do not lose your place while reading, and you remember what you read. (Concentration is difficult when you are immersed in grief.)
— You anticipate holidays with pleasure.
— You can begin to entertain people in your home again.
— You decide it is time to change jobs and meet some new people.
— You decide it is okay to date again.

Advice for the First Year

People often advise bereaved persons to refrain from making radical changes in lifestyle during the first year after a death. There is no question that this is a

> "After Wendy's death, it took me a number of years before I went from being alive to living again. The former being I just existed, and the latter being I started to open up to the rest of the 4-letter word called love. That took quite a long time. And not just intimate relationships but just all-around opening up to the universe again. It took almost 5 years for me."
>
> — Joanne

stressful time period and that all options may not be adequately considered. You will need to determine when you feel most comfortable with changes in your life, whether this is living conditions, jobs, or social engagements. Maintain your connections with the usual religious affiliations and any clubs you have actively engaged in over the years. Explore new options for solo activity in a gradual way. For example, you may want to go to a museum by yourself instead of staying home alone. You will see new things, get new ideas, and deflect some attention away from your grief. Try not to alter investments and other financial arrangements until you have thoroughly explored all the options and feel confident in your choices.

Toward the end of a year, or perhaps even sooner, you may feel restless to get on with some changes in your life. You may decide to change jobs, or move, or start dating again. When you can make a decision with comfort and confidence and wake up each day knowing that it is a good decision, you should be able to proceed with the plan without feeling anxious. This is a signal you have already begun to reconstruct your life.

Conclusion

It may be years before you are able to reflect on all the changes you make in your life and find confidence in your decisions. Gradual changes made with comfort probably reflect the best choices. Through a series of decisions, you exercise the strength of your own ideas and gradually discover a meaningful place to keep the memory of your loved one alive. The task of integrating your memories of the past life with the person you lost is important to constructing a future that feels whole.

Resources

Finding and getting the help you and your family need is a lot like going on a journey of discovery. The type of help you need may change as your circumstances change and the cancer progresses. The following national resources are a good place to begin your journey for help and support. Most of the resources can be contacted by telephone or e-mail. Many have Web sites. Many resources provide referrals to other organizations, including ones in your own community. Additionally, check with the many organizations that deal with your particular type of cancer, and don't overlook the department of social work at your local hospital.

Tips for Using Cancer Resources

- You may need help from more than one resource.
- You may have to make several calls before you get to the resource that fits your needs.
- Organize the information you get from resources in a notebook to help you remember.
- Be persistent: getting help is a process; it may not happen overnight.

General Cancer Resources

American Cancer Society (ACS)
1599 Clifton Rd., NE
Atlanta, GA 30329
Toll free: 1-800-ACS-2345 (1-800-227-2345)
Web site: http://www.cancer.org

The American Cancer Society (ACS) is the nation-wide community-based voluntary health organization dedicated to eliminating cancer as a major health problem by preventing cancer, saving lives, and diminishing suffering from cancer through research, education, advocacy, and service. Headquartered in Atlanta, Georgia, the ACS has state divisions and more than 3,400 local offices. The American Cancer Society provides educational materials, information, and patient services. A comprehensive resource for all your cancer-related questions, the Society can also put you in touch with community resources in your area.

American Psychosocial Oncology Society (APOS)
2365 Hunters Way
Charlottesville, VA 22911
Toll free: 1-866-276-7443
Phone: 434-293-5350
Fax: 434-977-0899
Web site: http://www.apos-society.org

This organization promotes the well-being of patients with cancer and families at all stages of disease. They provide clinical information, education, and a hotline for counseling and support services.

American Society of Clinical Oncology (ASCO)
1900 Duke Street, Suite 200
Alexandria, VA 22314
Toll free: 1-888-651-3038
Phone: 703-299-0150
Fax: 703-299-1044
E-mail: asco@asco.org
Web site: http://www.asco.org or
http://www.peoplelivingwithcancer.org

This organization has information about cancer doctors, research, treatment, and patient care. The ASCO-sponsored *People Living with Cancer* Web site provides information on types of cancer, coping, and patient support organizations.

Association of Oncology Social Work (AOSW)
1211 Locust Street
Philadelphia, PA 19107
Phone: 215-599-6093
Fax: 215-545-8107
E-mail: info@aosw.org
Web site: http://www.aosw.org/

Oncology social work is the primary professional discipline that provides psychosocial services to cancer patients, their families, and caregivers. Oncology social workers connect patients and their families with community, state, national, and international resources. AOSW and its members work to increase awareness about the social, emotional, educational, and spiritual needs of cancer patients through research, writing, workshops and lectures, and collaborations with other patient advocacy groups and national and international oncology organizations whose primary focus is access to quality care for cancer patients.

Cancer Care, Inc.
275 Seventh Ave.
New York, NY 10001
Toll free: 1-800-813-HOPE (1-800-813-4673)
Phone: 212-712-8080
Fax: 212-712-8495
Web site: http://www.cancercare.org

Cancer Care, a nonprofit social service agency for cancer concerns, provides counseling, guidance, and links to a wide variety of resources, information, and support. Their mission is to provide free professional help to people with all cancers. This is done in person, on the telephone, and via the Web site. Cancer Care also has information for children in families experiencing cancer.

National Cancer Institute (NCI)
NCI Public Inquiries Office, Suite 3036A
6116 Executive Boulevard, MSC8322
Bethesda, MD 20892-8322
Toll free: 1-800-4-CANCER (1-800-422-6237)
TTY: 1-800-332-8615
Web site: http://cancer.gov/cancerinformation.gov

This national organization is a reliable source of information on cancer in general and specific types of cancer, treatments, coping, support, and resources.

Oncology Nursing Society (ONS)
125 Enterprise Drive
RIDC Park West
Pittsburgh, PA 15275-1214
Toll free: 1-866-257-4ONS
Phone: 412-859-6100
Fax: 877-369-5497
E-mail: customer.service@ons.org
Web site: http://www.ons.org

The Oncology Nursing Society (ONS) is a professional organization of more than 30,000 registered nurses and other health care providers dedicated to excellence in patient care, education, research, and administration in oncology nursing. The overall mission of ONS is to promote excellence in oncology nursing and quality cancer care.

The Wellness Community
919 Eighteenth Street, NW, Suite 54
Washington, DC 20006
Toll free: 1-888-793-WELL (1-888-793-9355)
Phone: 202-659-9709
Fax: 202-659-9301
Web site: http://www.thewellnesscommunity.org

This organization provides support, education, and hope to people with cancer and their loved ones. They offer education, support, classes, and a wide variety of programs to help, regardless of the stage of the cancer. There are 20 facilities nationwide in addition to international centers.

General Resources

AARP (formerly known as the American Association of Retired Persons)
601 East Street, NW
Washington, DC, 20049
Toll free: 1-888-687-2277
Phone: 202-434-3740
Fax: 202-434-6483
Web site: http://www.aarp.org

This organization is a comprehensive source of information and links related to health and wellness, care, family, money, grief, and transitions.

American College of Physicians American Society of Internal Medicine
190 N. Independence Mall West
Philadelphia, PA 19106-1572
Web site: http://www.acponline.org/public/h_care/index.html

This organization provides a free book called the *American College of Physicians Home Care Guide for Advanced Cancer* to help caregivers deal with the

complex issues of caring for someone with cancer. The entire book can be viewed or downloaded from the Web site.

Eldercare Locator
Toll free: 1-800-677-1116
(available weekdays, 9:00 a.m. to 8:00 p.m. EST).
Web site: http://www.eldercare.gov/

The Eldercare Locator is a public service of the US Administration on Aging. The Eldercare Locator connects older Americans and their caregivers with sources of information on senior services. The service links those who need assistance with state and local area agencies on aging and community-based organizations that serve older adults and their caregivers. For example, resources include Alzheimer's hotlines, adult day care and respite services, nursing home ombudsman assistance, consumer fraud, in-home care complaints, legal services, elder abuse/protective services, Medicare/Medicaid/Medigap information, tax assistance, and transportation.

National Association of Area Agencies on Aging (N4A)
1730 Rhode Island Ave., NW
Suite 1200
Washington, DC 20036
Phone: 202-872-0888
Fax: 202-872-0057
Web site: www.n4a.org

The National Association of Area Agencies on Aging is the umbrella organization for the 655 area agencies on aging (AAAs) and more than 230 Title VI Native American aging programs in the U.S. The N4A's primary mission is to help older persons and persons with disabilities and chronic illnesses live with dignity and choices in their homes and communities for as long as possible.

National Association of Social Workers (NASW)
750 First Street NE, Suite 700
Washington, DC 20002-4241
Toll free: 1-800-638-8799
Phone: 202-408-8600
Fax: 202-336-8331
Web site: http://www.socialworkers.org/

The National Association of Social Workers (NASW) is the largest membership organization of professional social workers in the world. The NASW Register of Clinical Social Workers, available on the Web site under "Find a Social Worker," is a resource members of the public can use to identify social workers who are qualified by education, experience, and credentials to provide mental health services.

Palliative Care
(Including Pain Control, End of Life, and Hospice)

American Academy of Hospice and Palliative Medicine (AAHPM)
4700 W. Lake Avenue
Glenview, IL 60025
Phone: 847-375-4712
Fax: 877-734-8671
Web site: http://www.aahpm.org

This organization offers a wealth of information on topics such as hospice, palliative care, pain, and dying. It includes a comprehensive directory of related sites.

American Alliance of Cancer Pain Initiatives Resource Center
1300 University Avenue
Room 4720 Medical Science Center
Madison, WI 53706
Phone: 608-265-4013
Fax: 608-265-4014
Web site: http://www.aacpi.wisc.edu

This organization promotes the relief of cancer pain through advocacy and education. It provides information for patients about pain management.

American Chronic Pain Association
P.O. Box 850
Rocklin, CA 95677
Toll free: 1-800-533-3231
Phone: 916-632-0922
Fax: 916-632-3208
E-mail: acpa@pacbell.net
Web site: http://www.theacpa.org/

The American Chronic Pain Association offers support and information for people with chronic pain. Its mission is to facilitate peer support and education for individuals with chronic pain and their families, so that these individuals may live more fully in spite of their pain, and to raise awareness among the health care community, policy makers, and the public at large about issues of living with chronic pain.

American Pain Foundation
201 N. Charles Street, Suite 710
Baltimore, MD 21201-4111
Toll free: 1-888-615-PAIN (7246)
E-mail: info@painfoundation.org
Web site: http://www.painfoundation.org/

The American Pain Foundation is an independent nonprofit organization serving people with pain through information, advocacy, and support. Their mission is to improve the quality of life of people with pain by raising public awareness, providing practical information, promoting research, and advocating to remove barriers and increase access to effective pain management.

Americans for Better Care of the Dying
4200 Wisconsin Avenue, NW, 4th Floor
Washington, DC 20016
Phone: 202-895-2660
Fax: 202-966-5410
E-mail: info@abcd-caring.org
Web site: http://www.abcd-caring.org

This organization aims to improve end-of-life care by working with the public, clinicians, policymakers, and other end-of-life organizations to effect social and political change. The site delivers an electronic newsletter and includes updates on relevant public policy.

City of Hope Pain/Palliative Care Resource Center (COHPPRC)
1500 East Duarte Road
Duarte, CA 91010
Phone: 626-256-HOPE (4673)
Fax: 626-301-8941
Web site: http://prc.coh.org

This organization serves as a valuable resource for information and resources on palliative care, cancer pain control, and end of life.

Choice in Dying/Partnership for Caring
1620 Eye Street NW, Suite 202
Washington, DC 20006
Toll free: 1-800-989-9455
Phone: 202-296-8071
Fax: 202-296-8352
E-mail: pfc@partnershipforcaring.org
Web site: http://www.choices.org or
http://www.partnershipforcaring.org

Partnership for Caring is a national, nonprofit organization devoted to raising consumer expectations for excellent end-of-life care and increasing demand for such care.

Growth House, Inc.
Phone: 415-863-3045
E-mail: info@growthhouse.org
Web site: http://www.growthhouse.org

Growth House provides resources about life-limiting illnesses and end-of-life care, and information and referral services for agencies working with death and dying issues. The primary mission of Growth House is to improve the quality of compassionate care for people who are dying through public education and global professional collaboration. The Web site includes information on major issues in hospice and home care, palliative care, pain management, grief, death with dignity, and quality-of-life improvement, as well as a host of other resources, including the unique *Growth House Radio.*

Hospice Association of America
228 Seventh Street, SE
Washington, DC 20003
Phone: 202-546-4759
Fax: 202-547-6638
Web site: http://www.hospice-america.org

This national organization represents more than 2,800 hospices and thousands of caregivers and volunteers who serve terminally ill patients and their families. It is the largest lobbying group. It provides information about hospice care, a consumer's guide, and a Bill of Rights for hospice patients.

Hospice Education Institute
3 Unity Square
P.O. Box 98
Machiasport, ME 04655
Toll free: 1-800-331-1620
Phone: 207-255-8800
Web site: http://www.hospiceworld.org

This organization provides *Hospice Link*, a database and directory of all hospice and palliative care organizations in the United States. It is an independent organization that provides information and education about the many facets of caring for the dying and bereaved.

Hospice and Palliative Nurses Association (HPNA)
Penn Center West One, Suite 229
Pittsburgh, PA 15276
Phone: 412-787-9301
Fax: 412-787-9305
E-mail: hpna@hpna.org
Web site: http://www.hpna.org

The purpose of the HPNA is to promote excellence in end-of-life nursing, to promote understanding of the specialties of hospice and palliative nursing, and to study and promote hospice and palliative nursing research. Although mostly for professionals, the site includes a rich array of Web links as well as position statements on pain, palliative sedation, artificial hydration and nutrition, and other topics of interest.

Initiative to Improve Palliative Care for African-Americans (IIPCA)
P.O. Box 2491
New York, NY 10021
Phone: 212-639-6398
Fax: 212-423-4691
Web site: http://www.iipca.org/index.html

The IIPCA was formed to define and promote a research, education, and policy agenda for the improvement of care for African-American patients facing serious illness.

International Association for Hospice and Palliative Care (IAHPC)
5535 Memorial Dr., Suite F-PMB 509
Houston, TX 77007
Phone: 713-880-2940
Fax: 713-880-2948
E-mail: info@iahpc.com
Web site: http://www.hospicecare.com

IAHPC is a not-for-profit organization that provides a wide array of information about hospice and palliative care services, including articles, and a bookstore with books and videos. Also includes a discussion forum.

Last Acts Partnership (see Partnership for Caring)
Web site: http://www.lastacts.org

This national coalition's goal is to improve the care and caring near the end of life. They believe in palliative care, offer help with managing pain, and provide support and information. Of particular interest is Kit's Legacy, a personal and practical guide for preparing for death.

Moyers on Dying
Web site: http://www.pbs.org/wnet/onourownterms/index.html

Based on a highly acclaimed PBS TV series with Bill Moyers, this organization has become a national outreach movement to improve the way Americans die. The Web site includes information on end-of-life tools, care options, final days, therapy, and support.

National Chronic Pain Outreach Association, Inc. (NCPOA)
P.O. Box 274
Millboro, VA 24460
Phone: 540-862-9437
(available 8:00 a.m. to 6:00 p.m. EST)
Fax: 540-862-9485
Web site: http://www.chronicpain.org/

NCPOA is a nonprofit organization established to lessen the suffering of people with chronic pain by educating pain sufferers, health care professionals, and the public about chronic pain and its management. NCPOA operates an information clearinghouse that offers a wide range of publications and audio tapes for both pain sufferers and health care professionals; publishes a quarterly newsletter, *Lifeline*, which provides information on pain management methods and coping techniques; provides a Support Group Starter Kit for people who want to start their own local chronic pain support groups; provides referrals to health care professionals and medical facilities nationwide; and maintains a computerized registry of chronic pain support groups in the United States and Canada.

National Hospice and Palliative Care Organization (NHPCO)
1700 Diagonal Road, Suite 625
Alexandria, VA 22314
Toll free: 1-800-658-8898
Phone: 703-837-1500
Fax: 703-837-1233
Web site: http://www.nhpco.org

This organization is dedicated to providing information about hospice care, including a hospice locator by state and related links. This organization is committed to improving end-of-life care, expanding access to hospice care, and enhancing the quality of life for dying people and their loved ones.

National Institute for Jewish Hospice (NIJH)
732 University Street
North Woodmere, NY 11581
Toll free: 1-800-446-4448
Web site: http://www.nijh.org/

The mission of NIJH is to help alleviate suffering in serious and terminal illness. Advocates for quality end-of-life care for Jewish patients; counsels families, patients and caregivers; and provides locations of hospices, hospitals, health professionals and clergy of all faiths. Also provides booklets, books, and cassettes and monographs confronting such issues as truth telling and euthanasia, and provides insights into the art of hoping, the techniques of caring, and the understanding of pain.

National Resource Center on Diversity in End-of-Life Care (NRCD)
4201 Connecticut Avenue, Suite 402
Washington, DC 20008-1158
Toll free: 1-866-670-6723
Phone: 202-537-3599
Fax: 202-244-2628
E-mail: info@nrcd.com
Web site: http://www.nrcd.com

This organization is committed to improving the provision of and access to quality culturally appropriate care for all individuals with life-limiting illnesses.

Partnership for Caring, Inc.: America's Voices for the Dying
National Office
1620 Eye Street NW, Suite 202
Washington, DC 20006
Toll free: 1-800-989-9455
Phone: 202-296-8071
Fax: 202-296-8352
Hotline: 800-989-9455
Web site: http://www.partnershipforcaring.org

This organization raises consumers' expectations and knowledge for excellent end-of-life care by providing information and counseling regarding end-of-life care, living wills and medical powers of attorney, and treatment decision making.

Legal Resources

Cancer Legal Resource Center
Western Law Center for Disability Rights
919 South Albany Street
Los Angeles, CA 90015-1211
Phone: 213-736-1031
TDD: 213-736-8310
Fax: 213-736-1428

E-mail: wlcdr@lls.edu
Web site: http://wlcdr.everybody.org

This organization provides information and educational outreach on cancer-related legal issues to people with cancer, their families, friends, employers, and those who provide services to them.

Finances, Insurance, and Benefits

Centers for Medicare and Medicaid Services (CMS)
Department of Health and Human Services
7500 Security Boulevard
Baltimore, MD 21244
Toll free: 1-877-267-2323
TYY: 1-866-226-1819
Web site: http://www.cms.hhs.gov

This is a federal agency within the U.S. Department of Health and Human Services. The Web site provides information about different programs to assist with medical coverage.

Medicare Hotline
Department of Health and Human Services
Toll free 1-800-MEDICARE (1-800-633-4227)
Web site: http://www.medicare.gov

Call or visit the Web site to receive information about local services.

Medicare Rights Center
1460 Broadway, 17th Floor
New York, NY 10036
Phone: 212-869-3850
Fax: 212-869-3532
Web site: http://www.medicarerights.org/Index.html

Medicare Rights Center is a national, not-for-profit, non-governmental organization that helps ensure older adults and people with disabilities get good affordable health care. It provides telephone hotline services to individuals who need answers to Medicare questions or help securing coverage, and teaches people with Medicare and those who counsel them (health care providers, social service workers, family members, and others) about Medicare benefits and rights.

National Viatical Association
Toll free: 1-800-741-9465
Web site: http://nationalviatical.org

This organization provides information on predeath purchase of life insurance and cashing in existing life insurance due to a terminal disease.

Patient Advocate Foundation
700 Thimble Shoals Blvd., Suite 200
Newport News, VA 23606
Toll free: 1-800-532-5274
Fax: 757-873-8999
Web site: http://www.patientadvocate.org

This organization provides professional case managers who negotiate with cancer patients' insurers, employers and creditors for patients confronting insurance denials and employment discrimination. It also assists those needing help negotiating public assistance programs.

Social Security Administration
Department of Health and Human Services
Office of Public Inquiries
Windsor Park Building
6401 Security Blvd.
Baltimore, MD 21235
Toll free: 1-800-772-1213
TTY: 1-800-325-0778
Web site: http://www.socialsecurity.gov

This federal organization provides information about local services. You can apply for social security disability, obtain survivors' information, benefits, and other financial information. You can check on your benefits and even apply on the Web site.

Department of Veterans Affairs (VA)
Washington D.C. Regulatory Office
1722 I Street, NW
Washington, DC 20421
Toll Free: 1-800-827-1000
Web site: http://www.va.gov

Contact the VA for information on health benefits and services, compensation and pension benefits, life insurance benefits, burial and memorial benefits, and other services.

Family and Caregiver Support

The Center for Family Caregivers
Tad Publishing Co.
P.O. Box 224
Park Ridge, IL 60068
Web site: http://www.caregiving.com

This grassroots organization provides practical information on being a caregiver, managing the stress of caregiving, and solutions for caregiving situations.

Family Caregiver Alliance
690 Market Street, Suite 600
San Francisco, CA 94104
Toll free: 1-800-445-8106
Phone: 415-434-3388
Fax: 415-434-3508S
Web site: http://www.caregiver.org

This organization's mission is to support families caring for loved ones with chronic, disabling conditions through information, education, services, research, and advocacy. The site contains fact sheets, an online support group, and links to other resources.

Kids Konnected
27071 Cabot Road, Suite 102
Laguna Hills, CA 92653
Toll free: 1-800-899-2866
Web site: http://www.kidskonnected.org

This national organization offers groups and programs for children who have a parent with cancer. They provide information, referrals to local services, a newsletter, and grief workshops.

National Alliance for Caregiving
4720 Montgomery Lane, 5th Floor
Bethesda, MD 20814
E-mail: info@caregiving.org
Web site: http://www.caregiving.org

This organization is dedicated to providing support to family caregivers and to the professionals who help them. They provide public awareness, information on public policy, and lots of practical tips for the caregiver.

National Association for Home Care
228 Seventh Street, SE
Washington, DC 2003
Phone: 202-547-7424
Fax: 202-547-3540
Web site: http://www.nahc.org

This organization represents home care agencies, hospices, home care aid organizations, and medical equipment suppliers. It provides a service locator and information on how to choose a home care provider.

National Family Caregivers Association
10400 Connecticut Avenue, Suite 500
Kensington, MD 20895-3944
Toll free: 1-800-896-3650
E-mail: info@nfcacares.org
Web site: http://www.nfcacares.org

This national organization focuses on the caregiver. It provides information, education, public awareness, and advocacy.

National Respite Locator Service
Toll free: 1-800-7-RELIEF (1-800-773-5433)
Web site: http://www.chtop.com/locator.htm

Respite is a break for caregivers and families. It provides temporary care to the person with a chronic or terminal condition. This organization helps people locate respite services in their community.

Grief and Bereavement

AARP Grief and Loss Programs
601 East Street, NW
Washington, DC 20049
Toll free: 1-888-687-2277
Phone: 202-434-3740
Fax: 202-434-6483
Web site: http://www.aarp.org/griefandloss

One of the many helpful services of the organization formerly known as the American Association of Retired Persons, AARP Grief and Loss Programs help bereaved adults and their families cope with the loss of a loved one. Community programs at the local level offer bereavement outreach services, support groups, and educational events. Publications dealing with specific areas of grief support are available in English and Spanish. Information, online support groups, and facilitated discussion boards are available on the Web site.

The Compassionate Friends
P.O. Box 3696
Oak Brook, IL 60522-3696
Toll free: 1-877-969-0010
Phone: 630-990-0010
Fax: 630-990-0246
Web site: http://www.compassionatefriends.org

The Compassionate Friends is a nationwide self-help organization offering support to families who have experienced the death of a child of any age from any cause. It makes referrals to nearly 600 local chapters.

The Dougy Center, The National Center for Grieving Children and Families
P.O. Box 86852
Portland, OR 97286
Phone: 503-777-5683
Web site: http://www.grievingchild.org

This organization is a nonprofit support center to help grieving children, teens, and families.

Funeral and Memorial Service Planning

Funeral Consumers Alliance
33 Patchen Road
South Burlington, VT 05403
Toll free: 1-800-765-0107
Web site: http://www.funerals.org/

The Funeral Consumers Alliance is dedicated to a consumer's right to choose a meaningful, dignified, affordable funeral. FCA provides educational materials on funeral choices to increase public awareness of funeral options and serves as a consumer advocate for reforms. Also monitors the industry and provides consumer alerts, answers to frequently asked questions, and "how to" pamphlets.

National Funeral Directors Association
Headquarters
13625 Bishop's Drive
Brookfield, WI 53005
Toll free: 1-800-228-6332
Phone: 262-789-1880
Fax: 262-789-6977
E mail: nfda@nfda.org
Web site: http://www.nfda.org

This organization is a comprehensive source of information about how to plan funerals as well as on loss and grief.

Glossary

A

acetaminophen: a well-known nonopioid pain reliever effective against mild or moderate pain like an NSAID but does not reduce inflammation.

acute care: *see hospitalization.*

acute pain: severe pain that begins suddenly and lasts a relatively short time.

adjuvant therapy: treatment used in addition to the main treatment. It usually refers to hormonal therapy, chemotherapy, or radiation added after surgery to increase the chances of curing the disease or keeping it in check.

advance directives: legal documents that provide a forum for individuals to express their wishes about end-of-life care and decision making if they become too ill to speak for themselves. The term advance directive applies to two basic types of legal documents: the durable power of attorney for health care and the living will.

advanced cancer: cancer that has recurred and/or spread to vital organs in the body. Advanced cancer usually means that treatments no longer work and the cancer can't be cured. *See also metastatic cancer.*

alternative therapy: treatments that are promoted as cancer cures. They are unproven (they have not been scientifically tested) or were tested and found to be ineffective.

anticancer treatment: medical interventions directed against the growth and spread of cancer, regardless of whether they are delivered with curative or palliative intent. Also called anti-tumor treatment.

anticipatory grief: a grief process that precedes the actual death, in which a person begins to recognize the inevitability of the loss of a loved one, and anticipate how his or her life will change after the loved one dies.

anxiety: an overwhelming feeling of uneasiness, apprehension, and fear.

appointment of a health care agent: *see durable power of attorney for health care.*

artificial hydration and nutrition: the act of mechanically providing fluids or nutrition to a patient via intravenous lines or feeding tubes that go in through the nose or the stomach wall.

artificial nutrition: feeding through a tube in the stomach or through an intravenous line.

autopsy: a special examination of a body to determine the cause of death or the nature or extent of disease at time of death.

B

bedsores: *see pressure ulcers.*

beneficiary: a person who receives assets of a will or trust.

benefits and burdens: a commonly used guideline for deciding whether or not to withhold or withdraw medical treatments. However, a benefit from one point of view can be experienced as a burden from another and might be viewed differently by doctors, patients, and families. Discussions of the benefits and burdens of medical treatments should occur within the framework of the patient's overall goals for care.

benign: non-cancerous.

bereavement: the state of grief.

biopsy: a diagnostic process in which a sample of abnormal tissue is examined under a microscope to see if cancer cells are present.

breakthrough pain: a brief and often severe flare of pain that occurs even though a person may be taking pain medicine regularly for persistent pain. Breakthrough pain typically comes on quickly, lasts only a few minutes or as long as an hour, and requires the use of a rescue medication. Also called incident pain.

C

cancer: a group of related diseases that cause cells in the body to change and grow out of control.

carcinomas: cancers that begin from the surface of organs, such as the lining of the lung or colon.

chemotherapy: treatment with various medicines.

chronic pain: mild to severe pain that may last for a few weeks or may be ongoing.

comfort care: care aimed at relieving, controlling, or preventing symptoms. *See also palliative care.*

complementary therapy: supportive treatment methods that are used to complement, or add to, mainstream treatments. Complementary methods are not given to cure disease; rather, they may help control symptoms and improve well-being. Examples of complementary methods include meditation, yoga, massage, and acupuncture.

complete response: tests and examinations have not detected any remaining cancer cells.

constipation: a decreased number of bowel movements or difficulty moving your bowels.

contemporaneous record: a diary of events written as the events take place (as opposed to recorded after the fact).

continuous pain: *see persistent pain.*

coping: managing problems and difficulties and attempting to overcome them.

culturally competent care: care that is responsive to a patient's unique beliefs, behaviors, personal preferences, values, and ethnocultural traditions.

curative surgery: the removal of a tumor when it appears to be confined to one area.

cure: all cancer cells are gone and the cancer will not come back. Doctors rarely pronounce a patient "cured," and will often use the term "in remission" or "complete response" instead.

D

death: legally, the irreversible cessation of circulatory and respiratory function, or of all functions of the entire brain.

debulking surgery: the removal of as much of the tumor as possible.

dehydration: the body's loss of adequate fluid.

delirium: an advanced state of confusion.

depression: a condition characterized by persistent feelings of sadness, guilt, or helplessness and a combination of physical symptoms such as a change in weight and appetite, in sleep and energy, in thinking and ability to concentrate, in the desire to participate in social activities, overall mood, and interest in both people and surroundings.

diagnostic surgery: used to get a tissue sample (also called a biopsy) to identify your specific cancer and make a diagnosis.

dietician: *see nutritionist.*

DNAR order: *see do not attempt to resuscitate order.*

DNR order: *see do not attempt to resuscitate order.*

do not attempt to resuscitate order: A DNAR order is written by a doctor saying that a dying person will not have cardiopulmonary resuscitation (CPR) or be placed on a breathing machine before death. A DNAR order is not a "do not treat" order. Also called a DNR (do not resuscitate) order. *See also nonhospital DNAR order.*

do not resuscitate order: *see do not attempt to resuscitate order.*

donating your body to science: *see whole body donation.*

DPOA: *see durable power of attorney.*

durable power of attorney (DPOA): a legal document that designates someone to make decisions on your behalf if you are not able to do so because of poor health. *See also durable power of attorney for financial matters; durable power of attorney for health care.*

durable power of attorney for financial matters: a legal document that designates someone to handle financial matters for you if you are not able to do so because of poor health.

durable power of attorney for health care: a legal document that designates someone to make medical decisions for you if you become too ill to speak for yourself. Also called a medical power of attorney, a health care proxy, or an appointment of a health care agent.

dying: those who are likely to die within a few days to several months; those that have a fatal, terminal, or incurable illness or advanced progressive disease whose "timetables" for death are less predictable.

dyspnea: difficulty breathing; the feeling of not getting enough air, shortness of breath, or breathlessness.

E

end of life: the period of time before death; the target time period of most palliative care interventions.

estate: the sum of property a person owns, including all assets

euthanasia: the act of administering a lethal dose of a medication into a person, ostensibly to relieve suffering. Euthanasia is not legal anywhere in the United States.

F

fatigue: an unusual and persistent sense of physical, mental, and emotional tiredness that can occur with cancer or cancer treatment.

forgiveness: to give up a grudge.

formal caregivers: professional staff members in agencies, hospice organizations, and hospitals (doctors, nurses, health aides, social workers, and allied health professionals like physical therapists) that provide care.

functional capacity: a person's ability to move around and care for themselves; a way health care professionals assess the overall physical functioning of patients.

G

gene therapy: an experimental therapy that involves inserting a specific gene into cells to restore a missing function or to give the cells a new function. Because missing or damaged genes cause certain diseases, it makes sense to treat these diseases by adding the missing gene or fixing the damaged one.

grief: the emotional distress resulting from loss, such as the death of loved one.

guaranteed-access programs: *see risk pools.*

guardianship clause: a portion of a will that provides instructions and provisions for the care of children and other dependents.

H

health care agent: a person designated in a durable power of attorney for health care who negotiates on your behalf with doctors and other caregivers and is required to make decisions according to your directions

health care declaration: *see living will.*

health care proxy: *see durable power of attorney for health care.*

home health care aide: a health care professional who can assist with day-to-day household tasks such as bathing and preparing or feeding meals.

home health nurse: a nurse who can give medications in the home, teach patients how to care for themselves, and assess their conditions to see if further medical attention is needed.

hormonal therapy: drug treatments that change the hormone environment in your body or react with hormone-sensitive substances in the cancer cell.

hospice care: a model of care within which palliative care is delivered. It can be a place where end-of-life care is delivered (most often the home, but sometimes a hospital or other care facility), or an organization or system through which this care is delivered. The term is often used to describe the Medicare hospice benefit.

hospice: a care delivery system that takes place at home, in a hospital, or in a freestanding hospice care facility such as a nursing home; an organization or program that arranges, provides, and provides guidance on a variety of medical and supportive services for dying persons and their loved ones.

hospitalization: care that is typically engaged during health care crises, when a patient's medical needs cannot be met in another environment. Also called inpatient care or acute care.

I

immunotherapy: treatment that uses the body's own immune system to fight disease by stimulating it to work harder, or using an outside source, such as man-made immune system proteins.

incident pain: *see breakthrough pain.*

informal caregivers: family caregivers and the network of unpaid people who help with caregiving tasks on a day-to day basis.

inpatient care: see hospitalization.

insomnia: difficulty sleeping.

integrative therapy: the combination of evidence-based standard treatments and complementary therapies.

intestate: the legal state of dying without a will.

intravenous: delivery into your bloodstream through your veins, or "by IV."

L

last will and testament: see will.

letter of instruction: a document that includes information not covered in the will, such as how to distribute personal property with little economic value but important sentimental value.

leukemia: cancer that begins in the bone marrow.

life review: the process of looking back on one's life and remembering what was most important as life draws to a close.

life-sustaining medical treatment: in general, anything mechanical or artificial that sustains, restores, or substitutes for a vital body function and that would prolong the process for someone who is dying. Each state defines this term differently.

living will: a document that gives instructions about the use of medical treatments at the end of life. Its purpose is to guide family members and doctors in deciding how aggressively to use medical treatments to delay death. Also called a medical directive or health care declaration.

lymphoma: cancer that arises in the lymphatic system, which filters bacteria, fights infections, and carries fluid from the limbs and internal organs back into the blood.

M

making an anatomical gift: see whole body donation.

malignant: cancerous.

mechanical ventilation: the use of a ventilator, a machine that pumps air and extra oxygen into a patient's lungs through a special tube to assist with breathing difficulties.

medical directive: see living will.

medical power of attorney: see durable power of attorney for health care.

mental health directive: a document defining a person's choices about treatment in the event that he or she becomes seriously mentally ill and is unable to make health care decisions.

metastasis: the spread of cancer cells to distant areas of the body by way of the lymph system or bloodstream.

metastatic cancer: cancer that has spread to other parts of the body. Cancer is called metastatic even if only a small amount of the cancer has spread. Metastatic cancer may be classified as advanced if it has spread many places or has greatly harmed tissues and important organs and cannot be removed. See also advanced cancer.

mourning: the process by which a person adapts to a significant loss.

N

narcotics: see opioids.

nausea: queasiness.

neurologist: a doctor who treats diseases of the nervous system.

neuro-oncologist: is a neurologist with expertise treating brain tumors and the neurological complications of cancer.

nonhospital DNAR order: a physician's order not to attempt CPR designed to protect seriously ill or dying individuals who are being cared for at home from unwanted resuscitation by emergency crews or health care providers unfamiliar with that person's preferences for end-of-life care and treatment. See also do not attempt to resuscitate order.

nonsteroidal anti-inflammatory drugs (NSAIDs): medications used to relieve mild to severe pain and reduce inflammation.

NSAIDs: see nonsteroidal anti-inflammatory drugs.

nutritionist: a professional who assesses your nutritional state and recommends ways to eat that will help you deal with having cancer and cancer treatments. Also called a dietician.

O

oncologist: a doctor who specializes in diagnosing and treating cancer.

oncology clinical nurse specialist: a registered nurse who is an expert at caring for people with cancer. Oncology nurse specialists may administer treatments like chemotherapy, monitor patients, prescribe and provide supportive care, and teach and counsel patients and their families.

oncology social worker: a health care professional who coordinates and provides non-medical care to people with cancer and their families, especially counseling and assistance in dealing with financial problems, housing (when treatments must be taken at a facility away from home), child care, and emotional distress.

opioids: the strongest pain relievers available. Examples are morphine, fentanyl, hydromorphone, oxycodone, and codeine. Prescriptions are needed for these medicines. Also known as narcotics.

oral advance directive: a verbal statement made by a person who is physically unable to obtain a written living will or written power of attorney for health care. This statement is written by someone else and properly witnessed. *See also advance directive.*

organ donation: the process of removing organs from a deceased person in order for the organs to be used for transplantation to save or enhance the life of a person in need.

ostomy: an operation (such as a colostomy, ileostomy, or urostomy) to create an artificial passage for bodily elimination; the bag that collects this waste.

P

pain specialists: doctors or nurses that make recommendations about the best treatments for controlling different kinds of pain.

palliative care specialists: health professionals (usually members of a team consisting of a physician, a nurse, social worker, and chaplain, all of whom have special training in palliative and supportive care) who focus on providing comfort, controlling physical symptoms such as pain, and giving emotional or spiritual support to people with advanced illnesses and their family members, especially as end-of-life nears.

palliative care: a comprehensive approach to treating serious illness that focuses on the physical, emotional, spiritual, and social needs of the patient and his or her loved ones rather than on a cure for disease. Its goal is to achieve the best quality of life available to the patient by relieving suffering, controlling pain and symptoms, and enabling the patient to achieve maximum functional capacity. Respect for the patient's culture, beliefs, and values are essential components. Also called comfort care or supportive care, although professionals draw some distinctions among these terms.

palliative medicine: the study and treatment of patients living with life-limiting or advanced illness where care is focused on relieving suffering and promoting quality of life. Major components of this specialty are pain and symptom management, information sharing, advance care planning, and coordination of care, including psychosocial and spiritual support for patients and their loved ones.

palliative surgery: used to treat complications of advanced disease. It is not intended to cure the cancer, but can be used to correct a problem causing discomfort or disability.

pastoral care expert: a specially trained, non-denominational religious leader or counselor who provides spiritual care.

pathologist: a doctor who uses laboratory tests to diagnose and classify diseases like cancer. The pathologist determines whether a tumor is benign or cancerous, and, if cancerous, the exact cell type and grade.

patient-controlled analgesia (PCA): a system of delivering pain medications that allows the person in pain to control the dosage of medication on an as-needed basis.

performance status: a measure of how active a person is and how well he or she feels.

persistent pain: pain that is present for long periods of time. Also called continuous pain.

physical therapist: a health professional trained to educate and assist patients with exercises and other methods to restore or maintain your body's strength, mobility, and function.

physician-assisted suicide: the act of prescribing medicines by a physician that are intended to cause the death of a patient. The physician "assists" the suicide by making the medication available to the patient, but the physician does not administer it. Legal only in the state of Oregon.

postoperative pain: pain due to surgery.

pressure ulcers: sores that occur on the skin that overlies bony prominences due to pressure or staying in one place or position for continued periods of time. Also called bedsores.

preventive surgery: done to remove body tissue that is not cancerous but is likely to become so.

primary care physician: the doctor you would normally see first when a problem arises. Your primary care doctor could be a general practitioner, a family practice doctor, a gynecologist, or an internal medicine doctor/internist.

prognosis: a prediction of the probable course and outcome of a disease and an indication of the chances for survival.

progressive disease: the cancer has increased in size by 25 percent; the cancer is worse.

proxy: a person designated in a durable power of attorney who negotiates on your behalf with doctors, caregivers, and other individuals and is required to make decisions according to your directions.

psychiatrist: a medical doctor who specializes in mental health and behavioral disorders, provide counseling and can also prescribe medications.

psychologist: a health professional who assesses a person's mental and emotional status and provides counseling.

psycho-oncologist: a psychiatrist with expertise dealing with people who have cancer.

Q

quality of life: health as perceived and valued by people for themselves rather than by clinicians; a broad term that can involve physical, mental, and social dimensions, ability to fulfill daily roles and responsibilities (sometimes called role functioning), freedom from bodily pain, satisfaction with health care, and an overall sense of general health and well-

being. Simply put, a person's ability to enjoy life and perform his or her usual activities.

R

radiation oncologist: a doctor who specializes in radiation therapy given to treat cancers.

radiation therapy: x-ray treatment designed to prevent cancer cells from continuing to divide and multiply and spread.

reconciliation: an agreement between two people in which the offender admits to doing a hurtful thing, apologizes, repents, and asks for forgiveness, and the other person grants forgiveness.

recurrence: cancer that has come back after treatment. Local recurrence means that the cancer has come back at the same place as the original cancer. Regional recurrence means that the cancer has come back in the lymph nodes near the first site. Distant recurrence is when cancer metastasizes after treatment to organs or tissues (such as the lungs, liver, bone marrow, or brain) farther from the original site than the regional lymph nodes.

religion: a type of spirituality usually identified with adherence to a particular set of institutionalized beliefs or practices.

remission: tests and examinations have not detected any remaining cancer cells. Also called complete response.

rescue medication: medicine used to treat break-through pain.

respite care: relief for the person with cancer's at-home caregivers.

respite: help with or a brief reprieve from caregiving responsibilities.

response rate: an estimate of how likely the cancer is to get better with a particular treatment. A complete response means that the cancer completely goes away by physical examination and all diagnostic tests (x-rays, bone scan, etc.) and stays away for at least four weeks. A partial response means that all of the cancer shrinks by at least 50 percent and stays away for at least four weeks.

risk of recurrence: an estimate of how likely cancer is to come back.

risk pools: a method for states to provide comprehensive health insurance to residents with serious medical conditions who can't find finding affordable coverage in the private market. Also called guaranteed access programs, they provide a safety net for the "medically uninsurable" population.

S

sarcomas: cancers that begin in the bone and cartilage, joints, and muscles. Carcinomas are more common than sarcomas.

screening: the search for disease, such as cancer, in people without symptoms.

spinal cord compression: pressure on the spinal cord from cancer.

spirituality: a person's sense of peace, purpose, meaning, and connection to others and to the transcendent.

stable disease: the cancer has not grown bigger or smaller by more than 25 percent, and has not spread.

staging surgery: helps determine the extent and the amount of disease.

staging: the process of determining how far the cancer has spread.

statistics: the collection, study, and interpretation of facts and figures to learn more about a certain event, experience, or group of people.

supportive care: care aimed at relieving, controlling, or preventing symptoms. *See also palliative care.*

surgical oncologist: a doctor who specializes in cancer surgery; usually these doctors focus on one part of the body, like the abdomen or the head and neck.

survival rate: an estimate of how likely you are to live and for how long.

systemic therapies: treatment that can target multiple places throughout the body.

T

tissue donation: the process of removing tissues from a deceased person in order for the tissues to be used for transplantation to save or enhance the life of a person in need.

treatment with curative intent: treatment designed to cure cancer.

trust: a means of transferring property from you to another person or entity designed to help eliminate the probate process and minimize inheritance taxes.

trustee: a person or financial institution to whom another person has transferred ownership of property for management.

tumor: a cancerous lump or mass which can invade and destroy healthy tissue.

V

ventilator: a machine that pumps air and extra oxygen into a patient's lungs through a special tube to assist with breathing difficulties.

viatical: the sale of a life insurance policy to a third party for cash.

vomiting: regurgitation or throwing up.

W

whole body donation: the process of assigning your body to a medical school or research institution upon death to assist in research and education. Also called donating your body to science or making an anatomical gift.

will: a legal document that describes what happens to your property after your death. Also called a last will and testament.

withdrawing treatment: discontinuing (stopping) life-sustaining measures after they have been used for a certain period of time.

withholding treatment: forgoing life-sustaining measures.

References

General References

American Cancer Society and National Comprehensive Cancer Network. *Advanced Cancer and Palliative Care: Treatment Guidelines for Patients, Version I/December 2003.* Atlanta, GA: 2003.

Brookes T. *Signs of Life: A Memoir of Dying and Discovery.* New York: Times Books, 1997.

Byock I. *Dying Well: Peace and Possibilities at the End of Life.* New York: Riverhead Books, 1998.

Byock I. *The Four Things That Matter Most: A Book about Living.* New York: Free Press, 2004.

Doyle D, Hanks GWC, MacDonald N, eds. *Oxford Textbook of Palliative Medicine,* 2nd ed. Oxford; New York: Oxford University Press, 2004.

Enck RE. *The Medical Care of Terminally Ill Patients,* 2nd ed. Baltimore: Johns Hopkins University Press, 2002.

Ferrell BF, Coyle N, eds. *Textbook of Palliative Nursing.* Oxford: Oxford University Press, 2001.

Field, MJ, Cassel, CK, eds. *Approaching Death: Improving Care at the End of Life.* Committee on Care at the End of Life, Division of Health Care Services, Institute of Medicine; Washington, DC: National Academy Press, 1997.

Foley KM, Gelband H, eds. *Improving Palliative Care for Cancer: Summary and Recommendations.* National Cancer Policy Board, Institute of Medicine and National Research Council; Washington, DC: National Academy Press, 2001. Available at http://www.nap.edu/books/0309074029/html/. Accessed May 3, 2004.

Halpern SP. *The Etiquette of Illness: What to Say When You Can't Find the Words.* New York: Bloomsbury, 2004

Holder JS, Aldredge-Clanton J. *Parting: A Handbook for Spiritual Care Near the End of Life.* Chapel Hill: University of North Carolina Press, 2004.

Houts PS. *The American College of Physicians Home Care Guide for Advanced Cancer: When Quality of Life Is The Primary Goal of Care.* Philadelphia, PA: The College, 1997.

Houts PS, Bucher, JA. *Caregiving: A Step-by-step Resource for Caring for the Person with Cancer at Home,* revised ed. Atlanta, GA: American Cancer Society, 2003.

Joishy SK, ed. *Palliative Medicine Secrets.* Philadephia, PA: Hanley & Belfus, 1999.

Jenkins M. *You Only Die Once: Preparing for the End of Life with Grace and Gusto.* Nashville, TN: Integrity Pub., 2002.

Lynn J, Harrold J, and the Center to Improve Care of the Dying, George Washington University. *Handbook for Mortals: Guidance for People Facing Serious Illness.* New York: Oxford University Press, 1999.

McLeod BW, ed. *And Thou Shalt Honor: the Caregiver's Companion.* Emmaus, Pa.: Rodale, 2002.

McPhelimy L. *In the Checklist of Life: A "Working Book" to Help You Live and Leave This Life!,* 2nd ed. Rockfall, CT: AAIP Publishing Co. LLC, 1997.

National Consensus Project for Quality Palliative Care. Clinical Practice Guidelines for Quality Palliative Care. Available at http://www.nationalconsensusproject.org/guideline.pdf. Accessed May 5, 2004.

Nuland S. *How We Die: Reflections on Life's Final Chapter.* New York: A.A. Knopf; Distributed by Random House, Inc., 1994.

Preston TA. *Final Victory: Taking Charge of the Last Stages of Life, Facing Death on Your Own Terms.* Roseville, CA: Forum, 2000.

Rakel R, ed. *Textbook of Family Practice,* 6th ed. Philadelphia: Saunders, 2002.

Romer AL, Heller KS, Weissman DE, Solomon MZ, eds. *Innovations in End-of-life Care: Practical Strategies and International Perspectives,* volume 3. Mary Ann Liebert Inc. Publishers, 2002.

Solomon JR. *When The Journey of Life Ends: What You Need To Know and Do After a Death...An Information Guide to Assist Survivors.* Seekonk, MA: JRose Enterprise, 1998.

Tobin DR, Lindsey K. *Peaceful Dying: The Step-By-Step Guide to Preserving Your Dignity, Your Choice, and Your Inner Peace at the End of Life.* Reading, MA: Perseus Books, 1999.

Waller A, Caroline NL. *Handbook of Palliative Care in Cancer,* 2nd ed. Boston: Butterworth-Heinemann, 1996.

Introduction References

Doyle D, Hanks GWC, MacDonald N, eds. *Oxford Textbook of Palliative Medicine,* 2nd ed. Oxford; New York: Oxford University Press, 2004.

Field MJ, Cassel CK, eds. *Approaching Death: Improving Care at the End of Life.* Committee on Care at the End of Life, Division of Health Care Services, Institute of Medicine; Washington, DC: National Academy Press, 1997.

Last Acts. Some Basic Facts about Dying in America Today. Available at http://www.lastacts.org. Accessed January, 2004.

Milch R, Schumacher JD. Finding Our Way. There's Light at the End of the Tunnel for America's End-of-Life Care. Available at http://www.findingourway.net/Articles/article_current_reality.htm. Accessed December 12, 2003.

Nuland, S. *How We Die: Reflections on Life's Final Chapter*. New York: A.A. Knopf, Distributed by Random House, Inc., 1994.

Chapter 1 References

American Academy of Hospice and Palliative Medicine. Position Statements. Available at http://www.aahpm.org/positions/definition.html. Accessed January 24, 2004.

Doyle D, Hanks GWC, MacDonald N, eds. *Oxford Textbook of Palliative Medicine*, 2nd ed. Oxford; New York: Oxford University Press, 2004.

Field MJ, Cassel CK, eds. *Approaching Death: Improving Care at the End of Life*. Committee on Care at the End of Life, Division of Health Care Services, Institute of Medicine; Washington, DC: National Academy Press, 1997.

Jennings B, Ryndes T, D'Onofrio C, Daly MA. Access to Hospice Care: Expanding Boundaries, Overcoming Barriers. Available at http://www.thehastingscenter.org/pdf/access_hospice_care.pdf. Accessed March 31, 2004.

Last Acts. A Vision for Better Care at the End of Life. Available at http://www.lastacts.org/docs/publicprecepts.pdf. Accessed January 14, 2004.

Milch R, Schumacher JD. Finding Our Way. There's Light at the End of the Tunnel for America's End-of-Life Care. Available at http://www.findingourway.net/Articles/article_current_reality.htm. Accessed December 12, 2003.

National Hospice Foundation. Hospice Care: Comfort and Compassion When It's Needed Most. Available at: http://www.nhpco.org/files/public/NHF_brochure_green_Medicare.pdf. Accessed March 26, 2004.

Partnership for Caring. Glossary of Terms. Available at http://www.partnershipforcaring.org/Resources/glossary_set.html. Accessed February 4, 2004.

Portenoy RK. Finding Our Way. Care to Ease the Final Days. Available at http://www.findingourway.net/Articles/article_palliative_care.html. Accessed December 12, 2003.

Steinhauser KE, Christakis NA, Clipp EC, McNeilly M, McIntyre L, Tulsky JA. Factors considered important at the end of life by patients, family, physicians, and other care providers. JAMA. 2000; 284:2476-2482.

Chapter 2 References

American Cancer Society. Cancer Control State of the Science Guide. Atlanta, GA: 2003.

American Cancer Society. Choices for Palliative Care. Available at http://www.cancer.org/docroot/CRI/content/CRI_2_4_4x_Choices_for_Palliative_Care.asp?sitearea=. Accessed December 11, 2003.

American Cancer Society and National Comprehensive Cancer Network. *Advanced Cancer and Palliative Care: Treatment Guidelines for Patients, Version I/December 2003*. Atlanta, GA: 2003.

Foley KM, Gelband H, eds. *Improving Palliative Care for Cancer: Summary and Recommendations*. National Cancer Policy Board, Institute of Medicine and National Research Council. Washington DC: National Academy Press, 2001. Available at http://www.nap.edu/books/0309074029/html/. Accessed May 3, 2004.

Last Acts. Care Beyond Cure: Palliative Care and Hospice. Available at http://www.lastacts.org/files/misc/Hospice&palliativecare.pdf. Accessed January 2004.

National Cancer Institute. Home Care for Cancer Patients. Available at http://cis.nci.nih.gov/fact/8_5.htm. Accessed January, 2004.

National Hospice and Palliative Care Organization. Hospice and Palliative Care. Available at http://www.nhpco.org/i4a/pages/index.cfm?pageid=3254&openpage=3254. Accessed January, 2004.

National Hospice and Palliative Care Organization. Hospice Care: Comfort and Compassion When It's Needed Most. Available at: http://www.nhpco.org/files/public/NHF_brochure_green_Medicare.pdf. Accessed March 26, 2004.

Waller A, Caroline NL. *Handbook of Palliative Care in Cancer*, 2nd ed. Boston: Butterworth-Heinemann, 1996.

Chapter 3 References

American Cancer Society. *A Breast Cancer Journey: Your Personal Guidebook*, 2nd ed. Atlanta, GA: 2003.

American Cancer Society. Health Professionals Associated with Cancer Care. Available at: http://www.cancer.org/docroot/ETO/content/ETO_2_6x_Health_Professionals_Associated_with_Cancer_Care.asp. Accessed April 29, 2004.

American Cancer Society. Physicians Not Always Forthcoming with Accurate Prognosis Information. *CA Cancer J Clin*. 2001; 51:267-268. Available at: http://caonline.amcancersoc.org/cgi/content/full/51/5/267. Accessed April 29, 2004.

Lamont EB, Christakis NA. Prognostic Disclosure to Patients with Cancer near the End of Life. *Annals of Internal Medicine.* 2001;123:1096-1105. Available at: http://www.annals.org/cgi/content/full/134/12/1096. Accessed April 29, 2004.

Lynn J, Harrold J, and the Center to Improve Care of the Dying, George Washington University. *Handbook for Mortals: Guidance for People Facing Serious Illness.* New York: Oxford University Press, 1999.

National Cancer Institute. Your Health Care Team: Your Doctor Is Only the Beginning (Cancer Facts). Available at http://cis.nci.nih.gov/fact/8_10.htm. Accessed December 12, 2003.

National Cancer Institute. Understanding Prognosis and Cancer Statistics (Cancer Facts.) Available at: http://cis.nci.nih.gov/fact/8_2.htm. Accessed April 29, 2004.

Chapter 4 References

American Cancer Society. *A Breast Cancer Journey: Your Personal Guidebook,* 2nd ed. Atlanta, GA: 2003.

American Cancer Society. Communicating with Friends and Relatives about Your Cancer. Available at: http://www.cancer.org/docroot/ESN/content/ESN_2_1x _Communicating_with_Friends_and_Relatives_About _Your_Cancer.asp?sitearea=ESN. Accessed January 20, 2004.

American Cancer Society. Coping with Advanced Cancer. Available at: http://www.cancer.org/docroot/CRI/ content/CRI_2_6x_Coping_with_Advanced_Cancer. asp?sitearea=. Accessed December 11, 2003.

American Cancer Society. Finding Support. Available at: http://www.cancer.org/docroot/ESN/content/ ESN_2_3X_A_Message_of_Hope_Finding_Support. asp?sitearea=ESN. Accessed January 21, 2004.

American Cancer Society. Support Groups: General Information. Available at http://www.cancer.org/docroot/ ESN/content/ESN_2_3X_Support_groups_general_ information.asp?sitearea=ESN. Accessed January 21, 2004.

FamilyDoctor.Org. Cancer: Helping Your Family Help You. Available at http://www.familydoctor.org/ x2386.xml?printxml. Accessed January 20, 2004.

Mayo Clinic. Tips for Coping with a Cancer Diagnosis. Available at http://www.mayoclinic.com/ invoke.cfm?objectid=1D66B64D-F30C-436E- ABFFEC8971616F07. Accessed January 20, 2004.

National Cancer Institute. Advanced Cancer: Living Each Day. Available at http://www.cancer.gov/cancerinfo/ advancedcancer/TOC#. Accessed January 21, 2004.

National Cancer Institute. When Cancer Recurs: Meeting the Challenge. Available at http://www.cancer.gov/ cancerinfo/when-cancer-recurs/TOC#. Accessed January 21, 2004.

National Cancer Institute. Cancer Support Groups: Questions and Answers (Cancer Facts). Available at: http://cis.nci.nih.gov/fact/8_8.htm. Accessed January 21, 2004.

Chapter 5 References

American Cancer Society. What Is a Life-Sustaining Medical Treatment? Available at http://www.cancer.org/ docroot/MIT/content/MIT_3_2X_What_is_a_Life_ Self-Sustaining_Medical_ Treatment.asp?sitearea=MIT. Accessed February 4, 2004.

Emanuel LL, Danis M, Pearlman RA, Singer PA. Advance care planning as a process: structuring the discussions in practice. *J Am Geriatric Soc.* 1995; Apr, 43(4):440-6.

Landay DS. *Be Prepared: The Complete Financial, Legal, and Practical Guide for Living with a Life-Challenging Condition.* New York: St. Martin's Press, 1998.

Last Acts. Thinking Ahead: Advance Planning for End-of-Life Care. Available at http://www.lastacts.org/files/ misc/THINKINGAHEAD.pdf. Accessed February, 2004.

Living Legacy Foundation. Frequently Asked Questions. Available at http://www.livinglegacyregistry.org/ learn/index.html. Accessed March 31, 2004.

Lynn J, Goldstein N. Advance care planning for fatal chronic illness: avoiding commonplace errors and unwarranted suffering. *Ann Intern Med.* 2003; 138:812-818.

Meisel A, Snyder L, Quill T. Seven legal barriers to end-of-life care: myths, realities, and grains of truth. *JAMA.* 2000; 284: 2495-2501.

McLeod BW, ed. *And Thou Shalt Honor: the Caregiver's Companion.* Emmaus, PA.: Rodale, 2002.

Chapter 6 References

American Cancer Society. *A Breast Cancer Journey: Your Personal Guidebook,* 2nd ed. Atlanta, GA: 2003.

American Association of Retired Persons (AARP). Insurance. http://www.aarp.org/financial-insurance/. Accessed February 6, 2004.

American Cancer Society. Medical Insurance and Financial Assistance for the Cancer Patient. Available at http://www.cancer.org/docroot/MLT/content/MLT_1x_ Medical_Insurance_and_Financial_Assistance_for_the _Cancer_Patient.asp?sitearea=&level=1. Accessed March 15, 2004.

American Cancer Society. Caring for the Patient with Cancer at Home: A Guide for Patients and Families. Available at http://www.cancer.org/docroot/MBC/content/MBC_2_3x_Caring_for_the_Patient_with_Cancer_at_Home_A_Guide_for_Patients_and_Families.asp. Accessed March 15, 2004.

Association for Home and Hospice Care. Hospice Care FAQs. Available at http://www.homeandhospicecare.org/consumer/hospicecare.html. Accessed March 26, 2004.

Centers for Medicare and Medicaid Services, U.S. Department of Health and Human Services. Medicare Hospice Benefits (Publication No. CMS 02154). Available at http://www.medicare.gov/Publications/Pubs/pdf/02154.pdf. Accessed March 29, 2004.

Health Insurance Association of America. Guide to Disability Income Insurance. http://www.hiaa.org/consumer/disability.cfm. Accessed February 9, 2004.

Hospice Net. Medicare Hospice Benefits. Available at http://www.hospicenet.org/html/medicare.html. Accessed March 26, 2004.

Landay DS. Be Prepared: The Complete Financial, Legal, and Practical Guide for Living with a Life-Challenging Condition. New York: St. Martin's Press, 1998.

McLeod BW, ed. And Thou Shalt Honor: the Caregiver's Companion. Emmaus, PA: Rodale, 2002.

The Motley Fool. Insurance Center. Available at http://www.fool.com/insurancecenter/life/life01.htm. Accessed February 9, 2004.

National Hospice Foundation. Hospice Care: Comfort and Compassion When It's Needed Most. Available at: http://www.nhpco.org/files/public/NHF_brochure_green_Medicare.pdf. Accessed March 26, 2004.

Chapter 7 References

American Cancer Society. A Breast Cancer Journey: Your Personal Guidebook, 2nd ed. Atlanta, GA: 2003.

American Association of Retired Persons (AARP). End of Life. Available at http://www.aarp.org/Articles/a2003-12-02-endoflife-financialpower.html. Accessed February 6, 2004.

Health Insurance Association of America. Guide to Disability Income Insurance. Available at http://www.hiaa.org/consumer/disability.cfm. Accessed February 9, 2004.

Landay DS. Be Prepared: The Complete Financial, Legal, and Practical Guide for Living with a Life-Challenging Condition. New York: St. Martin's Press, 1998.

Chapter 8 References

American Cancer Society. A Breast Cancer Journey: Your Personal Guidebook, 2nd ed. Atlanta, GA: 2003.

American Cancer Society. American Cancer Society's Guide to Pain Control: Understanding and Managing Cancer Pain, revised ed. Atlanta, GA: 2004.

American Cancer Society and National Comprehensive Cancer Network. Advanced Cancer and Palliative Care: Treatment Guidelines for Patients, Version I/December 2003. Atlanta, GA: 2003.

American Society of Clinical Oncology (ASCO). Optimizing Cancer Care: the Importance of Symptom Management. Dubuque, IA: Kendall/Hunt Pub. Co., 2001.

Berger A, Portenoy RK, Weissman DE, eds. Principles and Practice of Palliative Care and Supportive Oncology, 2nd ed. Philadelphia, PA: Lippincott Williams & Wilkins; 2002.

Waller A, Caroline NL. Handbook of Palliative Care in Cancer, 2nd ed. Boston: Butterworth-Heinemann, 1996.

Chapter 9 References

American Cancer Society and National Comprehensive Cancer Network. Advanced Cancer and Palliative Care: Treatment Guidelines for Patients, Version I/December 2003. Atlanta, GA: 2003.

Berry P, Griffie J. Planning for the Actual Death. In Ferrell BF, Coyle N. (Editors) Textbook of Palliative Nursing. Oxford: Oxford University Press, 2001:390-391.

Block, SD. Perspectives on care at the close of life. Psychological considerations, growth, and transcendence at the end of life: the art of the possible. JAMA. 2001 Jun 13;285(22):2898-905.

Byock I. Dying Well: Peace and Possibilities at the End of Life. New York: Riverhead Books, 1998.

Byock I. The Four Things That Matter Most: A Book about Living. New York: Free Press, 2004.

Harwell A. Ready to Live: Prepared to Die. Wheaton, IL: Harold Shaw Publishers, 1995.

Spence L. Legacy: A Step-By-Step Guide to Writing Personal History. Athens, OH: Swallow Press/Ohio University Press, 1997.

Storey P, Knight C. Unipac Six: Ethical and Legal Decision Making When Caring for the Terminally Ill. American Academy of Hospice and Palliative Medicine (AAHPM), 1996.

Chapter 10 References

Byock I. *Dying Well: Peace and Possibilities at the End of Life.* New York: Riverhead Books, 1998.

Daaleman TP, VandeCreek L. Placing religion and spirituality in end-of-life care. JAMA. 2000 Nov 15;284(19):2514-7.

The Gallup Organization. *Americans More Religious Now Than Ten Years Ago, but Less So Than in 1950s and 1960s* (poll released March 29, 2001). Available at www.gallup.com/poll/releases/pr010329.asp. Accessed February, 2004.

Groopman JE. *The Anatomy of Hope: How People Prevail in the Face of Illness.* New York: Random House, 2004.

Holder JS, Aldredge-Clanton J. *Parting: A Handbook for Spiritual Care Near the End of Life.* Chapel Hill: University of North Carolina Press, 2004.

Koenig HG. *Is Religion Good for Your Health? The Effects of Religion on Physical and Mental Health.* New York: Haworth Pastoral Press, 1997.

Last Acts. Care for the Spirit: The Role of Spirituality in End-of-Life Care. Available at http://www.lastacts.org/files/misc/careforspirit.pdf. Accessed February 10, 2004.

Levin JS. How religion influences morbidity and health. *Soc Sci Med* 1996; 43:849-864.

Lo B, Ruston D, Kates LW, Arnold RM, Cohen CB, Faber-Langendoen K, Pantilat SZ, Puchalski CM, Quill TR, Rabow MW, Schreiber S, Sulmasy DP, Tulsky JA; Working Group on Religious and Spiritual Issues at the End of Life. Discussing religious and spiritual issues at the end of life: a practical guide for physicians. JAMA. 2002 Feb 13;287(6):749-54.

National Cancer Institute. Spirituality in Cancer Care (PDQ). Available at http://www.nci.nih.gov/cancerinfo/pdq/supportivecare/spirituality. Accessed February 10, 2004.

Rutlan-Wallis M, Maddry H. Finding Our Way. Spirituality and Faith: In Death, Spirituality Can Deepen Meaning of Life. Available at http://www.findingourway.net/Articles/article_spirituality_faith.html. Accessed December 12, 2003.

Sheehan, MN. Spirituality and care at the end of life. *Choices: The Newsletter of Choice in Dying.* 1997 6(2).

Smedes LB. *The Art of Forgiving: When You Need to Forgive and Don't Know How.* Nashville, TN: Moorings, 1996.

Chapter 11 References

Arno PS, Levine C, Memmott MM. The economic value of informal caregiving. *Health Affairs.* 1999;18:2:182-188.

Burns CM, Dixon T, Broom D, Smith WT, Craft PS. Family caregiver knowledge of treatment intent in a longitudinal study of patients with advanced cancer. *Supportive Care in Cancer.* July 26, 2003; 11:10:629-637.

Chalmers KI, Luker KA, Leinster SJ, Ellis I, Booth K. Information and support needs of women with primary relatives with breast cancer: development of the Information and Support Needs Questionnaire. *Journal Advanced Nursing.* 2001; 35:4:497-507.

Covinsky KE, Goldman L, Cook EF, Oye R, Desbiens N, Reding D, Fulkerson W, Connors AF, Jr., Lynn J, Phillips RS. The impact of serious illness on patients' families. SUPPORT investigators. Study to understand prognoses and preferences for outcomes and risks of treatment. *Journal American Medical Association.* 1994; 272:1839-1844.

Family Caregiver Alliance. Available at http://www.caregiver.org. Accessed September 11, 2003.

Foley KM. Supportive care and quality of life. In: Devita VT, Hellman S, Rosenberg SA, eds. *Cancer: Principles & Practice of Oncology.* Philadelphia, PA: Lippincott Williams & Wilkins, 2001:56:2989.

Gobel BH, Anxiety. In: Yabro CH, Frogge MH, Goodman M, eds. *Cancer Symptom Management.* Sudbury, MA: Jones and Bartlett Pub, 1999; 30:580-593.

Harding R, Higginson IJ, Donaldson N. The relationship between patient characteristics and career psychological status in home palliative cancer care. *Supportive Care in Cancer.* 2003; 11:10:638-643.

Iconomou G, Vagenakis AG, Kalofonos HP. The informational needs, satisfaction with communication, and psychological status of primary caregivers of cancer patients receiving chemotherapy. *Supportive Care in Cancer.* 2001; 9:591-596.

Lynn J. Learning to care for people with chronic illness facing the end of life. *Journal American Medical Association.* 2000; 284:2508-2511.

Much JK, Barsevick AM. Depression. In: Yabro CH, Frogge MH, Goodman M, eds. *Cancer Symptom Management.* Sudbury, MA: Jones and Bartlett Pub; 1999:30:580-593.

National Hospice Foundation. Hospice Care: Comfort and Compassion When It's Needed Most. Available at: http://www.nhpco.org/files/public/NHF_brochure_green_Medicare.pdf. Accessed March 26, 2004.

National Profile of Family Caregivers in Canada-2002: Final Report. CMA Research, Policy and Planning Directorate. Canada. Available at http://www.hc-sc.gc.ca/english/pdf/care/nat_profile02.pdf. Accessed March 15, 2004.

Nijboer C, Triemstra M, Tempelaar R, Sanderman R, van den Bos GAM. Determinants of caregiving experiences and mental health of partners of cancer patient. *Cancer.* 1999; 86:4:577-587.

Rabow MW, Hauser JM, Adams J. Supporting family caregivers at the end of life: "they don't know what they don't know." JAMA. 2004 Jan 28; 291(4):483-91

Roth AJ, Massie MJ. Psychiatric Complications in Cancer Patients. In: Lenhard RE, Osteen RT, Gansler T, eds. *Clinical Oncology*. Malden MA: Blackwell Science; 2001; 36:837-851.

Schulz R ,Beach SR. Caregiving as a risk factor for mortality: The Caregiver Health Effects Study. *Journal American Medical Association*. 1999; 282:2215-2219.

Schulz R, Beach SR, Lind B, Martire LM, Zdaniuk B, Hirsch C, Jackson S, Burton L. Involvement in caregiving and adjustment to death of a spouse: findings from the Caregiver Health Effects Study. *Journal American Medical Association*. 2001; 285: 3123-3129.

Sansone-Fisher R, Girgis A, Boyes A, Bonevski B, Burton L, Cook P. The unmet supportive care needs of patients with cancer. *Cancer*. 2000; 88:1:226-237.

Soothill K, Morris MS, Harman J, Francis B, Thomas C, McIllmurray MB. The significant unmet needs of cancer patients: probing psychosocial concerns. *Supportive Care in Cancer*. 2001; 9:597-605.

Soothill K, Morris SM, Harman JC, Francis B, Thomas C, McIllmurray MB. Informal carers of cancer patients: what are their unmet psychosocial needs? *Health Soc Care Community*. 2001; 9:6:464-75.

Spector W, Fleishman J, Pezzin L, et al. The characteristics of long-term care users. *Agency for Healthcare Research and Quality Research Report*. Rockville, MD. (AHRQ Pub. No.00-0049). August 2000:44.

Wagner DL. Workplace programs for family caregivers: good business and good practice. Family Caregiver Alliance. San Francisco: 2003.

Wingate AL, Lackey NR. A description of the needs of non-institutionalized cancer patients and their primary care givers. *Cancer Nursing*. 1989;12:4:216-25.

Wong RKS, Franssen E, Szumacher E et al. What do patients living with advanced cancer and their carers want to know? A needs assessment. *Supportive Care in Cancer*. 2002; 10:408-415.

Chapter 12 References

American Cancer Society and National Comprehensive Cancer Network. *Advanced Cancer and Palliative Care: Treatment Guidelines for Patients, Version I/December 2003*. Atlanta, GA: 2003.

Baker DC. *Studies of the inner life: the impact of spirituality on quality of life*. Quality of Life Research, 2003; 12(Suppl 1)51-57.

Block SD. Psychological considerations, growth, and transcendence at the end of life: the art of the possible. *Journal American Medical Association*. 2001; 285: 2898-2905.

Breitbart W. Spirituality and meaning in supportive care: spirituality- and meaning- centered group psychotherapy interventions in advanced cancer. *Supportive Care in Cancer*. 2002; 10:4:272-280

Cancer Care. Nurturing the spirit when cancer is advanced. Available at http://www.cancercare.org/ EducationalPrograms/EducationalPrograms.cfm?ID=345 1&c=381. Accessed March 15, 2004.

Chen H, Haley WE, Robinson BE, Schonwetter RS. Decisions for hospice care in patients with advanced cancer. *Journal American Geriatric Society*. 2003; 51:6:789-797.

Kelly B, Edwards P, Synott R, Neil C, Baillie R, Battistutta D. Predictors of bereavement outcome for family carers of cancer patients. *Psycho-Oncology*. 1999; 8: 237-249.

Lamont EB, Christakis NA. Complexities in prognostication in advanced cancer. *Journal American Medical Association*. 2003; 290:1:98-104.

Last Acts National Program Office. Means to a Better End: A Report on Dying in America Today. Washington DC: 2002.

Lepore SJ, Smyth JM. Eds, *The Writing Cure*. Washington DC: American Psychological Assoc.; 2003.

Levine SA, Boal J, Boling PA. Home care. *Journal American Medical Association*. 2003; 290:9:1203-1207.

Lunney JR, Lynn J, Foley DJ, Lipson S, Guralnik JM. Patterns of functional decline at the end of life. *Journal American Medical Association*. 2003; 289:18:2387-2392.

Lynn J. Learning to care for people with chronic illness facing the end of life. *Journal American Medical Association*. 2000; 284:2508-2511.

Lynn J. Serving patients who may die soon and their families: the role of hospice and other services. *Journal American Medical Association*. 2001; 285:925-932.

National Cancer Institute. End-of-Life Care: Questions and Answers (Cancer Facts). Available at http://cis.nci.nih.gov/fact/8_15.htm. Accessed December 12, 2003.

National Hospice and Palliative Care Organization. NHPCO Facts & Figures. Alexandria, VA: July 2003.

Ringdal GI, Jordhoy MS, Ringdal K, Kaasa S. Factors affecting grief reactions in close family members to individuals who have died of cancer. *Journal Pain & Symptom Management*. 2001; 22:1016-1026.

Schulz R, Beach SR. Caregiving as a risk factor for mortality: The Caregiver Health Effects Study. *Journal American Medical Association*. 1999; 282:23:2215-2219.

Chapter 13 References

American Cancer Society. Talking to Children about Death. Available at http://www.cancer.org/docroot/MBC/content/MBC_4_1X_Talking_To_Children_About_Death.asp?sitearea=MBC. Accessed May 3, 2004.

American Cancer Society and National Comprehensive Cancer Network. *Advanced Cancer and Palliative Care: Treatment Guidelines for Patients, Version I/December 2003*. Atlanta, GA: 2003.

Barrett R K. Psychocultural influences on African American attitudes toward death, dying, and funeral rites. In J. Morgan, ed. *Personal Care in an Impersonal World*. Amityville, NY: Baywood; 1993: 213-230.

Block SD. Psychological considerations, growth, and transcendence at the end of life: The art of the possible. *Journal of American Medical Association*. 2001; 285:22:2898-2905.

Brave Heart MYH, DeBruyn LM. The American Indian holocaust: Healing historical unresolved grief. *American Indian & Alaska Native Mental Health Research*. 1998; 8:60-82.

Casarett D, Kutner JS, Abrahm J. Life after death: A practical approach to grief and bereavement. *Annals of Internal Medicine*. 2001; 134:3: 208-215.

Catlin G. The role of culture in grief. *The Journal of Social Psychology*. 2001; 133:173-184.

Chan CLW, Mark JMH. Benefits and drawbacks of Chinese rituals surrounding care for the dying. In R. Fielding & C. L-W. Chan. eds. *Psychosocial oncology and palliative care in Hong Kong: The first decade*. Hong Kong: Hong Kong University Press; 2000: 255-270.

Christ GH. *Healing Children's Grief: Surviving a Parent's Death from Cancer*. New York: Oxford University Press; 2000.

Grabowski J, Frantz TT. Latinos and Anglos: Cultural experiences of grief intensity. *Omega – Journal of Death & Dying*. 1992; 26:273-285.

Ho SMY, Chow AYM, Chan CLW, Tsui YKY. The assessment of grief among Hong Kong Chinese: A preliminary report. *Death Studies*. 2002; 26:91-98.

Jennings B, Ryndes T, D'Onofrio C, Baily MA. Access to Hospice Care: Expanding Boundaries, Overcoming Barriers. *Hastings Center Report*, Supplement. March/April 2003.

Johnson JW. Gone down death. In MG Scundy. ed., *Trials, tribulations and celebrations: African-American perspectives on health, illness, aging and loss*. Yarmouth, ME: Intercultural press. 1991; 171-173.

Kagawa-Singer M, Blackhall LJ. Negotiating cross-cultural issues at the end of life: "You got to go where he lives". *Journal of American Medical Association*. 2001; 28: 2993-3001.

Kalish R, Reynolds D. *Death and ethnicity: A psychocultural study*. New York: Baywood. 1981.

Klass D. Solace and immortality: Bereaved parents' continuing bond with their children. *Death Studies*. 1993; 17, 343-368.

Klass D. Continuing bonds in the resolution of grief in Japan and North America. *American Behavioral Scientist*. 2001; 44:742-763.

Lynn J, Harrold J, and the Center to Improve Care of the Dying, George Washington University. *Handbook for Mortals: Guidance for People Facing Serious Illness*. New York: Oxford University Press, 1999.

National Cancer Institute. Loss, Grief, and Bereavement (PDQ). Available at http://www.nci.nih.gov/cancerinfo/pdq/supportivecare/bereavement/patient/. Accessed December 12, 2003.

Oltjenbruns KA. Ethnicity and the grief response: Mexican American versus Anglo American college students. *Death Studies*. 1998; 22:141-155.

Redinbaugh EM, Schuerger JM, Weiss LL et al. Health care professional's grief: A model based on occupational style and coping. *Psycho-oncology*. 2001; 10:187-198.

Shaprio ER. Grief in family and cultural context: Learning from Latino families. *Cultural Diversity & Mental Health*. 1995; 1:159-176.

Siefken S. The Hispanic perspective on death and dying: A combination of respect, empathy, and spirituality. *Pride Institute Journal of Long Term Home Health Care*. 1993; 12:26-28.

Smith SH. "Fret no more my child... for I'm all over heaven all day": Religious beliefs in the bereavement of African-American, middle-aged daughters coping with the death of an elderly mother. *Death Studies*. 2002; 26:309-323.

Waller A, Caroline NL. *Handbook of Palliative Care in Cancer*, 2nd ed. Boston: Butterworth-Heinemann; 1996.

Young G, Young K. *Loss and Found: How We Survived the Loss of a Young Spouse*. Calabasas, CA: Calabash Press; 2001.

Index

We Care About Your Opinions.

Please take a moment to complete this survey and fax it to *Books/Product Marketing Specialist* at **404-325-9341**, or email your comments and suggestions to us at **trade.sales@cancer.org**. *Thank you!*

PLEASE PRINT.

First Name _____

Last Name _____

Address _____

City _____ State _____ Zip _____

Email _____

1. Gender: ☐ Female   ☐ Male

2. Age: ☐ 20–39   ☐ 40–59   ☐ 60+

3. How many health books have you bought or read in last 12 months? ____

4. How did you find out about this book? (Please choose one.)
   ☐ Recommendation   ☐ Store Display   ☐ Online
   ☐ Advertisement   ☐ Catalog/Mailing   ☐ TV/Radio

5. Did this book meet your needs? _____
_____
_____

6. Is there a topic you feel should appear in the next edition of this book?
_____

7. What attracts you most to a book? (Please rank 1–4 in order of preference; 1 being most important.)
   ____ Title   ____ Content   ____ Cover Design   ____ Author

8. If you would you like more information about other books published by the American Cancer Society, please tell us how you prefer to be contacted:
   ☐ E-mail   ☐ Mail